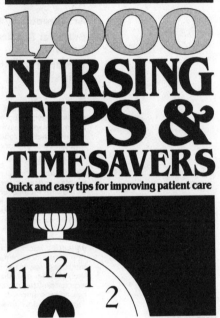

1,000 NURSING TIPS & TIMESAVERS

Quick and easy tips for improving patient care

SECOND EDITION

Springhouse Corporation
Springhouse, Pa. 19477

1,000 Nursing Tips & Timesavers

Editor: Regina Daley Ford, RN, BSN, MA

Clinical Editor: Marlene Ciranowicz, RN, MSN

Art Director: John Hubbard

Editorial Services Manager: David Moreau

Senior Production Manager: Deborah Meiris

ISBN 0-87434-034-9

The clinical procedures described and recommended in this publication are based on research and consultation with medical and nursing authorities. To the best of our knowledge, these procedures reflect currently accepted clinical practice; nevertheless, they can't be considered absolute and universal recommendations. For individual application, treatment recommendations must be considered in light of the patient's clinical condition and, before administration of new or infrequently used drugs, in light of latest package-insert information. The authors and the publisher disclaim responsibility for any adverse effects resulting directly or indirectly from the suggested procedures, from any undetected errors, or from the reader's misunderstanding of the text.

Library of Congress Cataloging in Publication Data

Main entry under title:
1,000 nursing tips & timesavers.

Rev. ed. of: 500 nursing tips & timesavers. © 1982.
"Nursing87 books."
Includes index.
1. Nursing—Handbooks, manuals, etc.
2. Nurses—Time management—Handbooks, manuals, etc. I. Springhouse Corporation. II. 500 nursing tips & timesavers. III. Title: One thousand nursing tips & timesavers. IV. Title: 1,000 nursing tips and timesavers.
[DNLM: 1. Nursing—handbooks. WY 18 Z99]
RT51.A16   1987   610.73   86-26055
ISBN 0-87434-034-9

CONTENTS

Foreword v

1. **Communicating** 1
   With the patient 1
   Patient information 6
   With the family and friends 12
   Staff information 15

2. **Teaching** 21
   The patient 21
   The family and friends 34
   The public 35
   The staff 39

3. **Adult patient care** 53
   Fluid and nutrition 53
   Surgery 59
   Mobility 62
   Restraints 64
   Physical care 65
   Comfort 68
   Emergencies 78
   Supportive measures 80

4. **Pediatric patient care** 85
   Fluid and nutrition 85
   Play therapy 86
   Mobility 92
   Physical care 93
   Comfort 100
   Emergencies 103
   Supportive measures 104

5. **Home care** 106
   Administering self-medication 106
   Fostering independence 109
   Improvising equipment and supplies 113
   Resolving elimination dilemmas 115
   Solving intake problems 116
   Improving physical care 116
   Performing emergency self-care 118
   Travel tips 118
   Pediatric measures 119

6. Assessment **123**
   Obtaining a history 123
   Information through examination 124
   Obtaining accurate measurements 128

7. Procedures **134**
   Performing mouth care 134
   Providing EENT care 135
   Cleaning equipment 137
   Preparing hot/cold therapy 139
   Positioning patients 141
   Making occupied beds 144
   Managing elimination and drainage 145
   Collecting specimens 154
   Securing tubes and drainage sets 158
   Applying dressings, bandages, and compresses 165
   Caring for the skin and wounds 169

8. I.V. therapy **176**
   Preparation 176
   Administration 179
   Maintenance 182

9. Medications **188**
   Preparation 188
   Administration 190
   Documentation 194

10. Safety **195**
   Patient safety 195
   Nurse safety 201

11. Cost and timesaver tips **204**
   Equipment 204
   Supplies 206
   Time 211

12. Personal grooming **220**
   Patient grooming 220
   Nurse grooming 224

13. Potpourri: A medley of suggestions **229**

Index **240**

FOREWORD

This year *Nursing87,* the world's largest nursing journal, celebrates 16 years of service to the nursing profession. And we know how precious a nurse's time is.

To help you make the most of your valuable time, the editors have collected, reviewed, and organized the best *Tips & Timesavers* published in the pages of *Nursing* magazine. We've looked for better ways to help you do your work, to save you money, and to make every minute count.

The tips included in this book show how to improve communications, keep accurate records, keep pediatric patients smiling, take the drudgery out of routine tasks, administer medication and I.V. therapy effectively, and increase your confidence in handling almost any situation.

From the time you spend with patients to the time you spend keeping up with the changing profession, this book will help you save time. That's what *Tips & Timesavers* is all about—saving time. And more time's something you can really use—isn't it?

The Editors

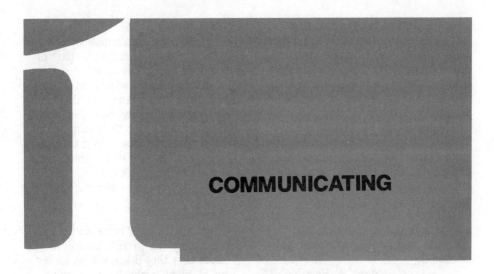

COMMUNICATING

WITH THE PATIENT

R*EAL* communication

Nothing is more frustrating than not being able to communicate, and being on a ventilator prevents normal communication. One solution to this problem is an electronic artificial larynx (EAL), a hand-held, battery-powered communication device. The patient on the ventilator holds the EAL against his throat and forms words with his lips, teeth, and tongue as usual. Electronic vibrations from the EAL mimic the natural vibrations of the patient's vocal cords, creating sound waves.

The EAL is available from local telephone companies and other manufacturers of communication devices for the speech-impaired.

Nancy Carole Munzig, RN

A toll call

When a quadriplegic patient was admitted to our acute-care hospital, we were concerned because he couldn't turn on the nurse's call light

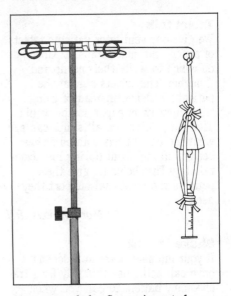

to summon help. So we invented a call system for him.

First, we stretched a sturdy wire coat hanger straight, except for the rounded handle end. Then, we wound the straight end of the hanger through the loops of a portable I.V. pole and taped the hanger to the pole for extra security. We tied one end of a piece of gauze to the hanger and tied the other end to the handle of a metal bell. Finally, we tied three *more* pieces of gauze to the bell's handle and tied and taped the loose ends of the gauze to the barrel of a small syringe.

We placed the I.V. pole near the head of the patient's bed and adjusted its height so the syringe hung near his mouth. With minimal head movement, he could grasp the syringe barrel and tug to ring the bell.

Our homemade call system made our patient *and* us confident that he could ring for help whenever he needed it.

Susan A. Harrison, RN

Tablet talk
We give our ventilator patients tablets of paper—not just scraps of paper— on which to write their needs and thoughts. The tablets stay at the patient's bedside, instead of being thrown away as paper scraps would. That way, nurses on all shifts can see what the patient has wanted or has been thinking about during his hospital stay. This helps us give these patients the emotional support they need.

Mary Winters, RN

Shake 'n' call
If your intensive care unit doesn't have call bells, use this way for a tracheotomy patient to call you when he needs assistance. Place pennies or paper clips in a small, plastic urine-specimen container. Then cap the filled container and tape it to one side rail of the patient's bed.

When the patient wants you, he just shakes his container.

Elizabeth McIntyre, BSN

Just whistle
A whistle can help a quadriplegic patient who can't move any part of his body except his mouth.

Attach a metal whistle to a piece of oxygen tubing and tape the tubing to the patient's face, near his mouth. He can then grasp the tubing with his tongue and blow into it to signal you. As a bonus, blowing the whistle also exercises his lungs.

Marsha Urben, RN

Baby alarm
When a baby goes home with a tracheostomy, his parents usually worry about how they'll know if he wakes up at night, since he can't cry. Suggest they get some tiny jingle bells—the kind toddlers wear on their shoes—and string them on ribbons to tie around the baby's wrist or ankle. Double-knotting the bells ensures that they won't come off so the baby won't swallow them.

Parents report that these "alarm bracelets" help *them* sleep better at night—at least until they hear the bells jingle.

Craig Uhler, RN, USN

Chime for the nurse
If you care for a patient who can't summon help, either by voice or call button, attach a wind chime to the I.V. standard built into the ceiling and fasten a long piece of twill tape to the chime clapper. The chime can also be attached to a regular I.V. pole. Then fasten the other end of the tape to the patient's ear with a rubber band. Thus, when the patient wants to call the nurse, he simply moves his head and the chimes ring.

The sound of the chimes is much more pleasant than banging on the side rails or clicking the teeth or other methods that patients in similar situations usually use. Both nurses and patients appreciate it.

Mae Paulfrey, RN, MN

Conversation cards

If you have patients with communication problems, such as aphasia or a tracheostomy, here's a way to help them. Write messages, such as "I am thirsty," "Please raise my bed," and "I want a drink of water," on index cards. Then punch holes in the cards and attach them to a large key ring so they'll be easy to locate. Patients can quickly communicate their needs or wishes by simply showing you the appropriate card.

You could make several sets of these cards for specific times. For example, mealtime cards might include such messages as "I'd like more

coffee" and "Please butter my bread." Cards for visiting hours might say "How is Sandra?" "Is there any mail?" "Who sent the flowers?" You can make other cards that meet a particular patient's needs.

These conversation cards can reduce frustration for both you and your patients.

Kathleen Cruzie, RN

Communicating mats

To make communicating with aphasic patients easier, one nurse illustrated patients' various needs on a placemat. The mat is divided into three sections: activities of daily living, primary needs, and rest and recreation. The activities of daily living section has a toilet, bath, and sink, for example. The rest and recreation section has a radio, bed, and chair.

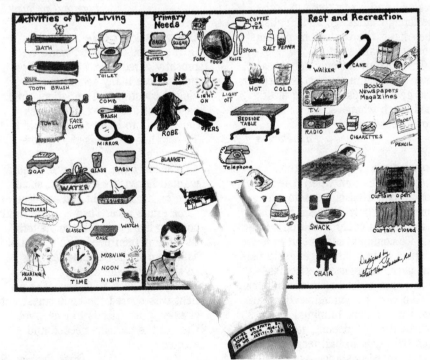

In all she illustrated 62 different needs on the 12″ × 18″ mat. The hospital then had 50 placemats printed and laminated. They're distributed to patients as needed.

Using the mat, the patient points to what he wants. Of course, the nursing staff still encourages aphasic patients to communicate on their own. But the mat helps improve communication between the staff and patient, thereby reducing the frustration so common among these patients.

Gail Van Tassell, RN

Bilingual poster

If no one on the staff can communicate with foreign-speaking patients, try a visual approach to the problem—a bilingual poster.

Choose a few important words, such as "bath," "pain," "food," and "water," and write them in both the foreign language and English. Then hang the posters in patients' rooms, in plain sight.

The posters not only help break down the communication barrier, but also give both patients and staff a good laugh whenever someone mispronounces a word.

Pam Barton, RN

Communicards

The obstetrics unit where I recently worked had a lot of patients who could speak only Spanish. But most of the nurses could speak only English. To communicate, we used a mixture of sign language, gestures, and facial expressions. Needless to say, this caused a lot of confusion.

To break the communication barrier, I made some bilingual, color-coded cards. I cut pink, yellow, and blue 3x5 cards in half lengthwise. I wrote questions and comments made during *labor and delivery* in English on the pink cards, with the Spanish translation underneath. (For instance, one card says, "You must breathe deeply" and underneath, "Hay que respirar profundo.") I wrote questions and comments made during the *recovery period* on yellow cards, and questions and comments made during the *postpartum period* on blue cards. Then I punched a hole on the side of each card, put a self-adhesive reinforcement around the hole, and used a metal ring to hold them together. I carried the cards in my pocket so they were readily available when I was assigned to a Spanish-speaking patient.

These cards could be adapted to any nursing specialty or language to help dispel patients' confusion and fears.

Loretta Thornton, SN

Grape juice code

In the hospital where I work, we recently cared for a 14-year-old patient whose many school friends visited constantly. The patient tired easily, but she didn't like to ask her friends to leave so she could rest. To help her, we devised a "grape juice code."

Whenever the patient was tired and wanted her visitors to leave, she'd turn on her call light and ask for some grape juice. Then a nurse would come to her room, tell the visitors that the patient needed to rest, and ask them if they'd mind leaving so she could take a nap.

Our code was a success. The patient was spared the embarrassment of asking her friends to leave, yet she got the rest she needed and wanted.

Dixie Burgess, SN

A questionable idea

A hospitalized patient and his family can think of a thousand questions for his doctor—usually when the doctor isn't around. If the patient doesn't call the doctor immediately, he may forget the question the next time the doctor comes to visit him.

To help your patient get the answers he needs, put a sheet of paper and a pencil on his bedside stand. Tell the patient (and his family) to write his questions on the paper and leave it on the stand. Then, the next time the doctor comes to the patient's room, he can read and answer the questions. (If the patient is asleep, the doctor can write his answers on the paper.)

Besides cutting down on the number of calls to busy doctors, the sheet ensures that the patient gets answers to his important questions.

Rosemary S. Martens, RN

Check the schedule

When a diabetic patient is admitted because his diabetes is out of control, he may be surprised to find that the hospital schedule for meals, insulin administration, and blood and urine testing is different—and stricter—than his at-home schedule. The difference could cause confusion and make following the new schedule difficult for the patient.

To avoid this confusion, post the schedule on the wall near the patient's bed. Here's an example:

7 a.m.	urine specimen (second voiding) for sugar and acetone test
7:30 a.m.	blood specimen for glucose test/insulin administration
8 a.m.	breakfast
11 a.m.	urine specimen (second voiding) for sugar and acetone test
11:30 a.m.	blood specimen for glucose test/insulin administration
12 p.m.	lunch
(and so on)	

The posted schedule should help clear up any confusion over verbal instructions. And it should encourage self-management, thus increasing compliance.

Michael A. Gibney, RN

Cardboard hang-ups

We made calendar-time boards to hang in the rooms of older patients who are confused as to date and time and can't remember the mealtime schedule. For each board, we covered a 22″ × 18″ piece of sturdy cardboard with light-colored cloth. We stapled three cardboard pockets across the top of the board and stapled the labels "month," "day," and "year" above the pockets.

In the pockets, we placed felt cutouts of all the months and dates. Each day we take out the right date and pin it to the pocket. We change the month and year as necessary.

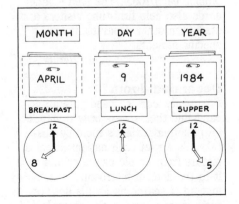

Across the bottom of the board, we stapled three cardboard clock faces, indicating mealtimes, and stapled the labels "breakfast," "lunch," and "supper" above the clock faces. We hung the board at eye level on the wall facing the patient's bed. These boards—with the patients' own clocks—have helped orient them to time and day.

Leola H. Cain, RN
Linda M. Hadyka, LPN

Current events calendar
To help a patient who has a poor memory for recent events, hang a large calendar in his room—the kind with a big block for each day. Then note daily happenings in the blocks. Some of your notes might read: "received card from daughter," "husband called," "chatted with nurse." The patient can refer to the calendar to recall events of recent days and weeks.

Holly Bennett, RN, NE

Photo finder
If elderly patients have trouble finding their rooms, tape a large color photo of the patient's face plus a name card printed in large black letters outside each room. The photo-name cards also help first-time visitors and staff from other departments find specific patients.

Nan Hernikl, RN

Decorated doors
Frequently, our confused patients can't find their rooms or will wander into another patient's room by mistake. So we let each patient select a picture from an old calendar and tape it to the door of his room. Then, instead of searching for his door or room number among the many look-alikes, the patient just searches for his picture. This makes good use of old calendars and magazines, too.

Sr. Huguette Blais, RN

PATIENT INFORMATION

Board and rooms
When hospital personnel needed to find a patient, they'd invariably stop at our busy nurses' station and ask for his room number. To eliminate these constant interruptions, we constructed a board, labeled it with all the unit's room numbers, and mounted the board next to the chart rack, out of public view.

Now when a new patient is admitted, we write his name, along with his doctor's, on a piece of tape and attach the tape next to the proper room number. This way the information's available to all personnel who need it, and they can get it themselves—without interrupting us.

Ron Yoder, RN

Put the card before the scan
Occasionally, patients undergoing a computed tomography (CT) scan have an allergic reaction to the iodine-based contrast dye administered during the scan. When this happens, I give the patient a card on which I write a message such as this:

Before performing an X-ray procedure or exam in which contrast dye is administered, please inform the doctor that on Sept. 11, 1984, John Smith had an adverse reaction to the iodine dye during a CT scan.

The patient can carry the card in his wallet and present it to the nurse or technician whenever he needs laboratory work done. A copy of the card also can be sent to his doctor, to be kept in the patient's medical record. Then, even if the patient forgets he's allergic to the dye, the card will remind the doctor and nurses to ask him about his previous reaction.

Carol L. Edwards, RN

Requisition reminder

To alert laboratory staff to be careful in handling specimens from a patient who has hepatitis, we put red stickers on all requisitions.

As a reminder, we also put a red sticker on the patient's Addressograph plate. When we stamp a requisition for that patient, we see the sticker and are immediately reminded to place another one on the requisition.

F. Carolyn Edmunds, RN, BSN

X-rays in a flash

Sending a patient who'd had a myocardial infarction (MI) to the X-ray department used to create problems. For example, he'd have to wait a long time for his turn, or he'd be asked to walk a long way because the X-ray department personnel were unaware of his condition. When he'd return to the unit, he'd be exhausted or, worse, have severe chest pain.

To avoid these problems, I now pin a red paper heart with the words "NO WALKING OR LONG WAITING" on the patient's robe before he goes to the X-ray department. When they see the red heart, the personnel know they should try to get this patient in, out, and back to the unit as quickly as possible.

Patricia Scully, RN

Stop, read, and follow

A stop sign makes people stop and take notice. So to make sure isolation precautions are noticed—and followed—nurses at Louisiana State

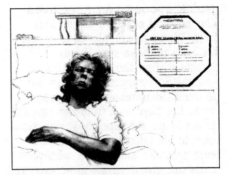

University Hospital, Shreveport, post a red stop sign outside the room or on the bed of a patient placed in isolation.

The sign is 10" × 10" and lists important information for visitors and staff. It tells at a glance how the patient's infection may be transmitted and what precautions may be needed. The sign emphasizes hand washing and checking with the nurses before visiting. It also has space for special instruction concerning the patient's isolation.

Before a nurse posts the sign, she assesses the patient and determines the type of isolation he needs.

To make sure nurses stop and refer to the isolation guidelines issued by the Centers for Disease Control (CDC), the sign is also printed on the cover of the CDC guidelines book. Nurses use the book (which is found on every unit) to determine the precautions needed and to fill in the other information on the patient's sign. They also assess the patient daily and update the information on the sign as needed.

They have found that the stop sign does indeed make people stop and think before they enter the patient's room.

Sue Crow, RN, MSN

Quick access can save lives

Our hospital serves a large rural area. When an ambulance is called, we have to make sure the driver is able to find the patient's house quickly. So I suggest that each patient in our cardiac rehabilitation program write the directions from the hospital to his home and tape those directions next to his telephone. Then if he ever needs an ambulance, whoever calls can give accurate directions, and no time will be wasted.

Gale Nunn, RN

Getting the message

Many of my private-duty patients have friends and business associates who often make surprise visits without considering the time of day or the patient's condition.

So with the patient's permission, I enforce certain visiting regulations by posting a note on his door with a message such as this: "Good morning. Mr. Jones has just completed some morning activities and is resting comfortably at present. He appreciates your stopping by and thanks you for letting him rest now."

The message, which I update according to the time of day and situation, is genial enough not to hurt any feelings. Yet it's direct enough so the visitor gets the message and my patient gets his rest.

Sandra Shute Hook, RN, BS

An I.D. to run with

If your patient jogs, tell him to save his hospital identification bracelet when he's discharged. Usually, it'll list his name, address, phone number, allergies, and doctor's name. If not, he can ink in the missing information, then attach the bracelet to the ties on one of his jogging shoes.

This way, he'll always have identification with him, which could come in handy in an emergency.

Kathleen E. Mason, RN

Leads on needs

All staff members at the nursing home where I work can't always check the cardex before giving patient care. So they might not know, for example, which patient needs a walker, soft restraints while sitting up in a chair, or help going to the bathroom.

To make all staff members aware of each patient's needs, I type a list of his basic and safety needs on an index card and post the card on the patient's bathroom door. I also include little reminders to be kind, gentle, give praise, and so on. I don't include any confidential information.

The staff members find the cards helpful. And patients and their families are pleased that *everyone* on staff remembers the needs of each patient.

Loretta C. Hopkins, RN, BS

Posting reminders

I post signs as reminders of patients' needs, too. For example, for a postoperative mastectomy patient: "No venipuncture or blood pressure on right arm" (or left, depending on which side the surgery was on).

As part of my preoperative teaching, I do tell the patient not to allow anyone to take blood pressure readings or perform venipunctures on the affected side. But since she's still sedated immediately after surgery, I post the sign as an added precaution.

Pauline Wagner, RN

Nurses, know thy patients

In our intensive care unit, we work 3

12-hour days, then have 4 days off. So when we return to work, we sometimes find that we don't know all of the patients. With everything else that's said and done during change-of-shift report, we may not get such information as the patients' symptoms on admission, past medications, history, and so on.

To learn about our patients quickly and to ensure continuity of care, we make a copy of the admission nurses' notes and place it on the cardex. It's easily accessible for change-of-shift report or for quick reference.

Deborah A. Woy, RN, BSN

Patient needs, at a glance

Nurses at the Riverview Unit of Windsor (Ontario) Western Hospital Centre have devised a system for reminding themselves of their patients' special needs. They use 3", color-coded paper disks tacked to a bulletin board that's affixed above the head of each patient's bed.

For instance, if the patient is allergic to a certain food, a green disk labeled with the allergy is tacked to the board. Or, if the patient needs two nurses to help him transfer from bed to chair, a pink disk with the number "2" written on it is used. Other colored disks refer to additional patient needs.

The disks are especially useful to registry and float nurses, who can determine at a glance what help the patient needs.

Anna Hayes, RN

Vitals under (Plexi)glas

When a number of people are working around a severely injured patient in our emergency department's (ED) trauma room, communication of vital signs becomes difficult. To solve this problem, we made a large construction-paper chart with columns for time, blood pressure, pulse, and number of I.V. bottles or units of blood. Then we covered the chart with Plexiglas and mounted it on an easily accessible spot on the trauma room wall.

Using grease pencils, we mark the patient's vital signs in their appropriate columns on the chart. This way—at a glance—we can check the patient's most recent vital signs and note any developing trends.

After the initial emergency is over, we transcribe the information from the chart onto the patient's permanent record. Then, when the patient leaves the ED, we simply rub off the chart, and it's ready to use again.

Our Plexiglas chart not only eliminates a lot of unnecessary verbal traffic, but it also lets us give our full attention to the patient.

Callie Jo Sandquist, RN

A noteworthy idea

I use the intake and output sheets that are posted on the doors of patients' rooms to write reminders to the nursing assistants on the unit. For example, I note any special dietary requirements and reminders for special procedures, such as "strain urine," "weight at 6 a.m.," or "gown for CT scan at 6 a.m." My notes help the assistants keep up with their work and assure me that these things will be done.

Tracey Rieben, RN

Patient hang-ups

Placing a 9½" × 17½" cork bulletin board beside each bed on the unit saves time and helps you give better patient care.

For instance, post patient informa-

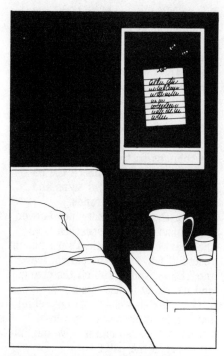

length as the real thing) in red ink, the sutures and staples in black, and the area of ecchymosis in blue. If the wound is draining, draw the drain and drainage on the tape in green. Then date and initial the tape and apply it to the top of the dressing.

This visual aid alerts staff to the exact type and size of the patient's wound and helps with patient teaching, too.

Sydney Anne Gambill, RN

Preventive charting
Patients can become constipated from the medications they receive for pain control. If this side effect occurs frequently, devise a chart to keep track of patients' bowel patterns and treatment modes. Keep the chart in the front of the cardex. List patients' names and room numbers in the first column. Head the rest of the columns with the date and divide into three vertical columns—one for each shift.

Use a simple legend: 0 = no bowel movement; B = bowel movement; E = enema; S = suppository. Fill in the chart at the end of each shift. It reminds you to administer treatment before constipation becomes a problem.

Catherine Haley, RN, BSN

tion, such as "limited fluids" or "blood pressure on *right* arm only," on the bulletin board, so nurses on all shifts will know immediately what precautions to take. When a patient is scheduled for a diagnostic procedure the next day, post that information plus whatever preparation is needed ("N.P.O. after midnight"). And when a patient must go out of his room for an X-ray or physical therapy, put a note on the bulletin board telling where he is.

Using these "patient hang-ups" reduces communication problems among staff, patients, and families.

Jenny Langlinais, RN

On the draw
Before dressing a wound, draw a picture of the sutured area on the tape that you will be using.

Draw the suture line (the same

Find a kid
The unit where I work has mostly adult patients, but pediatric patients are admitted from time to time. To help us locate the rooms of these young patients, we put plastic stickers next to their names and room numbers on the unit map at the nurses' station. The stickers, which are shaped like children, are colorful, reusable, and inexpensive. And they

tell us at a glance where our special patients are.

Karen Van De Loo, RN

Name that patient
In our skilled nursing facility, we post a name card at the *head* of each bed, instead of at the foot where it can't readily be seen. We also find out what the patient's favorite flower, pet, or hobby is and draw an appropriate symbol or paste a picture from a magazine on the card.

The patients enjoy their decorative identifiers. So do the visitors, housekeepers, and nursing students, who may not know the patients' names and interests.

Barbara Roehrenbeck, RN

On a first-name basis
Soon after a baby is admitted to our neonatal intensive care unit (NICU) and we're sure he is stable, we take a few moments to identify him. We make a sign for his warmer or incubator that says, "Hi! I'm Michael James," or whatever the baby's name is. Then we decorate the sign with colorful stickers.

The signs, which are large enough that we can see them from everywhere in the nursery, allow us to identify each baby at a glance—quite a feat in our busy NICU. And parents appreciate our familiarity with their babies' names when we're giving them a daily telephone report.

Wendy Kaveney, RN, BSN

One good turn
If many of your patients need to be turned every 2 hours, here's how to give good care and keep accurate records at the same time.

Put "turn books" by the patients' bedsides. These books are simply three-ring notebooks with columns for recording the time the patient was turned, position of the patient, date, and the initials of the turner.

Marjorie Kamtman, RN

Returning the call
When a patient's call light goes on and you respond over the intercom but get no verbal message from the patient, what do you do? Do you assume that the patient needs help or that the call button was pushed by mistake? Some patients, of course, can't respond because they can't speak or hear.

To make sure we don't ignore *any* call lights, we put colored dots on our intercom next to the room numbers of patients who can't respond. When a light flashes next to one of these dots, we don't wait for a response from the patient. Instead, we answer it by going to that patient's room. This is a great help to float nurses and others who aren't familiar with all the patients on our unit.

Fidelita Lim-Levy, RN

Easy access
Patients who frequent the emergency department (ED) may have charts as thick as encyclopedias. For instant access to essential information on such patients, nurses at the University of California Los Angeles Emergency Medical Center maintain a special cardex.

The cardex, a collection of 4" × 6" index cards, is kept at the triage desk. If a triage nurse recognizes a patient from previous visits, she pulls his card from the special cardex and immediately reviews the information listed under four headings:

• *Patient profile,* including personal information: the patient's occupation and marital status, plus pertinent observations such as "This patient frequently leaves against medical advice or becomes hostile if he's denied a request for narcotics."

• *Known medical problems,* including medical diagnoses taken directly from the patient's chart.

• *Suggested approach,* including directives as simple as "Immediately register this patient" or "Don't give this patient narcotics per Dr. Smith's order."

• *Resource persons and number of previous visits to the ED,* including the names of nurses, doctors, and others who've worked effectively with the patient, and dates of ED visits.

Cards are kept for patients who have chronic conditions that need emergency care, and for those who've made at least four visits to the ED within a 3-month period. During monthly triage meetings, the ED staff discusses these patients and suggests new or revised approaches to their care. If the patient's ED visits have decreased or management is no longer necessary, his card's removed from the cardex and placed in an inactive file. The special cardex also helps nurses identify people who abuse ED care and should be directed to a primary care doctor.

Journal of Emergency Nursing, July/ August 1982

Dear diary

Here's an idea that pediatric nurses can pass along to new parents: Suggest they keep a diary for their baby.

Of course, they can record the baby's achievements and developmental progress (first smile, first tooth, and so on). But they can also record medical information such as fevers, diarrhea, reactions to new food or medications, and even mood changes. Then if the child has a fever, the parents can refer to the diary and give the pediatrician an accurate description of the child's previous few days.

The diary will come in handy as the child grows older, too. And as more children come into the family, each of them should have his own diary. The diaries will document who had what childhood disease (mumps, chicken pox, measles) and when.

Katherine Link, RN

Night noises

The mother of a 6-year-old girl with cerebral palsy gave me this idea. Besides having to be suctioned two or three times a night, the girl had frequent seizures, so the mother had to check on her every hour or so. In between, of course, the mother slept fitfully, worried that her daughter might need her.

Then she bought a pair of battery-operated intercoms, put one in the corner of her daughter's crib and the other at the head of her own bed. Now she can listen to her daughter's breathing, coughing, and other noises that might indicate a problem— without having to get up every hour to check.

Lorna E. Stern, RN

WITH THE FAMILY AND FRIENDS

Calming calls

Family visits should have a calming influence on seriously ill patients, but in many cases they have the opposite effect. One obvious reason: an anxious family transmits its anxiety to the patient.

Ask doctors what they want the families of their patients to know. Then relay that information to the family on their next visit. Or, adopt the same routine, except phone each family every morning, telling them how the patient spent the night and what the doctor had to say.

Catherine Baden, RN, BS

"Baby-grams" for parents

If babies in the neonatal intensive care unit are brought in from rural areas, their parents have to travel long distances to visit or else make expensive phone calls.

Keep parents posted on their baby's progress by sending "baby-grams" on inexpensive postcards. On the card's message side, put the baby's footprint and a short note "from the baby."

The note can state the baby's weight and say something positive about his condition, if only to describe his curly hair or lusty cry. Parents love getting these cards and can add them to their baby books.

Nancy Hogg, RN

P.S. I love you

In the nursery where I work, premature babies aren't discharged until they tip the scales at 5 lb. That sometimes takes a while—especially if the baby's a real lightweight. But some new parents live far from the hospital and can't visit their babies as often as they'd like.

To keep parents up to date on their baby's progress, we send them postcards with good news. A typical card might read:

```
Dear Mom and Dad,  ☺
Today I weigh 4 pounds.
One more pound and I'll
be home with you.

          Miss you,
          Jessica
```

The price of the stamps and postcards is small compared to the lift the parents get from hearing about their baby.

Linda Jeronowitz, RN

Clockwork

After being on our unit for several months, an infant with congenital heart disease was ready for discharge. We were concerned about teaching his mother to manage his complicated medication and feeding schedules, because she was anxious and didn't speak the same language we did.

To teach her, I used colors rather than words: I made a color-coded medication/feeding schedule. First, I placed colored adhesive dots on the baby's medication bottles. I tried to use dots the same color as the medication—green for digoxin, yellow for Lasix, and so on.

Then I drew a large clock and placed colored dots (the same color as the dots on the medicine bottles) at the times the baby was to receive each medication. I also drew bottles of milk and placed them on the clock to indicate feeding times. I colored the a.m. medication/feeding times with a yellow marker and the p.m. medication/feeding times with a dark blue marker.

My system worked well. The mother was able to tell when to give the baby his medication and feedings and, at last report, both mother and baby were doing fine.

Barbara Marshall, RN, BSN

Phone-y idea

Procedures you easily demonstrate to patients in person may be difficult to explain over the phone. I learned this when the 13-year-old daughter of one of my diabetic patients called me because she couldn't arouse her mother and didn't know what to do. I told her to find the injectable glucagon, which she did. But she couldn't remember how to draw it up into the syringe or how to inject it.

To help *me* instruct her over the phone, I asked a co-worker (who was unfamiliar with injectable glucagon) to come into my office. As I explained the procedure over the phone, I demonstrated it to the co-worker in my office. If I became too technical, or if the girl didn't understand a particular instruction, my co-worker coached me by suggesting another less technical word or explanation. Together, as a three-person team, we successfully gave the patient her injection of glucagon.

David F. Kruger, RNC, MSN

Caring after death

Nurses at Hospice Nana in Bristol, N.H., don't stop caring after one of their patients dies. Instead, they make bereavement visits to the family 1, 2, and 3 weeks after the patient's death, then at 3 months, 6 months, and 1 year. They also visit at other times if they think the family needs it.

The hospice nurses have found that many families experience health-related problems within 6 months after a patient's death. That's when the cards have stopped coming, visits from friends have become less fre-

quent, and the death is supposed to be "a thing of the past." But family members, whose time was consumed by caring for the terminally ill person, find the loneliness difficult to bear. They become depressed and predisposed to illness.

The visits have helped the nurses offset the loneliness and detect illnesses early. They have, for instance, detected hypertension that developed in a widow 6 months after her husband died and severe depression in a mother whose child died of leukemia.

The nurses welcome the chance to support the family throughout the year following the patient's death—and families welcome the support and preventive health care they receive.

M. Dolan, RN

Hang-ups

We recently expanded visiting hours in our intensive care unit (ICU) but also began to enforce the "no visitors allowed" time more strictly than before. To help us inform visitors about the new policy, we made three large cardboard clocks (one for each shift) and hung them on our waiting room bulletin board. Each clock was marked as follows:

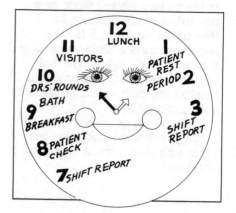

• busier times (such as change-of-shift report) when no visitors are allowed in ICU—in one color
• slower times (such as doctors' rounds or rest periods) when a phone call or nurse-family conference might be appropriate—in another color
• visiting hours—in still another color.

Next to the appropriate times on the clock, we noted what activity was taking place in the ICU. For instance, "9 a.m.: Breakfast," "10 a.m.: Doctors' rounds" (see illustration).

We also tacked sheets of paper below each clock so visitors can write down questions they think of while waiting and can ask the doctor or nurse later.

Our waiting room clocks have helped visitors by explaining what's going on in the ICU when they're not allowed in. They've also helped the nurses and patients by designating uninterrupted times to facilitate better care for the ICU patients.

Cynthia Brown, RN

STAFF INFORMATION

Attention-getter
Tape a square of washed X-ray film to the front of patients' charts to make a see-through pocket for messages or reminders to the doctor. Cut a large notch in the open end so notes can be inserted and removed easily. The pockets also serve as holders for identification plates of patients who are sent to surgery.

Diane Klaiber, RN

Forget-me-not
Keep a clipboard at the main desk. Write down questions as you think of them. Then before the doctors make rounds, they can check the board and

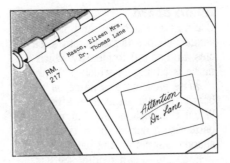

answer your questions.

Sharon Stevens, RN

Suggestions, please
Keep a suggestion box on each unit in which nurses can deposit suggestions for improvements in patient care. Each week, the head nurse can review the suggestions. Then she can list each suggestion on a flow sheet posted on the employee bulletin board, along with a follow-up plan of action. This provides feedback to the nurse who made the suggestion, so she'll know that her suggestion has actually been considered.

Not only does the system help provide better patient care, but it also helps build good employee relations.

Linda Kay, RN

Hang fire
Hang a red envelope marked "FIRE" on each nursing unit's bulletin board. Inside the envelope put 3" × 5" index cards, each listing one job that should be done during a fire or fire drill (for example, "shut all doors" or "report to central dispatch"). During drills, have each staff member take one card (or more, if you're short-staffed) for her assignment.

This system reduces the "who-does-what" confusion during fire drills.

Bonnie Shumaker, RN

All on board

Use a magnetic board and magnets in various shapes (squares, stars, circles, and so on) to identify which nurse is caring for which patient.

Write each nurse's name on the board and place a magnet after it. When the desk nurse assigns a patient to a nurse, she puts the same shaped magnet on the patient's chart.

Each nurse can readily see her assignments, and a doctor need only glance at the master board to see which nurse is caring for his patient.

Callie Sandquist, RN

Paperwork helpers

To help part-time and pool nurses who aren't familiar with our unit complete the paperwork for admitting and transferring a patient, I prepared some reference cards. I listed the step-by-step instructions for completing the paperwork on $5'' \times 8''$ index cards. The cards fit into the bottom of our cardex, so whenever a nurse needs help, she just has to reach for the appropriate card to proceed. The cards are a great timesaver.

Darlene Follett, RN

Get the message?

A pigeonholed wall cabinet marked with staff members' names works better than a cluttered bulletin board for getting messages and mail to the proper person. The cabinet neatly stores personal coffee mugs, too.

M.E. Glavin, RN

Manual labor

When I worked in a hospital, I found the procedure manual to be a great help as a quick reference guide. So I decided to write one for the doctor's office where I now work. The manual has clear, step-by-step instructions

for routine procedures such as taking a patient history, setting up for office surgery, ordering supplies, and so on. Both new and old staff members find the manual useful.

Lynne Tara, RN

Candid collage

Our medical/surgical unit supports the arts—with a gallery of candid photos of our staff. We make collages of the photographs and hang them at the nurses' station, in offices, and wherever there's room for them. We've even devised a unique conversation piece in our nurses' lounge by placing a collage on the coffee table and covering it with a piece of clear vinyl.

The collages help introduce new staff members to older ones and build a sense of belonging and camaraderie among the staff.

Rosalie Morrissey, RN

Pearls of wisdom

When I read especially useful suggestions in *Tips & Timesavers* (I call them "pearls"), I like to share them with our entire unit—via our "pearl board."

The pearl board is a large piece of construction paper hung in a central location. I clip the suggestions from the magazine and put them on the board, changing them periodically. For quick reference, I save old pearls in a double-pocket folder, also kept on the unit.

P. Gough, RN

Record-a-code

During a code, doctors sometimes order medications that don't get charted on the medication and code sheet. So we keep a cassette tape recorder on our crash cart.

As soon as a code is called, we start the tape recorder. Afterward, we play back the tape to see if we missed recording any medications—and to critique our handling of the code.

LtJG Peri Chapar, NC, USNR

A good sign

Bits and pieces of postoperative information (medication and lab study orders, patient allergies, and patient requests) frequently clutter the front of a patient's chart, and they're easily overlooked by operating and recovery room staffs. So we tape a bright red-and-white laminated stop sign to the front of each patient's chart, write the postoperative orders on white tape or a label, and attach the tape or label to the sign. With all orders together in *one* eye-catching spot, we're less likely to overlook them.

Later, when we return the patient to his room and all the orders have been noted and carried out, the floor nurses remove the tape and labels from the stop sign so the sign is ready for reuse.

Joan E. Lehan, RN

Taped reports—and then some

Almost every morning after we listen to our taped shift report, our head nurse spends another 5 or 10 minutes answering questions and giving us additional information not covered in the report. Unfortunately, nurses on the other shifts never heard this addendum to our reports—until we decided to tape it, too. The head nurse records the report addendum, then turns the cassette over so it won't be accidentally erased. Now none of the nurses on our unit

miss any important information.

Genevieve Milliken, RN

Question now, answer later

Our 30-bed surgical unit sometimes has patients from 11 different surgical services (orthopedic, vascular, general surgery, and so on). With all the routine, nonemergency questions and problems that arise, we spend a lot of time tracking down doctors for answers.

To organize our questions and decrease the number of times we must page the house staff, we've created a problem list—a sheet of paper divided into columns according to the different surgical services. In each column, we write the patient's name and room number and the question or problem we want to ask the doctor about. For example:

Orthopedic
Rm 648: Smith—I.V. orders $\bar{p}$ 3 p.m.
Rm 660: Johnson—renew Demerol
Rm 662: Jones—advance diet

Now when the doctors make rounds, they check the problem list, take care of the problems, and answer the questions.

Teresa Acquaviva, RN

An alarming reminder

On a busy unit, remembering to do certain tasks at certain times isn't easy. So we let an alarm clock at the nurses' station remind us.

For instance, when we must collect 2-hour urine specimens or return a patient to the X-ray department in 1 hour, we set the alarm for the time the task must be done and write the task and time on a note pad next to the clock. When the alarm sounds, the nurse who shuts it off reads the note, makes sure the task gets done,

and resets the clock for the next
task on the list.

Maureen Anthony, RN

Communication book

On our busy unit, staff communication
is a real problem—especially between
shifts. Sometimes we don't even
have time to bring up a question,
complaint, or suggestion. So to give
everyone a chance to speak up,
we use a "communication book."

This is a loose-leaf binder in which
staff members write their questions—
then sign and date their entries. As
soon as possible, the head nurse
or manager answers the questions,
writing each answer directly below
the question, then signing and dating
her answer. When indicated, she
takes action on the day's complaints
or suggestions and notes this, too.

Besides bridging our unit's communication gap, the book is also educa-
tional. We write a brief summary
of each inservice meeting and place it
in the book for the benefit of those
who couldn't attend.

Deborah Gibson, RN, MS

Cue cards

In our small, 42-bed hospital, a
cardiac arrest is a rare event. In the
past, no one was ever quite sure
what to do when it occurred, and we
lost valuable time deciding.

To clear up the confusion, at the
beginning of each shift we now
distribute five "Code Blue" cards:
cards listing specific duties the card-
holder will perform in the event of
a cardiac arrest. The five roles are
team leader, ventilator, compressor,
medication and recording nurse, and
runner.

Now we all know what our jobs are
before an arrest occurs, and we can

help the patient more quickly—
without losing time because of confusion and missed cues.

Jo Azzarello, RN

Assignments on board

Does your unit's assignment sheet
"wander" around the nurses' station?
If so, give the assignments a permanent home—on a bulletin board.

Across the top of the board make
four columns by posting these labels:
(1) room number, (2) patient's name,
(3) patient's doctor, (4) patient's nurse.

Under room number, post index
cards with the unit's room numbers,
one under the other. When a patient is
assigned to a room, print his name
on a card and post it in the second
column (patient name) next to the appropriate room number.

Then, post his doctor's and nurse's
name cards in the third and fourth
columns next to the patient's name
card.

Reserve a space at the top of the
board for a card naming the charge
nurse and a space at the bottom for a
card listing who has the day off.

Your assignments will be readily
available and clearly visible to more
than one person at a time; no one
will have to ask, "Who's in charge?"
or "Who's off today?" What's more,
you can change room or nursing
or medical assignments with just a
flick of a thumbtack.

E. Jane Mezzaontte, RN, MSN

Stickers to the rescue

One of our recent patients on the
orthopedic unit was an obese woman
who had several fractures, including
fractures of both acetabulums. Her
traction setups included three sets of
ropes and weights. Because her
weights had to be lifted every time

she was lifted, this meant several staff members had to be assembled. In all the commotion, we were never sure which weights went with which ropes. So whenever we moved her, we had to experiment in readjusting the weights; and in doing so, we caused the patient needless discomfort.

Finally, the patient came up with a solution. She asked us to put a different colored sticker on each weight and a corresponding sticker on that weight's rope. We could then see at a glance which rope went with which weight.

This patient's ingenuity saved *us* a lot of time and saved *her* a lot of discomfort.

Karen A. Taylor, RN

Checked charts

On the busy surgical unit where I work, our unit clerk routinely transcribes new doctors' orders from the patients' charts onto the cardex. Then the charge nurse checks the chart and cardex against each other and signs the chart if all is in order.

But too often the unchecked charts get mixed up with the charts that have already been checked. In all this confusion, we've missed some doctors' orders.

To solve this problem, we devised a way to flag charts that have new doctors' orders. We put a red check mark on a 1" piece of adhesive tape and attach it to the back of the patient's chart. After the unit clerk has transcribed the new orders onto the cardex, she moves the tape marker to the front of the chart. This alerts the nurse that the chart has orders to be checked. After checking the orders and signing the chart, the nurse moves the marker to the

back of the chart again.

Our markers have really put a check on missed orders.

Susan C. Steinman, RN

Nursing-home communicator

Communication among staff members in the nursing home where I work used to be a problem. But a loose-leaf logbook has helped bridge the communication gap.

At the beginning of each shift, the charge nurse writes the date and time in the logbook. Then she lists the staff members on duty, the doctors on rounds, the doctors' patients, sick residents, special events (such as a fire drill or special program), and so on. The next shift only has to read the logbook to see what happened during the previous shift. Part-time staffers, employees returning from vacation, and new employees can also keep up to date by reading the logbook.

Besides helping to communicate the daily events to staff members, our logbook is also a good legal record.

Katherine Link, RN

POPs are tops

If we held a formal inservice education session to introduce every new policy or procedure that affects the nursing department, we'd have little time for anything else. So to keep our staff up to date, we issue a "New POPs" (Policies or Procedures) sheet.

The New POPs sheet is one printed page with an easy-to-recognize banner headline. It highlights the new or revised policy or procedure and gives the source of this information, the effective date, and directions for finding further information.

Our nursing staff is enthusiastic about New POPs because they're getting the information they need without having to fit another inservice program into their already busy schedules.

Betty Thomas Daniel, RN, MSN

Temporary-help helper

The director of nursing service devised a handy and inexpensive way to orient temporary personnel to Brookview Health Care Facility, West Hartford, Conn.

She compiled a list of 16 "pool-personnel pointers" and had it printed on pocket-sized cards that were then laminated. She gives cards to temporary personnel when they first work at the facility.

The cards begin on a warm note: "Welcome to Brookview. We hope you enjoy your stay with us." Then, specific instructions are listed on how to use the phone, where to locate equipment such as oxygen and an emergency box, and what to do in case of a fire. General instructions cover directives such as the following:
• Know who the supervisor is.
• For newly admitted patients, take vital signs, order medications and laboratory work, and transcribe orders.
• Count narcotics when you start and end your shift; don't leave with the narcotic cabinet keys.

The cards help the new personnel adjust to the routine and reduce the time regular staff members devote to instruction.

Rosemary Schilling, RN

2

TEACHING

THE PATIENT

Rubber-band aid

Athletic patients don't always heed warnings about resting their sprained ligaments to give them time to heal. So use a teaching aid to help them understand why proper healing takes time.

A ½" rubber band with a small cut in the edge represents a sprained ligament in the ankle. When you stretch the rubber band, it tears even more—just as a ligament will tear if over-stretched by moving the foot.

This demonstration shows your patient how his ligament will have trouble healing unless he retires from the sporting world—for just a few days.

Robert W. Woodcock, RN

Cast care—for everyone

In our emergency department, we give patients instruction handouts to take home so they'll know how to care for their injury. For patients who get casts, we wanted an instruction sheet that would appeal to both children and adults.

We came up with a cast care sheet that combines simple instructions with eye-catching illustrations. For example, it has a drawing of an elephant wearing a leg cast and sitting in a chair. Crutches are propped against the wall. The instructions say, "Do not walk on your new cast for ____hours. Then, use crutches to help you walk."

Other drawings of animals with casts remind patients not to get the cast wet, to elevate the casted arm or leg on pillows, to observe the color and temperature of the skin at the edge of the cast, to apply ice to the cast to prevent swelling in the first 24 to 48 hours, and not to poke inside the cast to scratch.

The sheet has been a hit with our adult patients as well as our pediatric patients.

Gabrielle D. Schneider, RN

A wounderful lesson

To help a surgical patient understand the complexities of his wound, I use

a "wound box" made with the following materials:
• a small box that's open at one side (which represents the open wound)
• a piece of red felt (which represents the muscle tissue)
• a blue ribbon (which represents the blood vessels)
• a wad of white tissue paper (which represents fat)
• irregularly shaped pieces of material (which represent general cellular growth)
• a knee-high stocking (which represents the skin).

I place the felt, ribbon, tissue paper, and pieces of material in the box to show the muscle tissue, blood vessels, fat, and cells that are under the skin. Then I put the stocking around the box to show how the skin covers the wound. I gather the stocking at the top of the box to represent a suture line.

My teaching aid is inexpensive and really helps my patients (especially children) understand what's *under* the suture line.

Janeen F. Lloyd, GN

Group therapy
On our busy general surgical floor, we usually are only able to give brief *individual* preoperative instructions to our patients. But we supplement these individual conferences with a group session.

On the evening before their surgery, we invite patients to the lounge and ask them to bring their pillows and inhalation spirometers. After discussing basic preoperative events, we have the patients practice coughing and deep breathing. We also demonstrate the proper use of spirometers and how to splint incisions with pillows.

Besides ensuring that our patients know what to expect the next day, the group sessions also give them the chance to share their feelings about surgery and to encourage each other.

Donna Avallone, RN

Painless taping
Teaching patients or their families how to dress and redress wounds on hairy areas of the body can be a problem, because the tape sticks to and pulls the patient's hair when it's removed. Shaving the area helps, but the tape still gets caught on some of the hair. Solve the problem with pink hairdressing tape. It keeps dressings as secure as regular tape, but it lifts off easily and with less discomfort to the patient.

Nancy E. Dirubba, RN, FNP

Demo doll
To teach patients and new staff nurses how to care for a Hickman catheter, we use the chest cover from an old resuscitation manikin. We can simulate all Hickman catheter care procedures on the manikin: exit-site care, flushing, blood drawing, changing the injection cap, and clamping. Both staff and patients appreciate this "live" demonstration of Hickman catheter care much more than the textbook presentation we previously gave.

Pat Tobin, RN

Keep it simple
Sometimes simple teaching tools are as effective as sophisticated ones. I discovered this when one of my patients, scheduled for a bowel resection, didn't understand her doctor's description of the impending surgery.

To simplify things, I took a flexible drinking straw and asked that she think of it as her large intestine. The

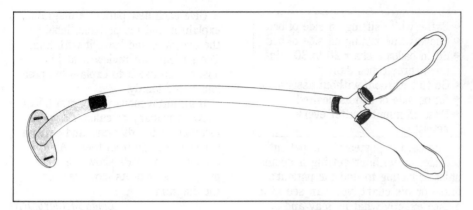

flexible part, I suggested, represented the tumor that had to be removed.

Then I performed the "surgery": I cut the straw on either side of the "tumor," removed the tumor, and taped the straw back together again.

"Now I understand," she said. That certainly pleased me—and even impressed the doctor.

Jane Grabenstein, RN

Teaching ventilation

If a baby on your unit has a tracheostomy and occasionally needs artificial ventilation when he becomes apneic and stimulation won't arouse him, you'll need to teach his mother how to ventilate him at home.

To help her practice, make a model respiratory system from the following materials: two finger cots, two rubber bands, a small Y-connector, some oxygen tubing, and a trach tube. Use the Y-connector to attach the finger cots to the oxygen tubing, securing them with the rubber bands. Then, attach the trach tube to the other end of the tubing. Finally, attach an Ambu bag to the trach tube.

Now the mother can practice gauging the amount and rate of pressure needed to inflate the finger-cot "lungs." When she becomes proficient in ventilating the model, she can take the baby home.

J. Thuman, RN

Say it with flowers

If you ever have to explain collateral circulation to a myocardial infarction patient and his family, compare your patient's injured vessel to the stem of a plant that's been accidentally broken off. When placed in a glass of water and given some time and care, the stem will sprout new roots. So, too, the patient's heart with proper care and rest will sprout new vessels.

Not only does this explanation bring a difficult subject into clearer focus, but it also gives the patient some much-needed hope for recovery.

Diana McLeod, RN

Cardiac cards

Our cardiac rehabilitation program has seven levels of activity through which patients progress before they're discharged. To remind the patient and staff members what the patient's activity level is and what he can and can't do, we've printed and laminated cards that describe each level.

For instance, activity level four is described as follows:

- Bathe while sitting on side of bed
- Shave while sitting on side of bed
- Sit in bedside chair 20 to 30 minutes, three times daily
- Go to bathroom without assistance
- Sit on side of bed as desired
- Rest 45 minutes after every activity.

The card is posted at the patient's bedside, so without getting a doctor's order or having to find the patient's nurse or his chart, you can see at a glance exactly what he may and may not do. It's also a constant reminder to the patient of how much he can do.

Sherry Gainey, RN

Inner view
Since many urology patients are unfamiliar with the anatomy of their kidneys and urinary tract, you may have trouble explaining their problem and treatment to them. To help teach them, have some anatomical diagrams printed.

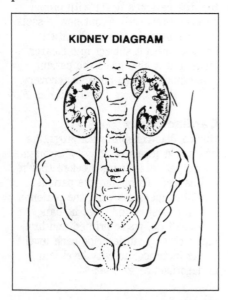

KIDNEY DIAGRAM

Give each new patient a diagram, explain it and his problem, label the diagram, and leave it with him. The patient can review it at his leisure and use it to explain his problem to his family.

If an intravenous pyelogram (IVP) shows a urinary calculus, show its location on the diagram and explain where it will go from there. Also, if subsequent IVPs show the stone's progression, plot its movement on the diagram.

Linda McClary, RN

Teaching tool for diabetes
To help my patients who have Type II diabetes understand what they can do to control their disease, I use an inexpensive teaching tool. I made the tool from the following materials:
- a large foam rubber ball (with holes cut into it) representing a *body cell*
- small foam rubber balls (with Velcro sewn onto one side) representing *glucose*
- foam rubber posts from a ringtoss game (cut in half, with Velcro sewn onto one end) representing *insulin*
- foam rubber rings from the ringtoss game (also cut in half) representing *fat*.

To use the teaching tool, I encircle the "cell" with the "fat" to show how fat blocks the cell's insulin receptor sites (the holes in the large ball). Then I attach "glucose" to the "insulin" (by pressing the Velcro strips together) to show how they're drawn together. But because fat blocks the receptor sites, the insulin and glucose can't enter the cell.

At this point I ask the patient how the insulin and glucose could get into the cell. Invariably, he'll say, "Take off the fat." So he sees that an

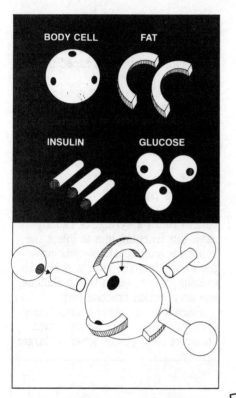

across the top of each card (the numbers represent the six food groups defined by the American Diabetic Association).

Under each number, list foods found in that group, varying some examples from card to card.

Next, cut enough blank paper disks to cover the squares on all the cards. Cut another set of disks and label each with one food mentioned on a card. Distribute the cards and blank disks to the patients and put the labeled disks in a container.

To play the game, one patient acts as caller, drawing a disk from the container and announcing the food listed on it. Each player must then recognize the appropriate food group and check to see if the food that's called is on his card. Additional disks

increase in insulin won't do the trick; rather, losing weight is the key to controlling his diabetes.

When patients can *see* the concept of fat interfering with diabetes management, they're better motivated to stick to their diet and get rid of the fat.

Susan Rush Michael, RN, MS

Do-it-yourself bingo for diabetics

Do you have difficulty teaching diabetics about an exchange diet? Solve the problem by devising a game called "Nutrition Bingo." Here's how to make the game:

Cut construction paper to make the bingo cards. Number from 1 to 6

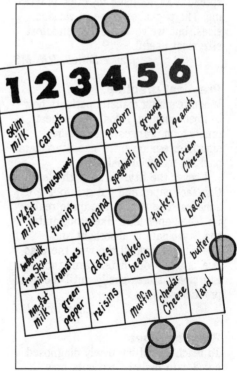

are drawn and called until one player achieves bingo by completing a line horizontally, vertically, or diagonally.

This game works well with groups of four to six patients, and a small prize can be given to the winner.

Marjorie A. Maddox, RN, MSN

Fruitless practice
With today's high cost of food, using grapefruit and oranges for practicing intramuscular and subcutaneous injections isn't practical.

But we've found a suitable substitute: a package of the blue gel that can be frozen and used to cool food in picnic hampers.

We can puncture the unfrozen package repeatedly, and it doesn't leak. We can also pinch it up or spread it for realistic injection practicing. The packages come in various sizes, but we've found the smallest size most useful.

Jeanne Sorrell, RN, MS

Practical practice
When teaching diabetic patients how to inject insulin, I don't have them practice on oranges or expensive simulator equipment; I use Styrofoam packing material instead.

I cover the Styrofoam with clear Con-Tact paper and cut it into 4″ × 4″ squares. The results are quite realistic. The paper feels like skin, and the Styrofoam is absorbent and doesn't roll around the way the practice oranges do. Afterward, the Styrofoam stores easily until the next practice session.

Jinny West, RN

Practice glove
To teach one of my newly diagnosed home care diabetic patients how

to inject her own insulin, I improvised a practice arm. I rolled two small hand towels, placed them inside an examination glove, and taped the end shut.

The towel-filled glove is so smooth and realistic that I use my on-the-spot improvisation as a standard teaching aid for all of my home care diabetic patients.

Joanne Cherry, RN

Practice pad
Teaching a newly diagnosed diabetic patient to fill a syringe is usually easy. But teaching him to inject the insulin is another story—jabbing the needle into the skin is scary. So, to help patients learn this technique, use an injection practice pad.

Place a foam rubber sponge, measuring 6″ × 8″ × 1½″, between two sheets of clear plastic about 1″ larger

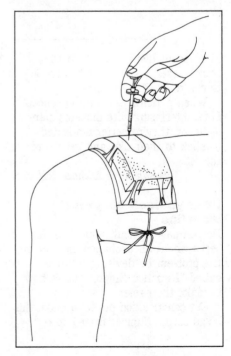

than the sponge. Seal the edges of the plastic with tape. Then, punch holes in the reinforced edges on each end and insert strings for ties. Finally, cut a large target hole in the plastic on one side. Then tie the pad snugly around the patient's upper thigh.

Using ½ ml of sterile water instead of insulin, the patient can practice injecting the needle through the sponge until he learns the proper direction and force. Placing the pad on his thigh also lets him practice at an actual injection site.

Make these pads in adults' and children's sizes and include one in each teaching kit supplied for diabetics by the central service department.

Marjorie B. Shaljean, RN

Rotation reminder
When teaching a newly diagnosed diabetic patient the importance of rotating injection sites, reinforce your lesson by marking the sites with a povidone-iodine swab. Since the povidone-iodine eventually washes off, give your patient a site rotation card as a *constant* reminder of his last injection site.

Elisa B. Bachrow, LPN

Mastering the mix
Ever have to show diabetic patients how to draw the right amounts of regular and NPH insulin into the same syringe without mixing the different insulins in their bottles? To help patients practice this, use sterile water and red food coloring to simulate the two kinds of insulins.

First, inject 10 ml of water into an empty insulin vial and label it "regular insulin." Then, inject 1 ml of red food coloring into a second vial, labeling it "NPH insulin."

When the patient draws the two "insulins" from the vials into a syringe, the color will tell him how accurately he's measured the correct amounts of "regular" and "NPH" insulin. Also, any food coloring in the vial of water or cloudiness in the food coloring vial will show that he's mixed the insulins the wrong way.

Nancy Schlossberg, RN

Trial vials
Newly diagnosed diabetic patients learning to take an insulin suspension sometimes forget to first rotate the vial between their palms to mix the insulin. So I put 2 or 3 ml of Maalox or Mylanta into their practice vials of sterile water. This makes the water look cloudy—much like their insulin suspension would—and they're reminded to rotate the vial.

I also label the practice vials with tape to ensure that they won't be used for the real thing.

Audrey Schupp, RN

Let your V be your guide
Recently, I was teaching a blind diabetic patient how to administer her insulin. When practicing, she'd often miss the injection site and stick her fingers (which were holding the skin taut) instead.

So I made an injection guide by taping two tongue blades together at one end to form a V. Then, just before she was ready to inject herself, she placed the tongue blades on her thigh, felt the outline of the blades, and inserted the needle—right on target— inside the V.

Theresa Gilliland, RN

Look...no hands
Teaching insulin injections to diabetic patients with blurred vision is always

a problem. Since they need both hands to work with the insulin bottle and syringe, they can't hold a magnifying glass, too. Use a magnifying glass holder that's easy to make and inexpensive.

Stack five paper foam cups upside down, one on top of another. Punch a hole the size of the magnifying glass handle through the center of all five cups. Then insert the handle through the hole. Put the insulin and syringe in back of the magnifying glass. You can adjust the height by placing books under the cups.

A tall, narrow-necked bottle can also be used as a holder.

Lee Korelitz, RN

Printed pointers for parents

At the hospital where I work, a new mother receives a lot of information (such as breast-feeding and car safety films, bath demonstrations, nutrition lectures) in a short period of time—especially if she's discharged within 24 hours after delivery. It's no wonder, then, that she's overwhelmed with all these new facts, figures, and explanations to remember.

We made up a folder to send home with the mother that contains information on parenting: resources such as the LaLeche League, for instance; a sheet with practical information such as cord care, how to take the baby's temperature, and what to do if the baby is fussy, has diarrhea, or is vomiting; a sheet describing the mother's physical condition during the postpartum period. New mothers appreciate the folder because it reinforces what we've already discussed with them during their short stay in the hospital.

Teresa Hays, RN

A balloon bust

We needed a breast model for our prenatal breast-feeding classes that was portable, pliable, realistic, *and* inexpensive. A small, inflated, oblong balloon met all these criteria.

The end of the balloon represents a nipple. (Or if we want to show a flat nipple, we hold the inflated balloon in the middle and force the air to the end.) We can demonstrate nipple preparation exercises and how to use a breast pump on our balloon breast model. And we always get a laugh when we pull out a green, orange, or multicolored breast model.

Janet E. Marshman, RN

Check it out

The doctors I work for have a large obstetric practice, and our patient-teaching program covers a lot of ground. To make sure we've given each patient all the necessary information and handouts, we've made a checklist.

During the initial interview with each patient, we rubber-stamp the inside cover of her folder with the following checklist:
__ 1. General information (nutrition, medications, activities during pregnancy, emergency department phone number, and so on)
__ 2. Fee policy
__ 3. Childbirth class information
__ 4. Breast-feeding books and class information
__ 5. Hospital preadmission form
__ 6. Labor and delivery information
__ 7. Insurance forms
__ 8. Last trimester and hospital information

After each prenatal office visit, we check off the information taught or items handed out. This way, we're sure the patient's well informed—on all fronts.

Linda J. Haugen, RN

A cord between home and hospital

Obstetric patients are being discharged from the hospital sooner than ever—many within 48 hours after an uncomplicated vaginal delivery. Concerned about how such patients manage at home, two nurses started a telephone follow-up service at the University Hospital in Denver.

The follow-up calls have four goals: (1) to determine if the care and instruction the patient received while hospitalized helps in the early postpartum period; (2) to identify new needs the patient has after she's discharged; (3) to provide follow-up teaching and referral if needed; and (4) to improve the teaching given to future patients.

Here's how the follow-up service works. On the day she's discharged, the patient is told about the service and asked to leave a number where she can be reached. Then, 2 days later, an obstetric nurse calls the patient. Using a printed form that lists specific questions, the nurse asks about the mother and the baby. She assesses the mother by asking about her breasts, vaginal discharge, elimi-

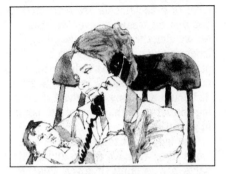

nation pattern, nutrition, and rest. She also asks about the mother's feelings and how she's getting along with the infant. The nurse assesses the newborn by asking about feeding, bathing, skin, and activity.

The conversation also gives the mother a chance to discuss any concerns she has. Some topics mothers have raised concerns about are exercise, colic, and sibling rivalry.

To improve the care of future patients, the nurse also asks which teaching was helpful, which was not, and what would been helpful if it had been offered.

How long does this follow-up service take? Calls to breast-feeding mothers average 17 minutes; calls to nonbreast-feeding mothers average 12 minutes. In most cases, a single call suffices.

The follow-up calls help the mothers by reinforcing what they've learned in the hospital, by preventing problems, and by dealing with problems that do occur. The calls help the nurses, too, giving them a sense of satisfaction for providing continuity of care after patients are discharged.

Chery Ann Hoffmeyer, RN, MS
Susan Pringle, RN

A better way to pass time

Patients hospitalized for premature

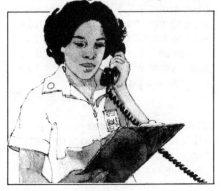

labor or preeclampsia are restricted to bed rest for weeks or even months. No wonder they can get discouraged, lonely, or just plain bored. To help patients through this tedious time, nurses at University Hospital, Seattle, distribute a weekly fact sheet describing the fetus at the appropriate point in gestation.

The fact sheet tells what the fetus looks like, what it's doing, and what parts are forming. It gives this information in a bright, nontechnical style the patient can easily understand. For instance, the sheet for the 24th week of gestation reads like this:

Although your baby is growing, her body is still very lean and her skin is wrinkled and red. The skin's wrinkled because the baby doesn't have much body fat yet. The skin's red because the blood vessels are close to the skin.

As the baby develops fat under her skin, she'll take on a pink color, the wrinkles will fill in, and she'll look plumper.

Besides describing the fetus's progress, the sheets describe changes the patient experiences. Here's what it says about the patient at 24 weeks:

Now that you're in your sixth month of pregnancy, you'll notice your weight increasing by about a pound a week. Remember, your baby needs good food from you to continue her steady growth. You may see stretch marks appearing on your stomach. These marks never go away completely, but they do become less noticeable after birth. You probably feel the baby moving. As she gets bigger her movements will become even more noticeable. Enjoy them!

Each patient looks forward to the next week to see what progress her fetus has made. The sheets also help the patient realize that the longer she keeps labor from starting, the more completely her fetus develops and the better its chances of surviving. Patients then understand how important their bed rest is, and they're more likely to comply.

Kathy Olney, RN

Infection detection

Discharge instructions may be overwhelming to patients who are leaving the emergency department after being treated for abrasions or lacerations. To make sure they remember the signs of infection, just remind them that "*P*eople *S*hould *R*eally *H*elp *P*eople":

> *P*ain
> *S*welling
> *R*edness
> *H*eat
> *P*us

This easy-to-remember mnemonic will help them learn what signs to report to the doctor.

Eileen M. Suraci, RN

A *proposition*

Next time you give a patient a sheet of discharge instructions for a self-treatment procedure (such as stoma care, insulin injection, or colostomy irrigation), make sure the instructions are written step-by-step in large block letters and are clearly numbered. Paste the instructions to the front of an $8'' \times 10''$ cardboard, easel-type picture frame. The patient can set the instructions in front of him and won't have to strain to read small print while he's learning to perform the procedure.

Marie O'Toole, RN, MSN

The learning game

When I give presentations on nutrition, infant and child care, dieting, or smoking, for example, to groups of patients, I try to make them more interesting by playing a game.

I divide the patients into two teams. Each team member takes a turn picking an index card from a pile of cards on which I've typed questions. The team member tries to answer the question on the card. If he can't answer it, his team pitches in and tries. If *they* can't answer it, the other team gives it a try.

The team that answers the question correctly scores a point. When all the cards have been picked and all questions answered, the team with the most points wins the game.

Besides adding an element of fun to my presentation, the game has prompted a lot of interesting, informative discussions.

Marion R. June, RN

Shoe-bagged pamphlets
Last time we cleaned out drawers in the clinic where we work, we found a lot of unused patient education pamphlets in disarray. We decided to display the pamphlets so patients would have access to them. To keep the pamphlets in order, we hung a clear, plastic shoe bag over the waiting room door and placed the pamphlets in the pockets.

Now the patients can choose the pamphlets they want, our work area is neat, and we find that patients—perhaps because of what they read in the pamphlets—are more informed and ask more questions about their conditions.

Ellen Pine, RNC, BS
Diane Squillace, RN

Class time...anytime
You're never too old to learn is the motto at the retirement home where I work. Each month, a number of our residents gather to learn about normal and disease-related aspects of aging. Some of the topics discussed have been causes and effects of arthritis, how aging affects the circulatory system, and how salt affects the body. Guest speakers have included dentists and dietitians.

The residents seem to be more conscious of preventive health measures since attending these classes. They tell us immediately when a problem occurs. And they really enjoy the classes, ask a lot of good questions, and encourage other residents to attend each month.

Ginny Knowles, RN

Labeling drug samples
In the doctor's office where I work, we frequently give sample drugs to patients to take until they can get their prescriptions filled. The samples, although clearly marked with the drug's name, don't have orders for how or when the drugs should be taken.

To help these patients remember how to take their new drugs, I devised this system: I place the sample in a small paper bag and attach a $2'' \times 4''$ label on the outside of the bag. On the label I write the date, the patient's name, the drug's name, its strength, when to take the drug, and what it's for. The label reinforces the verbal instructions the patient gets in the office.

As an added help, I staple a card with the patient's next appointment date to the folded bag. Now all his medical information is together in one place.

Lori Gross, RN

Posted pointers
In the pediatrician's office where I

work, we do supplemental patient and parent teaching this way: we make colorful posters on safety, nutrition, preventive health measures, and other subjects and display them on a bulletin board in the waiting room. (The board is hung high enough so little hands can't reach it, but low enough to read.)

Besides being a valuable teaching tool, the posters give our patients and their parents a little diversion if their appointment with the doctor is delayed a bit.

Toni Piller, RN

A drug tip-off

To help ensure that patients comply with their medication regimens at home, I keep a file of "drug tips." For example: Bactrim should be taken with a full glass of water, and the patient should drink plenty of water during the day.

When a patient is being discharged, I review with him the tips for his medications. If the patient is elderly or forgetful, I review the tips with a family member, too. Then, I write the tips on a card for the patient to take home with him. Even if such tips are printed on the drug containers, my teaching serves as one more way to ensure compliance.

Marianne Anderson, LPN

Album entrée

New patients sometime fear the unknown. To introduce newcomers to the radiation therapy department, take pictures of the treatment machines and of staff members at work. Mount the pictures in a photo album, and add a text that answers patients' most common questions.

The album is a useful aid to patient education. It is easy to design and

inexpensive to produce. And the idea can be readily adapted to other hospital departments.

Judith K. Stucke, RN

(Dis)charge cards

Writing and rewriting the same patient discharge instructions for many different patients is time-consuming. And if you write the instructions from memory each time, you may forget some important information.

That's why we use plastic plates (like credit cards) that are embossed with general discharge instructions. We just stamp an instruction sheet with the appropriate plate, individualize the instructions, and review them with the patients. Here are two examples:

Upper Respiratory Infection (Cold)

1. Return to the emergency department if you feel worse.
2. Drink 8 glasses of fluid a day.
3. Rest as advised.
4. Take aspirin or acetaminophen (Tylenol), 2 tablets every 4 hours as ordered.
5. Take other medicine as ordered.
6. Other: _____

High Blood Pressure

1. Follow your low-salt diet.
2. Avoid drinking alcohol and smoking.
3. Keep your follow-up appointment on

   _____

4. Take your medicine as ordered.
5. Return to the emergency department if you have dizziness, vision problems, headaches, or nosebleeds.

If a patient has multiple diagnoses, we stamp several sheets with the appropriate plates.

The plates make our discharge teaching a lot easier, and we're sure the patient gets complete discharge information.

Marcia Kiser Levitt, RN, BSN

Show the way
To teach a patient about his illness or treatment, do you usually give him a handout and a detailed verbal explanation? Why not use a photobook?

We made a photobook for our patients who are undergoing total hip replacement surgery. We wrote a simple explanation of each part of the patient's preoperative and postoperative care. Then with the help of the hospital photographer, we took pictures of traction equipment and other materials the patient would use, the way the patient would be moved, and so on. We put all the explanations and photos in a photo album. Now we give the album to each patient who will undergo this procedure so he can read about it and see what to expect.

This photobook seems to answer our patients' questions and alleviate their fears better than any of our other patient-teaching methods. And it proves that a picture really is worth a thousand words.

Deborah Estep, RN

Patient-teaching handouts
Fill a plastic loose-leaf binder with multiple photocopies of patient-teaching handouts on subjects such as low-salt diets, common disease symptoms, precautions for digitalis and anticoagulant use, cleaning respirators, and range-of-motion exercises.

Then when a nurse visits a patient, she has the handout he needs.

Do handout originals with a felt-tipped pen, using large letters. This makes for clear, legible photocopies—a feature welcomed by our elderly patients, especially those with poor vision.

Claudia Vepraskas, RN

A pocket book
My most successful patient-teaching aid is a $3\frac{1}{2}'' \times 5\frac{1}{2}''$ photo album. I fill each of the plastic envelope-like pages with information and pictures about a disease or condition and its treatment (for example, one album has information on juvenile rheumatoid conditions and anti-inflammatory drugs). When one of my patients is confused about his condition or treatment, I open my book and we review what he doesn't understand.

The inexpensive photo album holds 20 to 24 index cards or pictures. And it's small enough to fit in my pocket, so I can carry it everywhere.

Andrea Kovalesky, RN

Last things first
If you're teaching newly diagnosed insulin-dependent diabetic patients about their disease, begin by carefully assessing each patient's needs. Then decide which patients are ready for a self-injection practice session and which are better started off with films and literature.

This way, patients who are apprehensive about the "real thing" can get it over with quickly. After learning how to inject themselves successfully, they're much more receptive to the other information that remains to be taught.

Nancy Rufli Stepter, RN

Double-duty card
To reduce duplication of effort when teaching needs of diabetic patients, use a diabetic assessment card.

The front of the card provides space for patient identification.

The back of the card spells out the various responsibilities of staff nurse, inservice instructor, and dietitian.

The staff nurse's duties are to complete the patient assessment; have the patient listen to introductory teaching tapes; reinforce the inservice instructor's teaching; and chart the patient's progress in understanding his diabetic regimen.

The inservice instructor's duties are to provide teaching materials to meet the patient's specific needs; teach the patient individually or in a class; chart the patient's progress in understanding his diabetic regimen; and keep records of the patient's assessment and what he's been taught.

The dietitian's duty is to teach the patient his specific dietary needs.

The diabetic assessment card not only eliminates much duplication of effort but also ensures that patients' teaching needs *are* being met.
Jennifer Springer, RN, BSN

THE FAMILY AND FRIENDS

CPR: Keep it in the family
Most of our patients live in a rural community where an ambulance call usually takes 10 or 15 minutes to be answered. Those minutes are critical if someone has had a heart attack and family members don't know how to do cardiopulmonary resuscitation (CPR).

So our hospital and a local United Way agency established a program called CPR for Spouses. Here's how it works.

When a patient is identified as being at risk for having a heart attack, his spouse (or another family member) is offered the program. In six 1-hour segments, we teach spouses the American Heart Association's Heartsaver Program (one-rescuer CPR) and certain maneuvers performed to remove sudden airway obstruction. Our program ends with a "spouse talk" in which participants share their feelings about living with a person who has heart disease.

Besides getting a certificate at the end of the program, participants get peace of mind from knowing that they *could* save the person's life—if need be.
M. Cecilia Wendler, RN

Booties, bottles, and CPR
Here's an important tip to pass on to expectant parents. Suggest they fit a cardiopulmonary resuscitation (CPR) course in with all their other childbirth training, parenting lessons, and nursery remodeling projects. Such a course, with a focus on infant CPR and clearing an obstructed airway, *could* be the most valuable part of all their childbirth and parenting preparations.
Katherine Link, RN

A holding pattern
Giving eye drops to a squirming infant is never easy, but for the mother who must do this without someone to help restrain the baby, it's especially difficult. Here's a tip we give to mothers who take their babies home with a prescription for eye drops.

We tell the mother to sit on the floor with her legs apart and to lay the baby between her legs with his

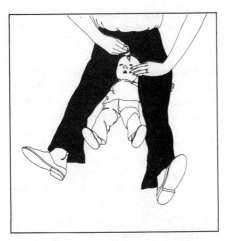

head toward her. Then she should place the baby's right arm under her right thigh and his left arm under her left thigh. She should hold the baby's head firmly but gently between her thighs. Then she can administer the drops.

This position frees both of the mother's hands while it immobilizes the baby's head. Thus, she'll be sure the eye drops go into the baby's eyes as ordered—not on his cheeks, nose, or chin.

Lenore Piccola, RN

Diabetic delights
A diabetic child doesn't have to sacrifice festive food at birthday parties and on special occasions. Tell his mother to substitute food he can have for the food he's not allowed. For instance, corn or apple muffins iced with unsweetened applesauce and decorated with raisins or nuts could be served instead of cake. Low-fat milk can be blended with vanilla extract and peaches, strawberries, or pineapple for a delicious cool drink. And instead of candy, serve vegetable sticks cut in various shapes.

Linda Jeronowitz, RN

Printed pointers for parents
We give handouts to new parents when they bring their baby to the pediatrician's office for checkups. Each handout tells how the child should be developing according to his age at the time of the office visit. And it describes certain developmental milestones that will probably occur before his next office visit. The handout answers questions that parents forget to ask during the office visit and those that come up before the baby's next visit to the doctor.

To personalize the handouts, we print the child's name, his height and weight, and the date of the office visit at the top of the sheet.

Wendy Kaveney, RN, BSN

Think THUNDER
One of my pediatric patients had chronic otitis media. To teach his parents the signs and symptoms to watch for, I developed the acronym "THUNDER." It stands for:
*T*emperature
*H*earing loss
*U*pper respiratory infections
*N*ausea
*D*izziness
*E*arache
*R*ed ears

I reminded the parents that otitis media feels like "thunder" in their child's ears, and I wrote the signs and symptoms on an index card for them to take home and keep as a reference.

Emoke Lukacs, SN

THE PUBLIC

Getting to show you
Does your family know what you do at work? Do your friends? Why not show them by holding an "open house"

on your unit, like the one held recently by the operating room (OR) staff at Hempstead (N.Y.) General Hospital.

A planning committee organized the event. Committee members selected the day (Sunday) and the time (11 a.m. to 1 p.m.). They also decided that the OR nurses would wear red carnations so they could be easily identified. The OR nurses then invited their families and friends.

Next, the committee members tackled some logistic problems: the recovery room area was set aside for any emergency surgery that might have to be performed during the open house. Scrub suits, caps, and booties were ordered for the 30 guests expected to attend.

On the appointed day, committee members arrived early to set up two ORs: one for a cholecystectomy and one for a hip pinning. They placed a Resusci-Annie on the table as a surrogate anesthetized patient, posted an X-ray of a gallbladder filled with stones, and displayed instruments, sponges, and other surgical equipment.

When the guests arrived, the OR nurses explained their work and answered questions. All guests— especially the children—enjoyed the hands-on experience of being hooked up to monitors, inflating cellulose sponges with water, and viewing a nylon eye suture under a microscope.

The nurses said the 2 hours they spent showing their families and friends the OR and the "tools of the trade" were worthwhile. Having guests in an area that's "off limits" to outsiders helped them feel a little less isolated—traditionally an occupa-

tional hazard among OR nurses.

Harriet Rosenman-Forman, RN, MPS, CNAA

More than just a "fair" idea

When 7-year-old Betsy went to the hospital to have her lacerated knee stitched, she impressed the nurses with her cooperation. Although Betsy had never been to a hospital before, she knew a lot about it. Why? Because she was one of the thousands of children who attended the Bronson Young People's Health Fair, sponsored by Bronson Methodist Hospital of Kalamazoo, Mich.

Like Betsy, children usually come to the hospital only if they're ill or injured. But once a year, the hospital comes to them. Hospital personnel take their equipment to a city park; here, children aged 4 to 18 can learn about health care and safety.

Nurses working at the fair involve the children through hands-on activities. For instance, one child stopped by the diabetes booth and told the nurse he was worried about his grandfather, who has diabetes. The nurse explained the disease to the child, telling him why his grandfather needed insulin injections. Then she had him inject "insulin" into an orange.

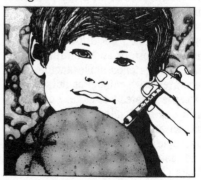

Nurses from all specialities work at the fair. An operating room nurse dresses in a scrub suit and shows children instruments and anesthesia equipment. She explains what happens during a tonsillectomy and shows a storybook that illustrates the operation. Respiratory care nurses help children into a mist tent and give them balloons that demonstrate how the lungs work.

Children aren't the only ones who benefit from the fair. The hospital nurses appreciate the chance to meet with healthy children and to teach them how to stay healthy. The nurses also mingle with representatives from community service organizations, such as the public health department, the American Red Cross, and the child abuse council. This makes them more aware of referrals they can make when a patient's being discharged.

The nurses who have worked at the fairs say the event is always well received. Children leave with no-smoking buttons, cancer prevention comic books, and balloons. But even more important, they leave with a keener awareness of good health and a positive feeling about the hospital and the nurses who work there.

M.E. Martelli, RN; A.M. Spaniolo, RN, MS; and B. Adams, RN

Healthy hearts

Mention Valentine's Day and what comes to mind? Hearts, of course. A nurse at Bellefonte (Pa.) Senior High School extends Valentine's Day into "Heart Week" to make students aware of their cardiovascular health. Her Heart Week program includes pamphlets, games, contests, and films.

Morning announcements and post-

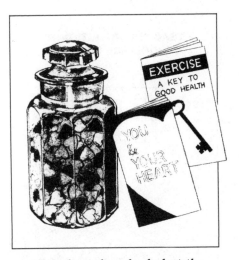

ers throughout the school alert the students to the program. They're invited to the health office to guess the number of candy hearts in a jar and to read the "Keep a healthy heart" bulletin board. They can also take pamphlets supplied by the American Heart Association and copies of crossword puzzles and scrambled-word games that emphasize the heart theme. During study periods, students view films on good nutrition, heart attacks, and strokes.

The nurse involves faculty members in the program by giving them lists of heart hints and heart facts to share with students. She also decorates a separate faculty bulletin board.

Other health maintenance programs offered throughout the year include high-blood-pressure prevention and control, the hazards of smoking, and how to do breast and testicular self-examinations.

Students and faculty respond well to these programs, and local newspaper coverage gets the word out to the community.

Joanna Lyons Mauger, RN, BS

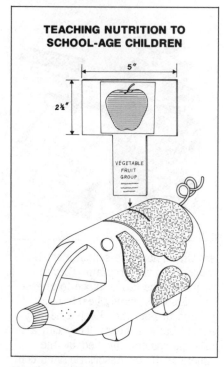

TEACHING NUTRITION TO SCHOOL-AGE CHILDREN

5"

2½"

VEGETABLE
FRUIT
GROUP

Hungry hound

Use flash cards and a toy dog to teach nutrition basics to first, second, and third graders.

To make the cards, you'll need the following:
• a 20″ × 54″ cardboard sheet
• 36 magazine pictures of junk foods and foods from the four basic food groups
• glue or paste.

Measure and cut the cardboard into 36 5″ × 6″ pieces, then cut each piece into the shape of a "T," 5″ wide and 6″ high (see illustration). Glue a food picture on the T's horizontal bar. On the vertical bar, print the name of the food group(s) represented by the picture and the words "Healthy for You" or "Not Healthy for You."

To make the dog, whom we named Hungry Hound, you'll need these materials:
• 1 empty gallon bleach bottle with cap
• 1 empty egg carton
• black or brown pipe cleaner
• black and brown felt
• glue.

Cut four rounded egg holders out of the egg carton. Glue them to one side of the bottle to represent Hungry Hound's feet—and to enable the bottle to stand.

Next, cut out three small black felt disks. Glue two of them into position as eyes; glue the third to the bottle cap for the nose.

Cut two pieces of brown felt in the shape of long, floppy ears, and glue these to the bottle sides.

Bore or punch a hole into the bottom of the bottle, and slide the pipe cleaner into the hole. Twist the pipe cleaner to make a curly tail.

Finally, set the bottle on its feet and cut a 2⅛″ slit into the top. You—or the children—can give Hungry Hound felt spots or decorations if you like.

To play the game, slide a T card into Hungry Hound's top so that only the food picture shows. Ask the children to name the food shown and to tell whether it's a junk food or to which food group it belongs. Pull the card out of the slot to check answers.

Children can play this game by themselves, in pairs, or as a class. But however they play it, they're sure to have fun *and* to learn about the foods they eat.

Leslie Grano, RN

Nutrition by the plateful

I have an effective, inexpensive tool

for teaching young school children the basics of nutrition: paper plates. I give each child a plate and ask him to draw two lines on the plate so it's divided into four equal "pie pieces." The children label each section with the name of a different food group and the number of servings needed each day from that group for adequate nutrition. Then they decorate the plates with a picture of each type of food and hang them on their classroom bulletin boards.

Betty Hedlund, RN, BSN

THE STAFF

Readin', writin', and arrhythmias

I work in a small, four-bed intensive care unit where we don't see many life-threatening arrhythmias. To be sure the staff will be able to recognize an arrhythmia when it occurs, about every 2 weeks I give each person a sheet of rhythm strips to study. Later we review the strips together. The staff finds the sessions helpful—especially when the next life-threatening arrhythmia actually does occur.

Margery Lebel, RN, CCRN

Get the rhythm

If you're just learning to interpret EKG rhythm strips, but you work on a unit where strips aren't readily available, how can you practice? Ask the nurses in the intensive care, cardiac care, or other monitoring units to save strips of interesting rhythms for you in a large envelope. If they write a brief description of the rhythm on the back of each strip, you'll have

ready-made flashcards for practicing interpretation.

Karen L. Foster, RN

Emergency practice

I work in a small hospital where we don't often have a chance to practice such procedures as cardiopulmonary resuscitation (CPR) or monitoring cardiac output. To be sure we'll know what to do and have all supplies and equipment on hand when we need them, we stage dry runs. We practice calling codes, performing CPR, setting up for Swan-Ganz catheter insertions, and so on. The doctors participate, too, so we'll all know how to proceed when a real emergency occurs.

Margery Lebel, RN, CCRN

Practice makes *CPR*fect

We have mock codes periodically to keep our staff's cardiopulmonary resuscitation (CPR) skills from getting rusty. After the code, we leave the resuscitation manikin in the room for those who want more practice. A certified CPR instructor stays with the manikin to supervise the practice. This gives everyone—not just those who directly participated in the code—a chance to polish CPR skills.

Kathleen Michael, RN, BSN

Crash-cart review game

To help nurses quickly locate any item on the resuscitation crash cart, turn your monthly crash-cart review into a game that helps the nurses learn and remember better.

Before playing the game, divide the nurses into teams of two and give each team a game sheet listing 20 emergency items. Then, one nurse

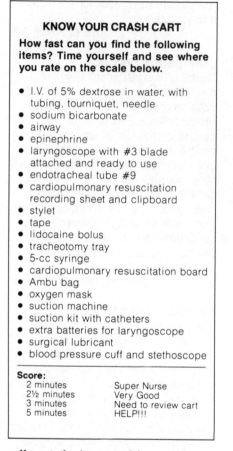

KNOW YOUR CRASH CART

How fast can you find the following items? Time yourself and see where you rate on the scale below.

- I.V. of 5% dextrose in water, with tubing, tourniquet, needle
- sodium bicarbonate
- airway
- epinephrine
- laryngoscope with #3 blade attached and ready to use
- endotracheal tube #9
- cardiopulmonary resuscitation recording sheet and clipboard
- stylet
- tape
- lidocaine bolus
- tracheotomy tray
- 5-cc syringe
- cardiopulmonary resuscitation board
- Ambu bag
- oxygen mask
- suction machine
- suction kit with catheters
- extra batteries for laryngoscope
- surgical lubricant
- blood pressure cuff and stethoscope

Score:

2 minutes	Super Nurse
2½ minutes	Very Good
3 minutes	Need to review cart
5 minutes	HELP!!!

calls out the items and keeps time, while her partner locates each item on the crash cart.

Carolyn Law, RN

Line finder

When it comes to assembling and setting up invasive monitoring lines, we wrote the book—a picture book, that is. We put together in a loose-leaf binder photographs of arterial lines, temporary pacemaker lines, cardiac output attachments, and intracranial pressure monitoring lines. The photos show all the equipment and how it's assembled as well as how it looks

in use. We also included a list of special equipment each doctor prefers.

The picture book helps us assemble and set up the different lines more quickly and accurately, and it's great for orienting new staff members to the unit.

Mary Larson, RN, CCRN, CNRN

A class tip

If you're demonstrating hemodynamic monitoring for an inservice class and want to produce some realistic waveform patterns, try this. Just as you'd insert an inside-the-needle catheter into a vein, insert the tip of a Swan-Ganz catheter into the rubber port of a 250-ml or 100-ml bag of 5% dextrose in water. Use a large-bore needle to introduce the catheter through the rubber port.

When the catheter's in place, re-move the needle, and you'll have a tight seal. Now squeeze the bag, and you'll create realistic waveform patterns—even, with practice, dicrotic notches.

Signe Prutsman, RN

You've gotta have heart

Nurses being oriented to cardiac care must thoroughly understand the heart's anatomy. Besides the usual teaching tools (lectures and slides), I use a real heart—a cow's heart. I dissect the heart in class, pointing out blood vessels, valves, chamber wall thickness, and so on. Cows' hearts are inexpensive and available from most meat markets. Best of all, nurses find this lesson the most meaningful part of the class.

Annmarie D. Campbell, RN

Show time

To familiarize new staff nurses with our unit, we give hands-on demonstrations of various procedures with used (but clean) equipment—Swan-Ganz catheters, fenestrated trach tubes, and endotracheal tubes, for example. These show-and-tell sessions are a welcome addition to our lectures and printed material, and they make orientation easier for the new staff *and* us.

Pamela Stuchlak, RN

Recycling Resusci-Annie

If you've ever had to teach mouth-to-stoma resuscitation, you know that finding a realistic teaching tool can be a problem. An inservice instructor at Huntsville (Ala.) Hospital tells how nurses there solved the problem by making some changes in an old Resusci-Annie.

They removed the head, neck, and air tube from the manikin and sepa-

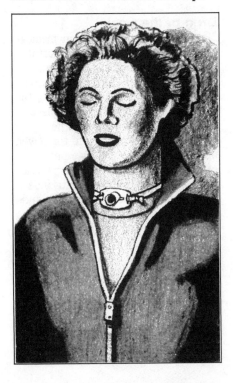

rated the face mask from the head. They cut a stoma-size hole in the neck and in the air tube that represents the trachea.

Then they put the face back on the head form and inserted a plastic tracheostomy tube through the holes, reconnected the air tube at the base of the head, and reattached the head to the body.

The nurses use the model to teach mouth-to-tracheostomy resuscitation and to show how to use an Ambu bag to ventilate a person with a tracheostomy. To demonstrate ventilating through a stoma, they simply cut off the tracheostomy tube at skin level.

Linda Dean, RN

Respiratory review

Nurses in the inservice education department at Northampton Accomack Memorial Hospital, Nassawadox, Va., found a novel way to review respiratory care. They offered a "respiratory review day" in a bazaar-type atmosphere.

First they announced the event on the bulletin board and in the monthly activities calendar. Then they gathered respiratory equipment for demonstrations and prepared handouts.

On the review day, they gathered in a central meeting room and hung posters showing postural drainage and other respiratory procedures. They set up three booths: one dealing with tracheostomy care; one with chest tubes; and one with postural drainage. Respiratory nurses or inservice instructors staffed the booths, which were open all day so nurses could stop by on their break or at mealtime.

An inservice instructor said the review day helped nurses become familiar with equipment and procedures they use only occasionally.

Bonnie P. Lewis, RN

The answer album

To conserve space in our emergency department drug cabinet, we don't keep package inserts with the drugs in stock. Instead, we keep a photo album (the kind with clear, plastic pages) on top of the drug cabinet. In the plastic pages, we slip a package insert for each of the drugs we commonly use. When we have a question about one of these drugs, we just flip to that page in the album.

Kathleen Rohrer, RN

It's in the cards

The drug reference book at our nurses' station was always disappearing, so we made a new reference—an index-card file. We listed the drug name, indications, and side effects on a card and filed the cards alphabetically according to the drug's classification. We also made an index of specific drugs.

We've discovered several advantages to using this system. For example, the card file can be chained to the desk so it won't disappear. The cards can be replaced or updated as often as needed. One or two cards can easily be taken to a patient's room for a patient-teaching session.

Best of all, the nurses who prepare and update the drug cards remember the drug information more readily than if they'd only read it.

Charlotte A. Thayer, RN, MSN

Pocket the info

With several new antihypertensive drugs recently placed on the market, we had to come up with a way to keep ourselves and staff members up to date. Our solution was to develop a pocket-sized reference guide on antihypertensive drugs.

The guide lists the three categories of antihypertensives (diuretics, adrenergic blockers, and vasodilators) and describes how each medication's supplied, its action, duration of action, dosage range, common adverse reactions, and contraindications. Several pharmaceutical companies contributed to the cost of printing the guide.

Our guide has become an invaluable aid, especially when we have to adjust a patient's dosage, change a drug regimen, or assess possible adverse reactions. What's more, we've distributed the guide to other hospitals in the area and they're equally enthusiastic about it.

Linda C. Moore, RN, MSN
C. Beth Pulliam, RN, MSN

Drug of the week

"How well do you know your medications?" That's the title of a colorful wall chart at our nurses' station. Under the title are two clear plastic pockets, one above the other. Into the top, smaller pocket, we put a piece of paper with the name of a new or unusual medication. Into the lower, index-card-sized pocket, we put a card with information on the medication's action, indications, contraindications, dosage, adverse reactions, and nursing implications.

Each week, one of our unit's staff members changes the cards and files the old ones for future reference. This way, each of us gets a turn at researching a drug. And we're all kept up to date on new medications.

Diane Boson, RN

In the cards

So many new chemotherapeutic agents

are being prescribed for cancer patients that you can be hard pressed
to keep up to date. Gather the information about dosage, route of administration, adverse reactions, and
specific nursing implications (if any)
for each new agent prescribed. Then
print or type this information on a
3″ × 5″ card and enclose it in plastic
to protect it. Keep these cards on
the cardex for easy access and quick
reference.

Carole W. Sweeney, RN

Crash cards

During an emergency you can easily
forget the correct medications and
procedures to use, in your rush to
help your patient.

That's why we list standing-order
emergency medications and procedures on cards and hang the cards in
a designated spot on our bulletin
board.

Then, if a patient goes into anaphy-
lactic shock, has an insulin reaction,
or a cardiac arrest, we can grab
the cards for a quick refresher course
in emergency nursing. We also color-
code our emergency drugs for easy
identification.

Of course, we study the cards any
chance we get; this way we're prepared before an emergency occurs.

Larry Asplin, RN

Drug of the month

I work in a newly opened recovery
room (RR) with staff members from
several different nursing backgrounds.
To help us all become familiar with
the many drugs used in the RR,
we've initiated a "Drug of the Month"
program.

Each month, one staff member
researches a drug (such as Sublimaze
or Innovar) and transcribes the fruits

of her research onto a colorful, eye-
catching poster. The poster is placed
in the staff lounge or kitchen where
nurses from all shifts can see it, read
it, and learn.

Joanna P. Couch, RN, CCRN

Thought for the week

To make sure our nurses keep up
with the latest in nursing care, I send
memos, hold mini-seminars, and
schedule regular one-to-one meetings.
But I also dispense information
with a "Thought for the Week" that I
leave in each nurses' rest room.

Each week's thought reviews a
nursing procedure (such as giving
heparin subcutaneously) or a patient-
teaching topic (such as what to teach
a patient about lumbar puncture or
taking nitroglycerin at home). The
nurses appreciate this quiet, uninterrupted opportunity to study and
look forward to the new thought each
week.

Paula Alamia, RN

UTI blitz

To reduce the number of urinary tract
infections (UTIs) occurring in patients, nurses from Ottawa General
Hospital took part in a "UTI blitz."

The blitz included a "UTI awareness
week," featuring daily speakers
discussing such topics as the need for
catheterization, indwelling versus
intermittent catheterization, and the
quality of a urine specimen. After
each talk, training manikins were
available for staff members to practice
male and female catheterization.

During the week, nurses received
handouts reviewing the general
principles of catheterization, catheter
insertion, and perineal and catheter
care. They also received a self-test
and a word-search game that included

terms related to the urinary system.

A nurse clinician at the hospital said the blitz helped the nurses become more aware of important catheter care principles.

Nicole Florent-Legare, RN

See how they grow
To teach staff members the importance of infection-control practices, have them conduct a clinical experiment: making their own cultures to see how quickly bacteria grow.

First, get four agar plates. Then have the staff take cultures from their hands, the bottom of their shoes, a bedside stand, and a patient's overbed table—especially one who places used tissues on the table rather than discarding them.

After taking the cultures and labeling the plates, take them to the laboratory to be incubated for 48 hours.

Later, share the report from the laboratory. The results will show the nursing staff the importance of maintaining cleanliness.

Cherry A. Karl, RN, BSN

Give her a hand
To demonstrate to staff members the importance of hand washing in preventing the spread of infection, try this. Rub a bit of water-soluble fluorescent poster paint into the hands of several volunteers. Tell them to imagine that the paint represents germs. Then ask them to wash their hands as they usually do after patient contact.

When the volunteers are satisfied that their hands are clean, wave a black light over their hands. Staff members are usually quite surprised when the black light reveals many remaining areas of paint. The mes-

sage—scrub hands thoroughly to get rid of germs—gets across.

Rosemary Sommers, RN, BSN, ANP

Bugging the bugs
A nurse epidemiologist from Madison (Wis.) General Hospital uses a "bug egg" to teach staff members good infection-control practices.

To make the bug egg, she glued a plastic ladybug to a plastic egg (the kind that holds panty hose). She puts in the egg cleverly written "infection alert" sheets. These sheets describe various contaminants or pathogens, where they can be found, and how to prevent them from endangering patients.

One such infection alert sheet is a letter from "Mr. Staphylococcus Epidermidis," who describes his recent change "from a bothersome contaminant to a major pathogen." He boasts of his accomplishments: prosthetic valve endocarditis, urinary tract infection, and conjunctivitis—to name just a few. Then he complains about practices that undermine his effectiveness: thorough hand washing, maintaining aseptic technique, and monitoring implanted devices.

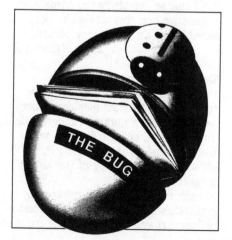

Another infection alert sheet is an ultimatum from "the president of the local bug union," who lists 15 conditions under which his members will strike. The "conditions," of course, are components of an infection-control program. The nurse places her plastic bug at various spots on every unit, so no one knows where or when it will turn up. She reports that staff members enjoy looking for it and profit from reading the advice it contains.

Llewellyn Haverty, RN, BSN

Senior class tips

In a course on aging, I learned some tips that might be helpful to other nurses working with geriatric patients.

For example, patients who have poor eyesight may have trouble reading your patient education handouts if you use blue paper. Use nonglare, yellow paper instead. Or if yellow paper isn't available, use a yellow highlighter to emphasize important points. If possible, have your printed materials enlarged so the letters, numbers, and words are easier to read.

Finally, because some of your patients may have a problem with short-term memory, frequently review and reinforce the points in your lesson.

Kay Preshlock, RN, BS

Staff development presentations

Looking for a new form of staff development presentation? Try the idea of poster packets now being used at Coatesville (Pa.) Veterans Administration Medical Center.

These poster packets, circulated by the nursing education department,

present staged photographs of staff members showing correct and incorrect methods of performing procedures, such as applying restraints. The photographs are mounted on 36" × 42" poster paper and accompanied by appropriate questions ("Is this restraint crisscrossed only at the back?" "What is the physiologic consequence of this procedure?"). Reference material is also suggested so nurses can read up on the procedures.

Each poster packet is spiral-bound and contains four laminated pages. A supplemental packet provides additional references, a description of related nursing procedures, and quiz sheets. Nurses complete the quiz sheets and send them to the nursing education department for credit.

The poster packets have many advantages over more traditional procedures for self-instruction. They're durable and large enough that they don't get lost. Nurses on all shifts can use them. They're fun to use because of the familiar faces in the photos. And the quiz is proof the nurses are using the packets and are accountable for the information they contain.

N. Yentzer; M. Kiernan

A shady aid

When preparing a staff program on ostomy care, I found few visual aids to help me. So I decided to make my own.

I bought a bright orange window shade and drew different types of colostomies on the shade with colored felt-tipped markers. During class I drape the weighted, pulled-out shade over a portable blackboard, then roll it up and put it away until the next class. (If all my classes were held in the same room, I'd install window-shade brackets on the wall.)

This inservice teaching aid is inexpensive, rolls up for easy storage, and can be adapted to many teaching situations. What's more, it's long lasting—mine's been around for 6 years.

Hedy H. Crapa, RN

Nurse librarians

The hospital where I work doesn't have a reference library, so our intensive care unit nurses decided to set up their own. We all contributed some of our textbooks and journals. Each nurse may borrow what interests her—after first signing a notebook and listing what she borrowed and when. Upon return of the material, the nurse crosses off her name and the title of the borrowed material.

As an added service for our staff, the borrower notes pages in the book or journal that she found particularly helpful. Then she writes a brief summary of these pages on an index card, titles the card according to subject, and files it in a topical index-card file.

Donna Roome, RN

Impromptu projecting

Slide presentations are effective—if done in a room specially set up with a screen and projector, at a time chosen well in advance. But I've discovered a way to make impromptu slide presentations that are just as effective.

I use a hand-held slide viewer. This smaller type of projector allows me to give presentations *whenever* and *wherever* I like: during break, on rounds, when giving report, at the patient's bedside for patient teaching (showing slides made from textbook illustrations), at the nurses' station, or on the floor.

Because it's so versatile and easy to tote, the hand-held slide viewer has become one of my most valuable teaching aids.

Shirley Moore, RN, MSN

Orientation—for everyone

Our nursing orientation programs aren't just for new employees. We also invite seasoned staff members to attend any sessions that interest them. Besides refreshing their memories, the orientation program is an excellent way for the seasoned staffers to meet the new staffers. And during the program, they can interject any pertinent information they've garnered from their own experience.

Teresa Gentry, RN
Charlyn Cassady, RN

Patient-teaching tip

Among the most common reasons nurses give for not completing—or even attempting—patient teaching is that they don't know how to go about it. But nurses working in cardiac rehabilitation at Cabell Huntington Hospital, Huntington, W. Va., know exactly where to start. Why? Because they use pocket folders that tell them.

The folders are packets of information that include behavioral objectives, a content outline, a list of suggested teaching aids, a discussion guide, review questions, and copies of handouts.

The folder on ischemic heart disease, for example, says the patient should achieve 11 objectives, such as defining ischemic heart disease, and listing what can bring on angina and what can relieve it. Included in the content outline is a review of the symptoms of heart attack and angina, how to tell the difference between the two, and indications for emergency treatment. The discussion guide is a script that tells the inexperienced teacher exactly what to teach. (More experienced teachers simply disregard the discussion guide and follow the content outline.) Review questions help the nurse to go over the material with her patient and evaluate how much he's learned. Finally, the folders contain a form to document the patient's understanding.

Improving on their idea, the nurses who prepared the folders are now color-coding the series of folders—for example, using red for cardiac rehabilitation, blue for congestive heart failure, and so on.

Robin Dennison, RN, MSN

Where can I find...?
If your unit frequently is staffed with nurses from a nursing pool who constantly have to ask where equipment and supplies are kept, try this. Make an alphabetical list of frequently used items and where they're stored. Post the list in clear view at the nurses' station.

When new pool nurses come to the unit, show them the key supply areas: central supply room, clean and dirty utility rooms, medication room, and so on. Then when they need anything, they can just refer to the posted list, go to the appropriate area, and get it themselves—without taking you away from your work.

Paula Shay, RN

Instrumental instruction
If some employees aren't familiar with all the commonly used medical instruments, start an *Instrument of the Month* game.

First, staple a plastic instrument holder to a manila folder. On the folder, write the name of the instrument and its pronunciation, what it's used for, and how to identify variations of the instrument. Place samples of the various instruments in the pockets of the instrument holder. Then post the entire display on a bulletin board in the nurses' lounge.

After presenting information about hemostats, scissors, and retractors, you may notice a change for the better in the staff's handling of the instruments.

Ellen L. Badger, RN

Show and tell in the ED
We have such a variety of supplies and instruments in our emergency department (ED) that keeping up with them becomes a problem. To help familiarize new staff members with these items, I made a poster titled "Instruments and Supplies of the Week" for the ED bulletin board. Each week, I place on the poster an index card describing a supply item or instrument. I post the item itself on the board under the poster. Some examples of items that have been displayed recently are a bone curette, packing forceps, Asch forceps, and Unna's paste boot.

New staff members quickly learn to recognize our equipment. Later, when they need a certain item in an emergency, they don't have to ask for help in finding or identifying that item.

Della Whipple, RN

OR aid
When I was studying operating room (OR) procedures, I had a hard time remembering some of the potential complications of surgery. So I devised a learning aid: the acronym "TAPS

for the VIP." It stands for:
T hrombophlebitis
A spiration
P neumonia
S hock

Loretta Thornton, GN

Hickman review

Nurses in our intensive care unit who
need a refresher in Hickman catheter
care procedures use a resuscitation
manikin for practice. An incision
is made in the manikin's chest next
to the nipple, and a catheter is inserted through this incision and
sutured in place.

The nurses practice cleaning the
insertion site, applying a dressing,
drawing blood from the catheter,
administering medications and blood
products through the catheter, and
changing tubings. Since the manikin
is kept on the unit, the nurses get
the practice they need and patients
are assured of competent care.

Sandra Fields, RN, BSN

Right in the pocket

To help new nurses become familiar
with hospital procedures, print a
booklet with information on medication times, surgical preparations,
admission and preoperative laboratory
work, and drug and I.V. drip-rate
formulas. A $2\frac{1}{2}'' \times 3\frac{1}{2}''$ booklet fits
into a uniform pocket—so the nurses
have a convenient reference source
near them at all times.

Marjorie M. Thomas, RN

Teaching tool for trach techniques

Here's how to make an inexpensive
yet realistic simulator for teaching
tracheostomy care techniques.

Get an inexpensive Styrofoam head

(the kind used to store wigs), and
cut a hole $1\frac{1}{2}''$ in diameter at the site
of the usual tracheostomy. Apply a
thin layer of clear nail polish around
the hole to prevent the Styrofoam
from crumbling. If you're artistically
inclined, you could paint a face on the
head.

You can use this simulator to teach
sterile dressing change technique,
removal and cleansing of the inner
cannula, sterile tie change technique,
and inflation and deflation of the
tracheostomy cuff. And you can apply
the various antiseptic agents used
in tracheostomy care to clean the
Styrofoam without causing it to dete-
riorate.

The simulator is so inexpensive
and easy to store that you might want
to get multiple heads to allow individual practice.

Rosemarie Moore, RN, BSN

Match test

Imagine you're looking at a large
corkboard on which are pinned empty
I.V. bags of different sizes. The bags
once contained dextrose 5% in water,
normal saline solution, dextrose 5%
in Ringer's lactate, hypertonic saline,
or other solutions. Also pinned to
the board are various doctors' orders,
laboratory test results, and diagnoses.

Could you match the doctors'
orders with the proper I.V. bag and
fluid? Nurses at St. Luke's Hospital in
Bluefield, W. Va., don't have to imagine taking such a test. The patient-
teaching coordinator asks nurses
to try their hand at matching the
orders and the fluids. A sample
matchup:

• *Doctor's order*—500 ml of normal
saline solution. (Nurse would select
appropriate I.V. bag.)

• *Diagnosis*—cardiac patient experiencing lethargy.

• *Laboratory test results*—serum sodium level of 119 mEq/liter.

In this case, the order for normal saline solution to be given to a cardiac patient seems unusual, but the low sodium level (normal is 135 to 145 mEq/liter) reveals why the doctor ordered what he did. To keep the nurses on their toes, the coordinator adds an extra I.V. bag, an inappropriate order, or an order that should alert the nurse that an I.V. solution is infusing too slowly or too rapidly. Above all, this clever match test helps remind nurses to check a patient's diagnosis and his laboratory test results before administering any I.V. fluids.

Sydney Anne Gambill, RN

Quickie card file

To keep track of important information you've read, try setting up a quick-reference personal card file.

After you read a pertinent article, list the subject, the source, and the page numbers at the head of a 5″ × 7″ note card. Then jot down the article's main points. If you need more cards for the same article, title each one and number them consecutively.

You can also photocopy most charts and tables and paste them on the cards. Then you can alphabetize the cards with dividers. The cards wear well, don't need much storage space, and can be easily reproduced for your clinical area. They're also great for a quick review.

Linda Weitzenkamp, RN

Who's got time to read?

To help nurses share the information published in nursing journals, Mt. Sinai Medical Center of Greater Miami has started a journal club. At the meetings, members receive copies of articles to discuss. They spend the first 20 minutes reading the articles and another hour or so discussing them. Before adjourning, they evaluate the meeting and suggest topics for future meetings. They discuss articles on aortic valve replacement and nursing's image in the media (enlivened by examples of how nurses are depicted in cartoons).

The nurse clinician in charge of the club says the meetings have helped nurses to keep abreast of interesting articles and to learn from each other.

Patricia Salome, RN

Boxed topics

We hold a staff-development conference on our unit every week to keep nurses up to date on patient education, equipment, and hospital policies and procedures. To make the conferences interesting, fun, and easy to conduct, we use a "conference box"— a large cardboard box that holds plastic bags filled with conference materials.

For example, if we want to have a conference on smoking, we put cigarettes, matches, and information on the effects of smoking in an 8″ × 10″ clear plastic bag. We write suggestions for discussion on index cards (such as "What are the effects of smoking on the adolescent, middle-aged, and elderly patient? On the fetus?" and "What is hospital policy on patient and visitor smoking?"). We place these cards in the bag, too.

Later, the nurse conducting the session opens a bag, spreads out the materials on a table, and reads the cards. We all participate in discussing the topic, and we all take turns adding, discarding, or updating topics as needed.

Nancy Lynn Grandovic, RN, BSN

Current events in a hurry
Here are three easy ways to help busy nurses on your unit stay up to date:

1. Each month, ask a different nurse to select an article from a nursing magazine, copy it, and post it on the unit bulletin board. When nurses have time, they can borrow the article, read it, and return it.

2. Choose a topic of special interest to nurses on your unit (perhaps something new or puzzling). Each month, invite a nurse who's well versed in that topic to give a presentation to the staff. Or get an audiocassette tape presentation that nurses can listen to whenever they have time.

3. Buy or make videocassette recordings of lectures given at nursing conventions or university medical schools. Hold screenings at different times during the month so most nurses on your staff can see it.

Katherine Link, RN

Word play
To help us keep up with developments in nursing, we play a word game.

Every day a different person from each shift writes a new or unusual nursing-related word on the assignment sheet, and the rest of us try to find out what it means.

Looking up the word takes time, but it's fun and everyone participates because we're actively searching out the word.

Betty Horvath, RN

Card tricks
I used to be discouraged when I found handouts left in the conference room or in the wastebasket after an inservice session. Then I started printing the main points of the sessions on both sides of $3'' \times 5''$ index cards. And voilà—the conference room was clean as a whistle after each inservice session.

The nurses tell me the index cards are easier to carry and store than the handouts; they can just put the cards in their uniform pockets or card files for handy reference, p.r.n.

Nancy Rhodenbaugh, RN

Portable study aid
If you can't find the time for the study and review you need for college courses or a new job, try this method. Instead of hitting the books, hit a button—the button on a battery-operated, pocket-sized tape recorder.

When you find a book or magazine article that pertains to your schoolwork or job, record its important points. Also tape the main ideas from your class notes—the notes from a one-semester course take only 3 hours to record. And if you attend a lecture that's especially interesting or helpful, the speaker's words are forever engraved on your pocket recorder.

Then, while driving to and from school and work, doing housework, or even just relaxing—you can study. And this extra time with the "books" makes you more confident on the job and more prepared for class.

Susan T. Rosen, BSN, CCRN

Towel trick
Here's an effective way for students to practice changing I.V. tubing. Half-fill a small, plastic trash bag with rolled-up towels, and knot the bag at the top. Then roll the bag into the shape of an arm and insert a catheter through a single thickness of plastic

and into a towel. Attach the catheter to I.V. tubing and attach the tubing to an I.V. bag filled with water.

Now students can practice changing and taping the tubing and learn how to regulate the flow clamp. What's more, they don't make a mess because the towels absorb the water.

Linda Schaffer Newman, RN

Less mess lesson

When nursing students practice using I.V. equipment with emesis basins to collect the solution, many times the tubing slips and the solution runs onto the floor, making a sticky mess. Solve this problem by having them use an empty, used I.V. bag to represent the patient's vein and collect the solution.

Just insert the needle from the tubing of the practice bag into the medication port of the empty I.V. bag. The tubing port of the empty bag can be clamped with a hemostat or plugged with an I.V. needle protector (which must be taped in place). Students can then regulate I.V. flow, check for backflow, remove air from the tubing, administer medications by I.V. push and piggyback, change I.V. tubing, and practice other I.V. skills with realistic results—and no mess.

Rosemary Fischer, RN

Ham 'n' legs

To teach my students how to bandage an amputee's leg stump, I use a dressmaker's ham. (That's a stuffed, fabric-covered version of a ham you'd buy in the grocery store. Dressmakers use it to press the sleeves and shoulders of garments.) One student holds the ham by the large end (which represents the amputee's thigh) while another student practices wrap-

ping the other end of the ham (the stump).

Florence Bradshaw, RN

What nerves

When I was in nursing school, I devised this number drawing to help me remember the 12 cranial nerves.

Beneath the drawing, I listed the nerves that correspond with the numbers in the picture. Then I named some of the actions or sensations controlled by those nerves. My list looked like this:
1. Olfactory—smell
2. Optic—vision
3. Oculomotor—iris and eye movements
4. Trochlear—eye movements
5. Trigeminal—upper and lower

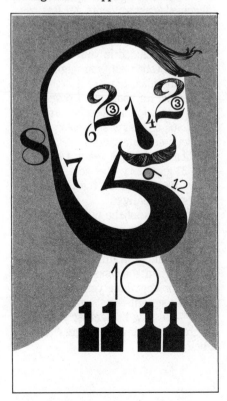

mouth and teeth, forehead, anterior half of scalp
6. Abducens—eye movement (lateral)
7. Facial—facial expression
8. Acoustic—hearing, balance
9. Glossopharyngeal—tastebuds on posterior part of tongue, throat sensations, saliva secretions
10. Vagus—swallowing, vocal cords, goes to abdominal organs
11. Accessory—head and shoulder movements
12. Hypoglossal—chewing, speaking, swallowing.
The drawing was a study aid in school, and it's a handy reference now.
Beatrice Humphris, RN

Pillow practice
Ever since I designed a special pillow "abdomen," my students get lots of practice in advancing Penrose drains and removing sutures. If these procedures are included in your state's nursing practice act, you might want to try this idea, too.

To make an abdomen, I cover a pillow-sized, foam-rubber square with about 36" of heavy, skin-colored, synthetic suede material.

When sewing the seam, I leave a 2" to 3" gap along one side. This allows me to replace the Penrose drain periodically.

On one face of the pillow, to the left side, I make a small slit through which the Penrose drain will protrude, to mimic a drain protruding from a patient's incision. To the right of this (or anywhere you wish), I make a long slit—or "surgical incision"—and sew it together with silk sutures. And for atmosphere, I add a belly button.

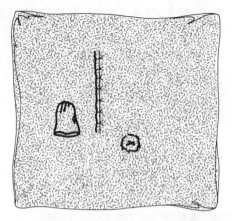

As students advance the Penrose drain through the small slit, the foam inside the abdomen offers a slight resistance, simulating actual drain advancement. Practicing this procedure and having the chance to repeatedly remove sutures helps give the students the confidence they'll need when they do the real thing.
Kay Segundo, RN

A puzzling lesson
To review indications for chest tubes with my nursing students, I use a "puzzle board." I draw an outline of normal lungs and a heart on a piece of white poster paper. Then I cut out puzzle-shaped pieces from blue and red paper to represent a pneumothorax and hemothorax. Students take turns placing the puzzle pieces over the appropriate areas on the puzzle board. (To show a hemopneumothorax, they place the blue and red puzzle pieces *together* on the board.)

Although puzzling at first, my teaching aid helps the students learn and remember the information.
Jayne Smitten, RN

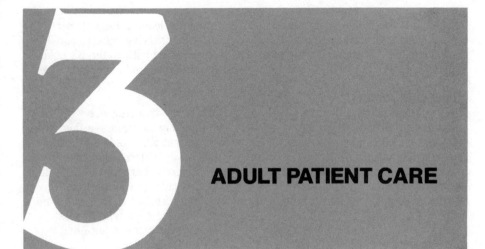

3

ADULT PATIENT CARE

FLUID AND NUTRITION

A good shake
When a patient wants—and *needs*—a high-calorie, high-protein bedtime snack, but the hospital's kitchen is closed, what can you do? Take a look at the snacks stored in your unit's refrigerator and improvise.

For example, you can mix a carton or two of any flavor of ice cream with milk for a quick, nutritious, and appetizing milk shake. (Let the ice cream soften slightly first for easier mixing.) Or mix some sherbert with a liquid elemental diet, such as Vivonex. Patients will like these shakes—and benefit from their nutritional value too.

Vicki Ephrou, RN

Supplemental selection
To spice up your patient's high-protein dietary supplement, don't use just the supplement's flavor crystals. Every now and then, substitute an instant drink mix and some sugar substitute instead. The mixes come in many flavors, so patients are much less likely to get bored with the selection.

Patricia Soukup, RN

Nutripops
When a patient needs a high-calorie, high-protein nutritional supplement, but is tired of the same old thing, try this recipe.

Mix one of the following combinations in equal amounts:
• strawberries, whipped cream, and vanilla Sustacal pudding
• chocolate Sustacal pudding and whipped cream
• vanilla liquid Sustacal, whipped cream, and several drops of peppermint extract.

Add pieces of banana, apple, or other fruit, according to the patient's preference. Then pour the mixture into 30-ml medicine cups, place a toothpick in the center of each cup, and put them in the freezer. When the mixture is frozen, remove the medicine cup and give the frozen "nutritional ice pop" to your patient.

These supplements keep well in the

freezer, so if you make plenty ahead of time, your patient can enjoy a tasty "nutripop" whenever he wants.

Jill Goulet, RN

Mixes that match

If your patient needs a dietary supplement, remember that instant breakfast mixes can substitute for drug-company supplements.

When prepared with whole milk, the mixes have nearly the same nutritional components as the supplements.

Besides, mixes are readily available in grocery stores, and, even when you include the milk, they cost about half what the supplements cost. (For more protein, you can add an egg to the mix.)

Caution: Before switching from a supplement to a mix, check the labels on both to make sure the nutritional components are similar. If not, keep looking until you find a suitable match.

Deborah-Ann S. Coleman, RN

Mixed drinks

To help your patient comply with his orders to drink a lot of fluids, try this: fill his plastic washbasin with some ice and several cans or cartons of his favorite juices or sodas. Place the basin at the patient's bedside, where he can reach it easily.

The patient will appreciate having a variety of fluids other than water on hand, and he'll be more likely to comply with his orders to "drink up."

Claire E. Mendenhall, RN

Watermelon magic

When a patient's treatment includes forcing fluids, do you find *yourself* doing the forcing? Solve the fluid

problem (at least in the summer months) by serving watermelon. The fruit is loaded with water, it's cold and nutritious, and patients love it!

Barbara Neale, RN

Pick from the bucket

Here's a way to encourage fluid intake for a patient who's ordered to "force fluids up to 3 liters/day." Ask the food service department to send up a plastic bucket (one for each shift) filled with ice and eight 4-oz plastic cups. Fill the cups with at least four different kinds of juice and cap with spillproof lids.

Leave the bucket at the patient's bedside. The patient will look forward to choosing his next drink from his juice bucket. You'll hardly ever have to remind him to take his fluids.

Jane S. McDermott, RN, BSN

The pop that refreshes

Patients on fluid restrictions have thirsts to satisfy, like anyone else. But small quantities of liquids that get swallowed in one sip aren't very satisfying.

To quench patients' thirsts and still keep accurate intake/output records, make "Popsicles" from juice or an allowed supplement. Pour the liquid into 30-ml cups, insert an orange wood stick in each, and then put the cups into a freezer. When you're ready to use the "Popsicles," loosen the cups by running them under warm water for a few seconds. Patients really enjoy these treats, and they stay within their fluid limits.

Mary Massaro, RN

Tube trick

If you have patients who must be tube-fed through a small jejunostomy tube, here's a way to set up a continuous system that's also nearly leak-proof. Remove the rubber top from a sterile eyedropper and discard the top. Insert the dropper end into the jejunostomy tube. Then connect a piece of suction tubing (about 4″ long) to the neck of the eyedropper. Connect the other end of the suction tubing to the adapter of the tube feeding setup, and the system is ready to go.

Wanda Tullier, SN

Colorful signals
When a patient with a tracheostomy takes fluids orally for the first time, do you worry about aspiration? Deciding which secretions he's coughing up—tracheobronchial or clear fluids in danger of being aspirated—isn't easy.

So, give colorful fluids, such as red gelatin or grape juice, instead of clear fluids. These colorful signals help identify the secretions and protect the patient.

Michael Couillard, RN

When it pumps, it pours
Some of our patients lack the strength and coordination to pour water or juice from a pitcher into a cup. To make sure they get their required fluids, we give each of them a "pump pot"—a small picnic jug with a spout that dispenses liquid when you push down on the lid.

Usually, patients can fill their cups themselves with the pump pots, so they're encouraged to take more fluids. We like the pots, too: they save us the time of refilling cups. And since they're insulated, we don't have to refill the pots with ice.

Jeanne Sorrell, RN

Free-flowing fluid
Helping a weak or debilitated patient take oral fluids can be frustrating. Holding a cup to his mouth gets more fluid *on* the patient than *in* him. And he may not have the strength to drink through a straw.

Instead, put a flexible straw upside down in his cup, so the short end is in the fluid; the flexible, ridged section rests on the rim of the cup; and the long end points down outside the cup.

By sucking just a little on the end of the straw, the patient can siphon the fluid into his mouth. He can easily regulate the flow of fluid with his tongue.

Jeff Lang, RN

A short cut
For a debilitated patient, taking liquids through a straw may require more effort than he can give. You can help him by cutting the straw to shorten the distance between the liquid and his mouth. Be sure, though, to place the cut end in the cup, so the rough edge won't hurt his mouth. And let hot liquids cool first—the patient may not expect to be able to drink so easily and he might burn his mouth.

Mary Ellen Palumbo, SN

Straw stretcher
Drinking without spilling isn't easy for a patient who must lie on his abdomen—even when he's using a straw. To help him, make a "straw stretcher."

Slide the tubing adapter of a 24″ length of I.V. tubing into the long straight end of a curved drinking straw. Put the I.V. tubing into the patient's glass and let him sip through the curved end of his straw. The tubing extension makes the straw long enough so the patient can drink without tipping his glass and spilling the contents on his bed.

Jean Sellers, RN

More pleasing by freezing
When a patient has trouble swallowing because of throat surgery or a hampered gag reflex resulting from a stroke, taking liquids may be a problem. But freezing liquids is helpful. Patients can swallow high-protein and high-calorie items such as Sustacal, milk shakes, and eggnog much more easily when they're in a semisolid state. Another advantage: freezing makes less-desirable liquids more palatable.

Barbara D. Mizenko, RN

Seal 'n' sip
Many patients who lack complete hand control and need to be fed express the desire to feed themselves. Here's how they can drink from a cup without assistance.

Tupperware sells a "sipper seal," which is 85% spillproof. A set of two seals and four mouthpieces costs about $1. The seals fit over inexpensive Tupperware cups. Patients may drink right from the mouthpieces or through a plastic straw inserted in the mouthpiece.

Victoria Paul, LPN

Gripping solution
Many patients with arthritis in their hands have trouble gripping eating utensils, pens, and pencils. To enlarge the grip on these and other slender items, use foam cylinders from hair curlers. A package of about 10 costs approximately $1, and they're available in many drug and department

stores. Just slip the foam cylinder off the plastic curler spindle and onto the slender pen or handle.

Evelyn Rossky, OT

Put a lid on it
Some bedridden patients spill more than they drink whenever they use a cup or glass. So ask their families to bring in an empty pint-size jar with a screw-on lid. (A mayonnaise jar is a good example.)

With a nail that has about the same diameter as a straw, punch a hole in the middle of the lid. Then pour the liquid into the jar, screw on the lid, and put a straw through the hole. The patient can drink away—and not spill anymore.

Deann Meyers, RN

Heads up
Sometimes a stroke patient has trouble holding his head up while sitting, which makes feeding him difficult and limits his view of his surroundings. Here are two solutions to this problem, depending on the patient's needs.
1. Refold a 3" × 4" folded dressing lengthwise to make it 1½" × 8", and put it across the patient's forehead like a headband or sweatband. Then, run a piece of 1" tape across the headband and fasten it to the back of the chair behind the patient's head. Although the tape holds the patient's head up, it doesn't touch his skin— and the "headline" supporting him isn't obvious to passersby.
2. Apply a cervical collar, perhaps cut a bit narrower than standard width. The collar especially helps if the patient's mouth droops on one side. With his chin resting on the soft collar, the patient can keep his mouth

comfortably shut, lessening drooling.

These supports lift a patient's morale as well as his head.

Elizabeth Gavula, RN

Lip service
A great gift idea for a patient who can't eat or drink anything is an assortment of different-flavored lip balms. The pleasant taste of the lip balm will help satisfy the patient's craving for flavor, while the moisturizing emollients will help soothe his parched, cracked lips.

Paula Brenton, RN

Decarbonation
For a patient who needs fluids and would like to have a soda but can't tolerate its carbonation, try stirring about ¼ teaspoon sugar into the soda. The sugar will neutralize the carbonation. Patients who've had throat surgery or radiation therapy, as well as ulcer patients, will appreciate this tip.

Judith Snow, RN, CMS

Spray thirst away
Do you have patients on restricted fluid intake? You can help them quench their thirst while using only a small amount of their allotted liquid by using a plastic squeeze bottle with a spray top.

Here's how. At the beginning of your shift, check to see what the patient's allotted amount of fluid is. For example, if he's allowed 50 ml of fluid during the shift, he may wish to use half his allotment in the water spray bottle. Then fill the bottle with 25 ml of water and let the patient spray his mouth as he feels the need. At the end of your shift, measure the remaining amount of water in the bottle. If, for instance, it

is 5 ml, you would record an intake of 20 ml from the spray bottle, plus whatever other fluid intake he's had during your shift.

Chris Christgau, RN

Refreshing squirt
A patient with second- and third-degree burns on his face has lips so sensitive that he can't put a straw or the rim of a cup against them. He can, though, use a syringe to squirt liquids into his mouth without touching his lips.

Fill several 50-ml sterile syringes with juice, milk, or water and leave them in ice at his bedside. Then, when he wants a drink, he can serve himself.

Melody L. Ziobro, RN

Mastectomy care #1
Frequently, the doctor orders a sterile towel to be draped over the patient's incision after the original dressing

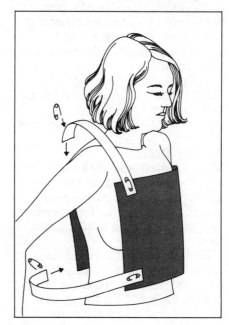

and drains are removed. But by this time, the patient is moving and exercising, so the towel just won't stay taped in place.

To solve this problem, hold the towel in place over the patient's incision and pin a strip of ½" gauze to one of the top corners. Bring the gauze over her shoulder and the opposite corner of the towel around to her back. Pin the gauze to this corner. Then pin some gauze to the bottom corner of the towel in front, bring the gauze around to the back of the patient's waist, and pin that end of the gauze to the bottom corner of the towel in back.

Now the towel will stay in place while the patient has enough freedom to move and exercise comfortably.

Judith Curry, RN

Mastectomy care #2
One of my patients who'd had a mastectomy developed some flap necrosis. To get rid of the odor from the necrosis, I soaked some pieces of gauze in oil of wintergreen and pinned the gauze near the neckline of her pajamas.

The patient loved her fragrant "sachets" and the clean, fresh feeling they gave her.

Pam Kirk, RN, BSN

Postop straw
When a patient who's had nasal surgery needs oxygen but can't use an oxygen mask, we make special oxygen tubing for him. Ingredients: Oxygen tubing and a flexible plastic straw.

First, we cut off the end of the tubing that would go to the patient's nose. We insert one end of the straw into the cut end of the tubing, bend the straw, and insert it into the

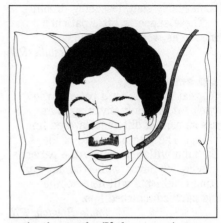

patient's mouth. (If the straw is too long and misses the patient's mouth, we snip a bit off its ends.) Then we tape the straw and tubing to the patient's cheek.

To make sure we never come to our "last straw," we make several special oxygen tube–straw sets ahead of time.

Mabel Rumbaugh, RN

Go for the goal #1
"Walk, walk, walk" is our constant chant to postoperative patients. But verbal prodding doesn't seem to get them moving as quickly as a visible goal.

So we hung a bulletin board at the nurses' station with the heading "You've come a long way." We posted pictures on the board of patients walking with I.V. poles, drainage bags, and various encumbrances. Then we attached a sheet of paper and a pencil so patients can sign their names on their first postoperative walk to the nurses' station. The sheet provides a goal for patients to work toward and shows the world (or at least the staff and other patients) that they've gone the course.

Maureen J. Dew, RN

Go for the goal #2

To encourage our postoperative patients to get up and walk after surgery, we use positive reinforcement. We set up a juice-and-ice cart in the hall. When the patients want a drink, they can walk to the cart and help themselves.

Terri Fleming, RN, BSN

SURGERY

Easy and painless

One of the most painful tasks for a patient with a bilateral mastectomy is raising herself to get out of bed. I've devised a way to make getting up easy—*and* painless besides.

When making the patient's bed, I lay a drawsheet over the top half of the bed. When the patient wants to get out of bed, I ask her to fold her arms under her chest area for comfort, and I raise the head of the bed as far as it will go. Then I grab the top of the drawsheet on both sides of the patient and pull it up toward me. As the patient rises, she swivels sideways and puts her legs over the side of the bed. After she rests there a minute or so, I again pull the drawsheet toward me to help her to her feet on the floor.

The drawsheet gives a patient the boost she needs without any painful tugging or pulling.

Norma Mecham, LPN

A basket cover

My mother had a radical mastectomy with extensive muscle and skin autografting over her entire right chest area. Her doctor didn't want any fabric (even a hospital gown) to touch the grafted areas, but he did want her to get out of bed and walk.

To help my mother comply with the doctor's orders—and retain some degree of modesty—we used a plastic laundry basket. We cut a hole large enough for her head in the bottom of the basket, taped gauze around the edge of the hole, and pinned sheets to the gauze. Then we put the basket over my mother's head so it rested on her shoulders. The sheets covered her, yet the basket held them away from her body.

This laundry basket cover could also be used for burn patients (if they're not on a "sterile dressing only" regimen).

Boni L. Ives, RN

A support report

A patient recovering from a unilateral mastectomy usually feels better if the remaining breast has some support. But a regular bra irritates the sensitive, sutured mastectomy area.

So I cut the unneeded cup and shoulder strap from the patient's old bra. What's left is a supporting cup for the remaining breast and an elastic band and fasteners, which usually pass under the sutured area without causing irritation.

Betsy Schrader, SN

Cut for comfort

For patients who've had radical neck surgery, hospital gowns just won't do. They're too tight around the patient's neck, causing pressure on suture lines and Hemovac sites, and they cover the tracheostomy opening, obstructing the patient's airway.

Unsnapping or untying the top fastener helps—but the gown may then fall off the patient's shoulders.

So make a slight alteration—cut a $4'' \times 4''$ section out of the front of the neckband—and rehem the band.

These altered hospital gowns serve patients well.

Rita Sauer, RN

To top it off

We used to give craniotomy patients a paper cap from the operating room to wear after their sutures and dressings were removed. But most patients didn't like the caps because they were too stiff or too big. As a substitute, I got some 8" wide tubular stockinette and cut off a 14" long piece. Then I rolled a cuff on one end and gathered the other end with a rubber band. The result? A soft, comfortable cap that fits.

Cheryl Gormbard, RN

Reflections on positioning

After retinal reattachment surgery, a patient may have to lie prone for 24 to 48 hours. To help him maintain this position without developing neck stiffness, facial irritation from the sheets, or boredom, try this.

Remove the headboard from his bed and put an overbed table between the wall and the bed (leave some space between the table and bed). Pad the table with a towel and position the patient with his forehead resting on the table so he'll be facing the floor.

Place a mirror on the floor beneath his face; this way, the mirror reflects the wall-mounted television screen or other room activity. Visitors can make eye contact with the patient by looking into the mirror. When the patient's eye needs to be examined, just raise the bed a bit, so the examiner can squat down—and look up.

Marilyn Burchett, RN

Propping pads

When a postoperative patient tries to get out of bed without assistance or without an overbed trapeze, he leans on one of his elbows for leverage. After he does this several times, he develops a sheet burn on his elbow.

To prevent this problem, give your patient elbow protectors. With his elbows comfortably protected, he'll be encouraged to get out of bed more often.

William T. Child, RN, BSN, MA

Warm therapy

The operating rooms in our hospital are usually cool. So a patient whose incisional area was exposed for a long time during the operation may be quite cold by the time he reaches the recovery room. To help the recovering patient warm up quickly, we cover him with heated blankets. And because a great deal of body heat is lost through the head, we wrap his head with a warm blanket, too.

Marci Smith, RN

Homemade care

One of our patients who had a gastrostomy showed me how his wife solved the problem of what to do with the tube. Rather than letting it hang loose or taping it to his abdomen, she made a small, soft, fabric bag for the tube. With the tube tucked into the bag and the bag carefully pinned to the patient's undershirt, the tube stayed in place and the patient's skin didn't suffer from tape irritation.

Diane M. Otte, RN, MS, ET

Support hose

A good, inexpensive means of abdominal support for the patient who's had abdominal surgery is an old pair of panty hose (with the legs cut off). The panty hose that provide extra "tummy control" are especially good. The support helps ease pain and encourages mobility.

Margaret Teufel, RN

Tea service
The unit where I work has many patients who've just had abdominal surgery and suffer from gas pain. Our care plan for them includes progressive diet; rectal tubes, p.r.n.; and mint tea (if the doctor okays it). The patients enjoy the tea, and it helps them expel the flatus.

Joanne Breden, RN

A splinted idea
After abdominal surgery, if the patient finds that splinting his incision with a pillow is awkward, suggest he try this: fold a bath blanket or sheet lengthwise and wrap it around himself. He can easily twist the ends together as tightly as necessary for the right amount of support. And he can do this while sitting or standing.

Kim Waters, RN, BSN

Sitting comfortably
If you're caring for patients who've had rectal or perineal surgery, here's a way to help them to sit up straight and to increase sitting time without added pain.

Get a piece of foam rubber measuring about $14'' \times 18'' \times 4''$. Cut out a circle in the center. Place the foam pad in a pillowcase and let the patient carry it with him from place to place for his sitting comfort.

Patients claim this type of pad is more comfortable than pillows or rubber rings, and it's less expensive than many commercially made decubitus pads.

Marie Ray Knight, RN

Resection redressed
Patients recovering from an anal-perineal resection need a dressing that's comfortable, stays in place, and that they can easily change by themselves. We've found that applying a sterile sanitary napkin over the dressing and holding it in place with a sanitary belt or T-binder works well. The patients tell us the napkin holds the dressing in place, is comfortable to sit on, and absorbs well. If we need to check the color and amount of drainage, the patients can just put the dressing and napkin in a plastic bag.

When the dressing is no longer needed, patients can use the sanitary napkin by itself.

Cindy Peterson, LPN

Laceration lubrication
If a scalp laceration is hard to suture because the patient's hair gets entangled in the suture material (even though the wound area has been prepared), try this technique. After you've shaved the area, apply Lubafax, or a similar sterile, water-soluble lubricant, around the hairline of the laceration. This will hold the hair down, preventing it from getting entangled in the suture and providing a more sterile field. The lubricant can be easily washed out after suturing.

Linda Drain, RN
Cheryl Westbay, RN

Nickel's worth
After eye surgery, a patient may have dressings over both eyes and have trouble finding the nurses' call button

on the bedside console. Tape a nickel on top of the button to help the patient identify it. Then he need only run his fingers over the console until he feels the familiar coin, and press the button.

Daryl Seifert, RN

Cool it
An elevated temperature is a common problem of postoperative patients on a surgical unit. Once proper infection-control procedures have been instigated (blood specimen sent to laboratory for culture and sensitivity, antibiotic therapy begun), here's how to lower the patient's temperature while waiting for an aspirin order.

Using a fracture bedpan as a water basin, have the patient place both hands in ice-cold water intermittently for 20 to 30 minutes. This technique has reduced temperatures nearly 2 degrees F. in just 30 minutes.

This procedure is ideal for the patient who's sensitive to aspirin; is more comfortable for the patient than alcohol rubdowns; takes less nursing time; and doesn't require a doctor's order.

Sue Jennings, RN

Cove*ring*
Do you use surgical tape to secure a patient's ring to his finger before surgery? If so, do you find a sticky, hard-to-remove film on the ring's stone when you take the tape off?

Next time, use a Band-Aid (with the gauze pad over the stone) to secure the ring. When you remove the Band-Aid, the stone's beauty will be unblemished.

N. May, RN

A cleaning trachnique
When a patient gets a tracheostomy that will be permanent, you know his

trach care must be performed with sterile technique at first. During this time, save the cleaning brush from his tracheostomy care kit. Later, when sterile technique is no longer necessary, you can continue to use the brush to clean his cannula. Make sure you sterilize the brush each time you use it, though.

Vicki Cornish, RN, BSN

MOBILITY

Skid-proof shoes
For the stroke patient who is just becoming ambulatory, firm, laced shoes with crepe or rubber soles are recommended. But if the patient doesn't have such shoes, you can make his own leather-soled tie shoes skid-proof. Just fit a pair of foam rubber hospital slippers over the patient's shoes and anchor them with adhesive tape. This will provide both the support and the friction the patient needs to keep from slipping or sliding.

Renee Berke, RN

One size fits all
Custom-fit disposable sponge slippers to a patient's foot size. Just tie a rubber band around the excess sponge at the slipper's heel, and it fits perfectly.

Peggy Young, RN, BSN

Nonslip slippers
Shiny hospital corridors can be hazardous to unsteady, recently postoperative or elderly patients. To help keep them from skidding—and boost their self-confidence—attach skid-proof bathtub appliqués to the soles of their slippers. Or you can put stockinettes on the patient's feet and attach the appliqués to the bottoms.

For pediatric patients, apply the appliqués to the bottoms of pajamas that cover the feet. To reinforce the appliqués so they'll withstand several washings, sew all around the edges.

And here's an even more economical tip—buy sheets of rubber that have an adhesive backing and cut out your own appliqués. Children love choosing their own designs—and they're a big boost to safety.

Ellen Roben, RN

Stocking up on exercise
After a mastectomy, the patient is usually instructed to exercise her arm and chest muscles by raising and lowering her arms. An easy way to do this is to put an old nylon stocking over the shower curtain rod, hold the two ends, and pull it in a seesaw motion.

Since the stocking doesn't hurt the rod or the patient's hands, it's a good motivator for *daily* exercise.

Holly M. Rook, RN

Briefly speaking
To make an inexpensive leg-lift or arm-lift exerciser, sew together the waistband of a man's cotton briefs. Then slip a 5-lb bag of sugar (or whatever weight the doctor orders) into the briefs through one leg hole. (Instead of a bag of sugar, you can also use a plastic bag filled with rice or flour.)

Have the patient put his leg through one leg hole of the weighted brief and out the other. Then have him balance the weight on his ankle (or wrist) and begin lifting it up and down. The brief's soft cotton will protect his skin and he can change

the weight as his exercise program progresses.

Marge Kempf, RN

From spool to exerciser
Don't throw away those empty traction-cord spools. They make great grip exercisers for patients with spastic or flaccid paralysis of the hands.

Trim a spool's round cardboard ends to within ½" of the spool core, then cover the ends' raw edges with adhesive tape to protect them. Pad the core by winding cast padding or cotton batting around it several times. Secure the padding or batting with a layer of Elastikon, Coban, or other soft adhesive material.

Thread a long piece of gauze through the core's open center. Position the gauze so an equal amount extends from both sides of the core.

Now you're ready to attach the spool-become-exerciser to the patient's hand. First, pad your patient's wrist with a sponge dressing. Then put

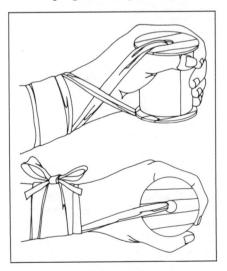

the core into his hand, cross the two gauze ends under his wrist, bring the ends up above his wrist, and tie them in a bow.

Depending on your patient's needs, you can use the exerciser one or more times daily.

Kathryn Calamita, RN

Versatile bulbs

I use a bulb syringe for a hand exerciser. I place the bulb in the patient's palm with the opening between the patient's thumb and index finger. Then I tie or wrap the bulb in place with gauze. The bulb helps keep the patient's hand from contracting and his fingernails from digging into his palm.

Dottie Williams, LPN

Inside pocket

Ambulating patients with a Hemovac can be a problem. The solution? A secret inside pocket.

Pin a washcloth to the inside of the patient's robe to form a pocket. Then tell the patient to *drop* (not pin) the Hemovac into the pocket when he gets out of bed.

This way, the Hemovac is out of sight and safe from being pulled out.

Linda Mitchell, RN

A handle on hand

Patients who have chest tubes in place needn't remain bedfast. With your help, they can get up and move around easily. Just attach the two metal bed hooks on the disposable chest drainage set to a package handle (the kind some department stores attach to heavy packages). Then the patient (or you) can carry the drainage set as he walks about.

Virginia R. Carlson, RN, CCRN

Hook the bag

Have trouble ambulating a Foley catheter patient by youself? Ask a hospital maintenance man to put a hook on the lower part of each movable I.V. pole. This hook holds the catheter bag more securely than a pin on the patient's clothing. Also, the patient can hold on to the I.V. pole for stability—and you can ambulate him by yourself.

One caution: Make sure the catheter tubing doesn't hang low between the patient and pole. Otherwise, the tubing could get caught under the pole's wheels.

Charlene Forvery, LPN

Traveling tongue blades

If your patient has an I.V. *and* a urinary catheter with a drainage bag, you can make mobility easier for him this way.

Place two tongue blades together and tape their bottom halves to the bottom of a portable I.V. pole. Then hook the drainage bag behind the top, untaped portion of the tongue blades. The bag's hung low enough for an adequate gravity flow, and the patient can push his I.V. pole and walk easily—without having to juggle his drainage bag, too.

Kathleen A. Seraphin, RN

RESTRAINTS

Strapped no more

Soft strap restraints used to keep patients from pulling out their I.V.s, nasogastric tubes, and Foley catheters don't always work well. Some patients wiggle free of the restraints, while others get confused and agitated because their movements are restricted. Sometimes the restraints even inhibit circulation to the patient's fingers.

Instead of straps, pull a stockinette over the patient's hand and up his arm as if it were a sleeve. Then secure the stockinette bottom around the patient's wrist with adhesive tape, being careful not to tape too tightly.

Next, put a sponge ball (the soft kind children play with) into the patient's hand, pull the stockinette back down his arm and over his taped wrist and hand, and tie a knot in the stockinette close to his fingers. Finally, repeat the procedure for the patient's other hand.

With both hands filled, the patient can't get hold of the I.V.s and other tubes. Still, he has freedom of movement—and he can squeeze the balls to exercise his fingers.

Kimberlee A. Hull, CVN

Restraining pants

Patients may try to slip out of vest or belt restraints and may end up with the restraints around their necks or faces.

So, try a fashionable approach to the problem. Buy inexpensive cotton slacks and insert ties made of heavy twill tape (such as venetian-blind tape) into the side seams at hip level. These ties replace the restraints and keep patients in place effectively. What's more, they look better, too.

Sharon Maylock, RN

Restraining discomfort

When a patient needs limb restraints, use pieces of egg-crate–like foam rubber to pad the restraints. Cut each piece about 3″ wide and long enough to fit around the patient's arm or leg. Place the smooth side of the foam against the patient's skin, the egg-

shaped side facing outward. Apply the restraint over the foam in the channels between the eggs. The eggs keep the restraint secure, while the foam cushions the skin and keeps the restraint from becoming too tight when it's pulled.

Regina S. Schuch, RN, BSN

Give 'em a boot

Give your patients with temporary transvenous pacemakers a boot—a Buck's traction boot, that is.

Simply place the patient's arm and the pulse generator in the boot, and fasten the straps to keep the arm immobile. If the patient's arm is longer than the boot, cut open the end of the boot. And, with confused patients, tie the boot to the bed with the attached traction rope.

The boot's metal strip keeps the arm straight but less rigid than it would be with a conventional arm board. Also, the pulse generator can be kept alongside rather than on top of the arm, adding to patient comfort.

Keep a Buck's traction boot on your pacemaker cart, since it's just the boot some patients need.

Joan Belisle, RN

PHYSICAL CARE

Maintaining dignity

When a patient is restless or confused and kicks off his covers, protecting his modesty becomes a problem. How can you keep him covered?

Just put another hospital gown on him—but put his legs through the armholes of this one. (The bottom edge of the second gown extends to the patient's chest.) Tuck the gown's sides under the patient, and you'll spare him, his visitors, and staff members the embarrassment of an unintended view.

Theresa Costin, RN

Sip tip

If you don't have enough hands or help to wrestle with a glass of water *and* a reluctant patient while you insert a nasogastric tube, try this. Have the patient just sip on a straw. This action directs the tube into the esophagus rather than the trachea. That achieves the desired result—with no water going to the N.P.O. patient, and no wet gowns, either.

Mary Jane Craig, RN

Aspirating solution

When a patient dies after a massive gastrointestinal bleed or esophageal varices, I aspirate all the lavage solution *before* I remove his nasogastric or intestinal tube. Removing excess fluid this way prevents possible regurgitation later, making morgue care easier.

Becky L. Squires, RN

A clear chaser

To hasten vomiting after administering a dose of ipecac syrup, offer the patient a clear soft drink such as ginger ale or 7-Up. The soft drink is more palatable than the warm water that's usually given, and its carbonation makes the patient feel full. A word of caution, though: The soft drink produces results quickly—so be prepared.

Grace Redheffer, RN, BSN

Stay-put pad—stay-dry bed

To keep an under pad in place on a patient's bed, tape it to the sheet. Then even if the patient tosses and

turns, the pad stays put, and the bed stays dry.

Katherine Link, RN

Controlled relaxation

The controlled-relaxation techniques for labor and delivery taught in prepared childbirth classes can be used prenatally and postpartum, too. For example, women who have difficulty falling asleep during late pregnancy may find that controlled relaxation helps induce sleep in a short time.

Also, nursing mothers who are tense or nervous at feeding times may find that controlled relaxation works just as well as a glass of wine or beer.

Muriel A. Zraning, RN

Isolation reminder

When a patient is in isolation, tape a plastic-covered 8½″ × 11″ chart to the door of his room. In the first column, list the different types of isolation: respiratory, reverse, enteric, and so on. Across the top of the chart, list equipment you'll be using when working with the patient.

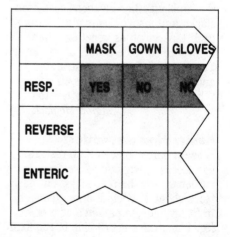

	MASK	GOWN	GLOVES
RESP.	YES	NO	NO
REVERSE			
ENTERIC			

If the patient is in reverse isolation, mark that row with a colored marker; if he's in enteric isolation, mark that row. Then, indicate which equipment requires isolation procedures by writing *yes* or *no* in the square that pertains to the type of isolation and the item.

This door guide reminds you at a glance which procedures you must follow with each patient in isolation.

Peg Koppmann, RN

Ringing reminder

On the busy acute care unit where I work, we sometimes lose track of time. This can lead to problems when a patient needs nursing care at a specific time—for example, for peritoneal dialysis. So we keep an ordinary kitchen timer on the unit. When we have a patient on peritoneal dialysis, we set the timer for the length of dwell time ordered by the doctor. When the timer rings, we're reminded to go back to that patient and continue his treatment.

Dottye Edwards, RN, BS, CRNA

When seconds count

When suctioning an artificial airway, you shouldn't apply suction for longer than 15 seconds at a time. But how do you know when the seconds have passed? Use this technique from cardiopulmonary resuscitation (CPR).

During CPR, you count—"one, one thousand; two, one thousand; three, one thousand"—to mark off the seconds. Similarly, in suctioning, you can count, "one, one thousand; two, one thousand;" and so on until the seconds have elapsed. Then remove the suction catheter.

Robert Hutson, RRT, EdD

A fitting idea

For a comfortable fit, don't give an obese patient *one* hospital gown—give him *two*. You'll have to do some "tailoring" first, though.

Here's how. Place the two unfolded gowns back to back and tie the neck tapes of one gown to those of the other. Now you'll have one gown with spaghetti shoulder straps and a roomy neckline.

Put the gown over the patient's head and position one gown in front of the patient and one in the back. Then tie the lower tapes at waist level for a belted effect.

You can turn the sleeves inside out and pin them to the gown's inside, if you wish. But even if you don't, you'll probably be surprised at the gown's good—almost Grecian—look.

Angela Tegarder, LPN

Gastrografin made easy

Many of our patients scheduled for abdominal computerized tomography (CT) scans have difficulty swallowing and keeping down the two large glasses of Gastrografin. So they spend an unusually long time in the radiology department trying to drink the bitter preparation.

To remedy this, we now flavor the Gastrografin with a low-calorie powdered fruit punch. The patients find it easier to swallow, and the added flavoring doesn't affect the CT studies.

Lorraine K. Smith, RN

Buttons 'n' sews

When a restless or confused patient continuously throws off his sheet, he may embarrass visitors and give himself a chill. With just a needle, a bit of thread, two $8'' \times 2''$ strips of

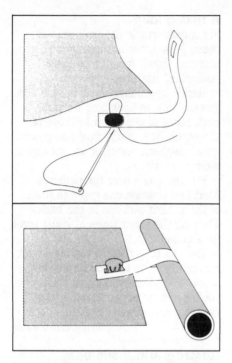

heavy cloth, and two large buttons, you can easily fix the sheet so it'll stay put.

Sew a button onto the end of one of the cloth strips. Make a buttonhole in the other end. Slip the side edge of the sheet (at a point near the top of the sheet) over the button, bring the cloth strip around the bed's side rail, and pull the button—with the sheet covering it—into the buttonhole. Make another cloth strip with button and buttonhole and attach it to the other side of the sheet the same way.

The sheet will stay over the patient now—no matter how restless he is.

Arlene McCully, RN

COMFORT

Stirrup comfort
As any woman knows, those ob/gyn examination-table stirrups can be cold, hard, and uncomfortable.

To minimize this, simply slip a pair of knitted or disposable foam slippers, bottom side up, over the stirrups.

The slippers will certainly help your patients relax. They may even prompt some patients to thank you for your thoughtfulness.

Faith Kahly, RN

No more complaints
If patients complain that they dread the cold speculum during their gynecological examination, here's a way to end the complaints. Keep a jar of warm water in each examining room. Just before the doctor goes into a room, put the speculum in the water. When the doctor's ready to do the vaginal examination, he'll remove the speculum. The warm speculum helps the patient relax, and the water serves as a lubricant to make insertion easier.

Karen Starling, RN, PHN

Warm 'n' ready
To help ensure a patient's comfort during a vaginal examination, warm up those specula.

Put a heating pad into a pillowcase, place both on the examining cart, and turn the pad to a low temperature. Then, set various-sized specula on the pillowcase and cover them with a small towel.

This guarantees your patient a bit more comfort during her examination. It also saves time because the equipment's always at the right temperature whenever you need to use it.

Catherine Lawer, RN

Jelly warm-up
To help patients relax during sigmoidoscopies and digital examinations, warm the lubricating jelly before you

apply it. Place the tube upside down in a pitcher of warm water for about 10 minutes. Then when the jelly's applied for the digital examination or sigmoidoscopy, the patient doesn't get as tense as with a cold touch.

Darlene Arnston, LPN

Prep talk

In preparation for GI diagnostic studies, a patient may need to drink castor oil or magnesium salts. To diminish the unpleasant taste of these preparations, give the patient some hard candy or gum between swallows. This sweet break also helps prevent nausea, so the patient can drink all of the liquid. If the patient is diabetic, use sugar-free candy or gum.

Wendy A. Simon, RN

A pajama parting

To protect patients from embarrassing exposure during colonoscopies and proctosigmoidoscopies, we use a pair of pajama bottoms altered as follows.

Starting 2″ above the crotch seam, we open the rear seam about 6″. Midway, we make a horizontal cut 4″ across. Then we fold back the four points of material and sew them down. This diamond-shaped opening gives the surgeon easy access, and the reusable pajama bottom saves the hospital the expense of using surgical drapes.

Eunice Kartheiser, Endoscopy Aide

Durable leg warmers

Some of our women residents in wheelchairs suffer from cold legs. Their dresses don't cover their legs, and their stockings are too thin to be warm. Lap robes don't help much either; they're constantly sliding off

and don't even cover the backs of the legs.

But we've found a solution to this chilling problem in leg warmers—those long footless socks that are so popular now, but were formerly worn only by dancers. Leg warmers are inexpensive, durable, and available in a variety of colors. Besides warming the lower leg, they extend well up over the knee, and stay there (yet they're not so tight that they impede circulation). And the patient doesn't have to bother taking them off when using the bathroom.

We keep several pairs of leg warmers on hand and suggest to residents' families that they make great gifts.

Nadine Hardage, CNA

Out of the cribs of babes

Crib blankets or coverlets are a perfect size for covering the laps and legs of people in wheelchairs. They're soft, washable, colorful—and they protect your patients' legs from cold and drafts.

Mary Hendela, RN

Lap rap

In the nursing home where we work, some residents in wheelchairs have trouble keeping their lap robes in place. So we glued a strip of Velcro to each side of the wheelchair and sewed corresponding Velcro strips on two edges of the lap robe. When the Velcro on the lap robe is attached to the Velcro on the wheelchair, the robe stays in place. Yet the robe can be pulled off easily if the patient must be transferred.

Sandra Magana, RN

Arm warmers

When a patient complains of cold arms but can't put on a long-sleeved gown or robe because of an I.V. line in his arm, give him some leg warmers (long socks with no feet)—for his arms. You can push the leg warmers up or down for I.V. insertion or inspection. And you can easily apply restraints over them, too.

Beryl Cleary, RN
Sue Pickering, SN

Who wears sweatpants?
In the extended care facility where I work, most of our elderly residents get out of bed and dress every day. But the men don't wear regular trousers; they wear sweatpants with a drawstring waist. Besides being easy to put on and take off, the sweatpants are warm, comfortable, inexpensive, and easy to launder.

Joanne Breden, RN

A roll(er) call
One of the chief complaints of a patient in labor is back pain. To help relieve this pain, try "massaging" her back with a medium-sized paint roller. Just move the roller up and down her back; it's less tiring for you than massaging with your hands and quite effective for the patient— the pain just rolls away.

Karen Mitchell, RN

Rolling pin relief
Here's a practical and effective way to treat women suffering from back labor. Use two rolling pins—the hollow kind that can be filled with water. Keep one in the placenta freezer and the other at the nurse's station ready to be filled with hot water.

Place a towel on the patient's back to protect her from the extreme temperature of the rolling pin. Then, with the help of the expectant father,

roll one of the pins over the woman's back. The combination of heat or cold and the gentle pressure from the rolling motion seems to give relief.

Rae K. Grad, RN

Cold comfort
To curb swelling and pain following delivery, tear an opening in one end of a "preemie" disposable diaper and insert a frozen "hot-and-cold pack" between the diaper's plastic and absorbent material. Then apply the diaper's absorbent side to the mother's body.

The hot-and-cold pack stays colder longer, the diaper absorbs any drainage, and the cold can penetrate through the diaper to the patient without giving her freezer burn.

Adia F. Mehus, RN

The heat's on
Here's how we ease the sacral discomfort of a woman in labor. We place a damp, $8'' \times 10''$ folded towel in the center of an opened Chux pad (plastic side down). Then we fold and tape the Chux around the towel—envelope style—and place it in a microwave oven. After 2 minutes, we take the Chux out of the oven, put it into a pillowcase, and place it against the woman's sacrum.

The pack stays hot for 30 minutes, can be reheated in the microwave oven, and, best of all, gives immediate, soothing relief to the patient in labor.

Jill Romm, RN

Numb mum
A new mother who wants to breast-feed her baby but whose nipples are sore might appreciate this suggestion from you.

Just before breast-feeding, tell her to wrap some ice chips in a cloth and apply it to the nipple. In a minute or so, the nipple will be numb, the baby can start sucking, and the mother won't feel the soreness that usually accompanies the first few moments of breast-feeding. (The cold also makes the nipple more erect, so it's easier for the baby to grasp.)

Maureen A. Storey, RN

Toasty toes

Toes extending from a foot cast can get awfully cold in the winter. To keep them warm and cozy, cover them with a baby's hat, tying the hat's strings around the ankle to keep the hat in place.

Marilyn McGarry, RN

A *legacy*

When a patient has a cast on one leg, his other leg may need attention, too. That's because he may inadvertently rub his cast against the uncasted leg, especially when he's asleep. To protect the leg, wrap a piece of sheepskin around the cast and tape it in place. Then, thanks to your *complete* attention, the patient's uncasted leg won't suffer while the other one heals.

Alice Svedjan, RN

Cool relief

Itchy skin under a plaster cast is a real problem for orthopedic patients. But a hand-held blow dryer, set at the cool temperature and aimed at the problem area, readily relieves the itching.

Debbie Almes, RN

For plastered itches

Sticking things down into the cast to scratch itchy spots bunches up the padding and makes uncomfortable lumps. So place a hand vibrator on the cast over the itchy spot. It relieves the itching without disturbing the padding.

Donna Hawkins, RN

Take a powder

Moisture can build up uncomfortably in an arm splint, even when the patient regularly takes his splint off and washes his arm. To prevent some of this moisture buildup, tell your patient to spray his arm with a powdered spray antiperspirant before reapplying the splint. He'll stay drier and feel better, too.

Deanna Jenkins, RN, MEd

Extra comfort

A patient who's had a total hip replacement and whose leg is now in a Kodel sling hip exerciser needs some extra comfort. Send some his way by putting a piece of a foam egg-crate-like mattress in the sling under his leg. The foam will comfortably pad the exerciser without interfering with the patient's movement.

Merle Haney, RN

Color that collar

Anyone who's had to wear a cervical collar knows it's disheartening enough without having to cope with a soiled or itchy stockinette cover.

Use smooth types of knee socks in cheerful colors to coordinate the collar with the patient's clothes. After cutting off the toe and pulling the sock on over the collar (with the heel inside, next to the patient's neck), put small pins on the front, or have the patient wear scarves that also match the clothes.

Being smoother, the sock prevents irritating rashes and, most important, is a big boost to morale.

Chloe Stewart, LVN

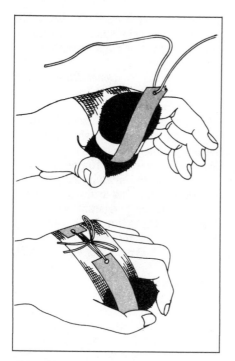

A hand towel

When a patient needs a hand splint, I make one that doesn't irritate his skin with a lot of tape. I just roll a small towel and tape it so it retains its rolled shape. Then I attach two Montgomery straps—one on each end of the roll. I place some gauze on the back of the patient's hand, put the rolled towel in his palm, and fasten the Montgomery straps over the gauze.

Besides being more comfortable for the patient, my hand towel splint is easier to manage than the taped-on variety.

Margie Downs, RN

Neat belt

Here's a way for a patient to wear a transcutaneous electrical nerve stimulator (TENS) unit without getting the wires tangled between his legs, on the furniture, or in his clothes every time he moves. Make a belt for the TENS unit from two catheter leg bands (the kind with Velcro tabs and catheter supports).

Attach the Velcro tabs of the two bands together to make one long belt. Put the belt around the patient's waist. Clip the TENS unit to the belt and fasten the wires inside the catheter support tab.

The wires will stay untangled while the sturdy belt holds the TENS unit securely—it won't pull down as it would if attached to the patient's clothing.

Barbara Panske, RN

Up and away

A patient with diabetic gangrene may complain of discomfort from the pressure of the covers about his foot. If a foot cradle isn't available, lay a lightweight aluminum walker on the bed to support the covers.

Shirley A. Brinson, RN

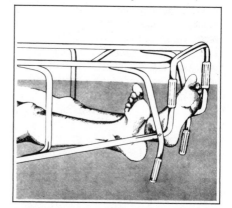

Beltless is better

Sanitary belts with metal or plastic hooks can cause undue pressure and irritation to female paraplegics. Since these patients lack sensation, they may be unaware that an ulcerated area is forming, especially in the sacral or coccygeal areas.

So instead, use tampons or feminine napkins with an adhesive strip that attaches to the undergarment.

Lois Pinnow, RN

Have a heart

If you use telemetry to monitor cardiac patients, you know that finding a comfortable way for them to wear their transmitters can be a problem. Solve it by having heart-shaped pockets sewn on the center of the patients' gowns. The transmitters fit neatly in the pockets. An added advantage is that when cardiac patients go to other departments, such as X-ray, they can be readily identified.

Diane Brown, RN

Double bed

If you're caring for a severely obese patient who's just too wide to turn in any hospital bed, ask the maintenance department to attach two beds and put an outer side rail on each, creating an extra-wide bed. Then, place a foam egg-crate-like mattress on top of each regular mattress. To make the bed, use two regular-sized bottom sheets, and one regular-sized top sheet. Making the bed takes a few extra minutes, but the patient can turn himself quite easily.

Paula Rees, RN

Water bed for the head

Concerned about the back of a patient's head when he must spend a great deal of time on his back? To relieve discomfort, fill a hot water bottle with 2 cups of water and press out all excess air. With the water pillow under his head, the patient is more comfortable.

Myrtle L. Little, RN

Taping tip

Here's a way to lessen discomfort to patients when you must remove tape from their skin to change dressings, stabilize tubes, and so forth.

When you first apply the tape, fold over one end (sticky sides together) to make a tab. Then when it comes time to remove the tape, you can grasp the starter tab. No need to pick at the tape (and the patient's skin) to get the strip started. You can save still more time and frustration if you leave a tab on the end of the roll of tape for quick access the next time you need it.

Diane Mahoney, RN

Water rings

Does your patient need an air ring? Give him a water ring instead. Just fill about three fourths of the ring with water, expel the air, and close the cap. The water-filled ring stays soft and is more comfortable than an air ring.

In cold weather, though, you might warm up the ring in a warm-water washbowl before having the patient sit on the ring.

Pauline Seibel, RN

No-friction fracture pan

Before giving a fracture pan to a patient, apply some body lotion to the pan rim. The lotion will decrease the friction—and the pain—of using the pan.

Deborah Wood, RN
Helen Kelsey, RN

Cuff cushion

When patients need frequent blood pressure readings, the repeated inflation and deflation of the cuff on the electronic monitor irritates the skin. So we put a piece of stockinette under the cuff. The soft stockinette cushions and protects the patient's skin.

Margery Lebel, RN, CCRN

Remade masks
Many patients refuse to wear their one-size-fits-all oxygen masks because these masks are simply too large and uncomfortable: The plastic rim juts into the patient's eyes and allows air to escape.

To tailor the mask, trim the top edge a bit and cover it with cloth tape. With a comfortable custom-fit mask, the patients become more compliant with their oxygen therapy.

Jerene Maune, RN

Skin cushion
A patient on long-term oxygen therapy may experience discomfort from the pressure of his nasal cannula on his upper lip, his cheeks, and behind his ears. But a clean pipe cleaner and some cotton can come to his rescue.

Layer the cotton around the pipe cleaner in a thin, tight roll. Then cushion the pipe cleaner between the cannula and the patient's skin, molding the pipe cleaner to the shape of the cannula, and tape the two together.

Diaphoretic patients and those with sensitive skin will especially welcome this comforting measure. And the pipe cleaner is light enough not to compromise the oxygen flow.

Eileen C. Connor, LPN, SN

Music to promote sleep
In our busy—and sometimes noisy— intensive care unit, many patients have trouble sleeping. I have found that a cassette player with earphones, brought from home, helps drown out

the noise for these patients. And when listening to their favorite music, they relax and fall asleep easier.

Capt. Marie Baudreau, USAF, NC

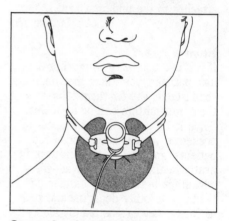

Stomahesive revisited
If a patient with a tracheostomy complains that the tube's faceplate rubs uncomfortably against his skin, try this. Cut a piece of Stomahesive in the shape of a "C." Apply the Stomahesive to the patient's skin around the stoma. (If you cut small slits along the inside edge of the Stomahesive, it will lie smoothly.) Besides cushioning the skin, the Stomahesive also acts as a barrier against secretions.

Madge Levy, RN, ET

What a mesh
I recently cared for a patient who had a Broviac catheter inserted at the sternal area. Securing the dressing at the catheter site presented more than a few problems. First, because of the patient's large breasts, there wasn't enough room on her chest to place and anchor the tape smoothly. Second, she was allergic to tape; third, she perspired so profusely that even hypoallergenic tape wouldn't stick.

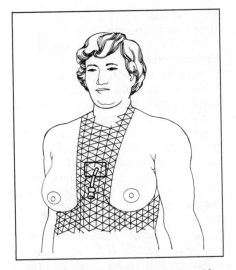

Our solution was to put a 10″ wide piece of Spandage (a mesh bandage usually used for burn patients) over the patient's head and cut a slit on each side for her arms and breasts. This armless "blouse" beat all the odds—and worked. It held the dressing in place without tape. And as a bonus, the holes in the mesh allowed perspiration to evaporate. The patient could wear a bra and a real blouse over the mesh.

Florence Bull, RN

Odor orders
If your patient gets nauseated from certain odors or cooking smells, tell him to put a small amount of Mentholatum Ointment or Vicks Vaporub just below each nostril. Then instead of the offending odor, the patient just smells the inoffensive camphor and menthol.

Ann Cooney, RN

Perfumed room
Recently we cared for a patient who had burns on 40% of her body. Several days after admission, she began to complain about the odors exuding from her burn dressings and wounds.

To alleviate this problem, the patient asked her husband to bring her favorite bottle of perfume to the hospital. He did, and each day he or a staff member sprayed the perfume into the air around her, making sure none of the perfume settled on the patient's burn sites.

We noticed several positive effects from the perfume treatment. First, the patient wasn't bothered by the odor from her wounds anymore. Second, she was buoyed by the control she exerted over her environment. Third, her husband felt a sense of participation in his wife's care.

Sue Hendricks, RN
Reginald L. Richard, PT, MS

No more numbness
When treating a patient's sore throat with an anesthetic antiseptic like Chloraseptic, you can easily get some of the spray on the patient's tongue. Then the patient's throat may feel better, but he has the discomfort of a numb tongue.

To prevent a numb tongue, invert the bowl of a teaspoon over the patient's tongue and then spray his throat. The spoon not only protects his tongue from the spray, but also depresses his tongue so you can see the area of his throat that's red and sore.

Linda Barker, RN

Soothing solution
Here's one way to relieve mouth soreness when patients undergo chemotherapy or radiotherapy. Give them yogurt. Chilled or frozen yogurt soothes the mucous membranes while providing a high-protein snack. (Both regular and diet yogurt contain 8

to 10 g of protein/8-oz container.)
Thus, yogurt also helps supply the
additional energy patients need when
undergoing chemotherapy or radiotherapy.

Connie Danser, RN

A cling thing

Flotation mattresses are beneficial to
the patients lying on them, but they
can be a real nuisance to the nurses
trying to keep the mattresses from
slipping off the bed.

To avoid slippage, place a rubber
mattress cover over the regular mattress with the reverse (rubber) side
up. The plastic covering on the flotation mattress clings to the rubber,
so the mattress stays in place. What's
more, the patient is more comfortable,
and the bed is easier to make.

Kathy Jennison, LPN

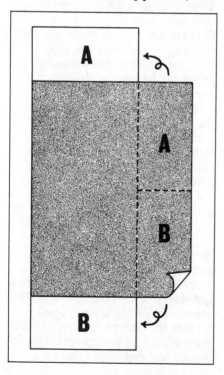

Neat sheet

Here's an alternative to rigid, wrinkled, uncomfortable plastic sheets
that don't stay tucked in. Use a
flannel-backed, rectangular vinyl
tablecloth. To make it fit the bed
properly, make some minor alterations.

First, cut about one third off the
longest side of the cloth. Then cut this
piece in half and sew one half to
each end of the tablecloth. Attach
these pieces so that the flannel side
of the tablecloth and the vinyl sides of
the two extensions are all facing
the same direction.

Now the patient rests comfortably
on the flannel side of the machine-
washable, waterproof sheet, and the
ends stay tucked under him *and*
his bed.

Maureen C. Organ, RN

What a lift

When we use a Hoyer lift to transfer
a patient from his wheelchair to
the toilet, we leave the lift's canvas
seat (which has a hole in it) under
him. However, some of our patients
used to complain that the canvas was
scratchy.

To make the seat more comfortable,
we sewed a piece of sheepskin (with
a hole cut in the middle) to the
canvas seat. The patients appreciate
the soft seat, and we like it because
the entire seat—canvas and sheepskin—can easily be taken off the lift
and laundered.

Diane Chamberlin, RN
Janet McMahill, Occupational Therapist

Bagged belongings

When transferring a patient in a
wheelchair from the intensive care
unit to another unit, do you pile
his personal belongings on his lap for
the trip?

If so, try this instead: Slip one side of a large, plastic trash bag's open end over the wheelchair's handles (so the bag hangs down the back of the chair), and put the patient's belongings in the bag. Without all the clutter on his lap, the patient will be more comfortable during his transfer.

Julia Ann Young, RN

On the level
If long-term patients picnic on hospital grounds, finding level surfaces for their paper plates, cups, and utensils can be a problem.

To solve this problem, obtain a large supply of empty fabric-bolt cores from a local yard goods store. Then cover the 30″ × 18″ cores with colorful adhesive-backed plastic paper. The result: lightweight, easy-to-clean, and easy-to-transport lapboards, usable by both wheelchair and ambulatory patients.

Ada M. Massa, RN

Skin lotion warm-up
Here's one way to avoid applying cold skin lotion to a patient after his bath: Place the lotion bottle, with the cap tightly closed, in the patient's bathwater. As the patient warms up, so does the lotion.

This warm-water treatment also keeps the lotion from thickening.

Gail Lew, RN

Drip no more
For patients receiving chemotherapy, an ice pack applied to the scalp is standard procedure to help minimize hair loss. But these ice packs are drippy and messy, so we've modified the procedure.

We place the patient in a high or semi-Fowler's position and gently dampen his hair roots with warm water. Then we get three cold gel packs and tape a washcloth around each.

We place the slightly pliable packs around the patient's hairline in a circle and tape them together to keep them in place. Then we put an ice bag on the uncovered crown of the patient's head. To make sure the ice bag and gel packs stay put, we secure them with Kerlix or Kling in turban style.

Besides eliminating the drippy mess, this type of ice cap allows the patient to sit up and read or even walk around.

Terrilynn M. Fox, RN

Relieving pain—contralaterally
Looking for a noninvasive way to relieve the pain of a bone marrow aspiration? Try giving an ice massage to the site *opposite* the aspiration site. That's what nurses at the Veterans Administration Wadsworth Medical Center in Los Angeles did—and it worked.

The nurses didn't apply the ice directly to the aspiration site because it would have interfered with the procedure, besides invading the sterile field. But knowing that *both* sides of the body influence pain impulses

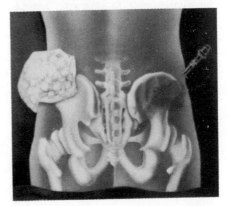

passing through the spinal cord, they decided to apply the ice contralaterally.

The patient was scheduled to have bone marrow aspirated from his right posterior iliac crest. For 5 minutes before the aspiration, the nurses massaged the area above the *left* posterior iliac crest with ice. Then they prepared the aspiration site, draped it, and injected lidocaine. The doctor inserted the aspiration needle into the right iliac crest, but before he actually aspirated the marrow, the nurses again massaged the contralateral site—this time for 1 minute. The doctor then performed the aspiration.

And what did the patient feel during all this? Nothing—no pain at all. Only the ice and pressure.

The inpatient head nurse of the hospice program at the medical center said they've also used contralateral ice massage to relieve postoperative pain. The medical center's research committee, she added, has verified that contralateral ice massage is an ingenious method of pain relief.

Barbara Hudziak, RN

That old smoothie

You've probably heard about using a satin pillowcase to save your hairdo, but here's another idea for that old smoothie, satin.

For arthritic patients, just turning over in bed at night can be a real problem. Suggest that a satin drawsheet be made for their beds.

First, buy enough satin for the width of the bed. Then sew a strip of terry cloth or a bath towel on two ends to tuck under the mattress. Being a coarser texture, the terry cloth keeps the satin from slipping.

Roberta Steele, RN

Vacuum power in the ED

Use a small, battery-powered vacuum cleaner to remove tiny glass particles from auto accident victims' hair and clothing. The vacuum is more effective than combs and brushes. As an added bonus, it keeps the glass from falling on the floor.

Richard P. Kirschke, RN

EMERGENCIES

Lead keeper

Lead wires from cardiac monitors often get tangled and are difficult to place on a patient when you're in a hurry. So to keep them straight, attach the leads to a tongue depressor with a piece of tape and label the tape accordingly. Now, when you need

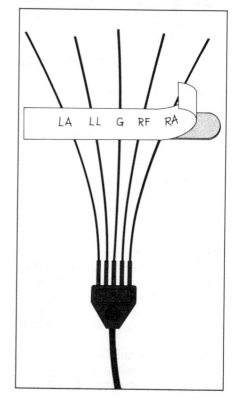

to monitor a patient, quickly remove the tongue depressor and place the lead on the patient. This technique can eliminate some of the confusion that occurs during emergencies.

Mary Eggen, RN

Bee ready

Here's a way to make life easier for patients who are allergic to bee stings and must carry an anaphylaxis kit. Tell them a plastic travel toothbrush case holds the equipment compactly. Especially convenient for children, the case fits into a back pocket so it can be carried easily outdoors.

To alert others to the patient's prescribed dosage, a prescription label can be attached to the case.

Linda Dattolico, RN

Crash box

Place a "crash box" of emergency supplies on each floor in a place where you can reach it quickly. Each crash box—a clear plastic box about the size of a shoe box—should contain:
- oxygen mask
- oxygen nasal cannula
- instant ice
- airway
- vial of sterile water
- smelling salts
- syringe with needle
- flashlight
- sterile gauze
- tape.

To be sure the boxes are always ready, someone on each shift should check all items, make any necessary replacements, and sign a sheet near the box.

Carolyn Bidwell, RN

Ventilation preparation

Picture this: A patient with a laryngectomy is admitted to the ICU.

You soon learn that he hasn't worn his laryngectomy tube for years, and the respiratory therapists can't insert a tube. So you worry that if the patient has a cardiac arrest, you'd have only one way to ventilate him—mouth to stoma resuscitation. You couldn't place him on the ventilator or deliver any high oxygen concentration to him.

The solution? Place an endotracheal tube into his stoma just far enough to get a seal. This will allow you to ventilate him with a manual resuscitation bag or place him on a mechanical ventilator.

Marti Brown, RN

Snip 'n' shrivel

For the patient with a Sengstaken-Blakemore tube in place, the possibility of the esophageal balloon's slipping upward, causing the patient to suffocate, poses a threat. As a safeguard, keep a pair of scissors taped to the head of the bed for emergencies. If immediate deflation becomes necessary, cut the inflation tube and release the pressure. Although this happens rarely, life hangs in the balance, so be prepared.

Brigid Jaynes, RN

Put it on tape

When your patient has an arteriove-

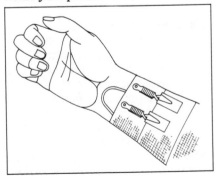

nous shunt, his cannula clamps should be easily accessible, especially in an emergency. To make sure they are, wrap stretchy roller bandage around the patient's shunt, as usual. Then fold two pieces of paper tape over the edge of a bandage row (see illustration). Place the clamps on the paper tape.

Now you can reach for the clamps in a hurry, and they won't get stuck in the bandage's gauze fibers.

Sue Drogos, RN

Sealed for safety

Do you keep a crash cart between medical units, where it's easily accessible? And during routine equipment checks, do you occasionally find that someone borrowed an item and forgot to replace it?

With the help of the maintenance department, insert heavy-duty staples into the frame of the cart, below each of the drawers. Then wrap 10" wire around the staples and the drawer handles to seal the drawers shut.

The wires break with very little exertion, so the drawers are still easy to open. But now you know at a glance whether they've been opened and if crucial supplies might be missing.

Nancy Bonne, RN

Keep in good spirits

Allowing one or two family members to stay with an anxious patient in the emergency department helps calm the patient. But sometimes a family member becomes ill or faints. To handle such "visiting emergencies," keep two ampules of spirits of ammonia on double-backed tape within easy reach in each cubicle. The faster you revive the visiting patients, the sooner you can get back to the "real" patients.

Mary Kennedy Eggen, RN

Feel the way

If the beds on your unit are equipped with a panel of buttons for turning on the TV, calling the nurse, and so forth, vision-impaired patients may have trouble: turning on their TVs instead of calling you, for instance. That increases frustration, especially in an emergency.

Tape finger cots over all the *call buttons*, and patients can feel their way to the right button. They'll be pleased with the added convenience, and you'll be confident they can reach you when they need you.

Lesley Golden, LVN

SUPPORTIVE MEASURES

Extra strokes for special folks

Valentine's Day is the time to show your affection for people you care about. But all year round, staff members at Crowell Memorial Home in Blair, Neb., show their affection for residents through a program called "Extra Strokes."

Each week the staff selects four residents, one from each of the home's four areas, and gives them "extra strokes of affection."

The residents selected are those with special problems. Perhaps they're ill or new to the home. Or their spouse may have died recently.

The staff posts the names of the four residents in every area so all personnel will know who's selected for that week. Then they discuss the selected residents at daily conferences and shift reports. They take a close look at these residents' problems, review their health care, assess

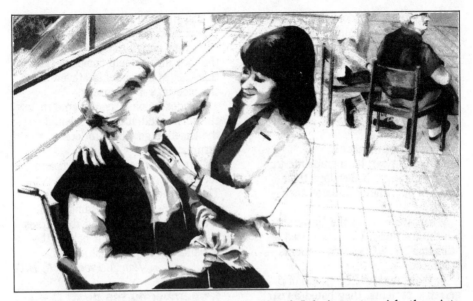

their interactions with other residents and staff members, and examine their life-styles since coming to the home. At the heart of the program is the attention the staff lavishes on the selected residents. They give them extra hugs and take time to sit with them and just chat. All personnel go out of their way to greet the residents and give them special attention.

The extra strokes of affection program has been in effect for more than a year. Manipulative residents, says one of the nurses, become less demanding because their need for attention is satisfied. Lonely residents appreciate having someone care for them and someone they can care for in return. Residents with Alzheimer's disease, she notes, respond especially well to this extra loving attention.

Barbara Dunlop, RN

The healing feeling

When my nursing home patients are angry, sad, frustrated, or disap-

pointed, I don't try to cajole them into a better mood. Instead, I encourage them to vent their feelings through "low moan therapy."

I gather several patients into a group and lead off the session by talking about something that might be bothering me, such as the building's broken air conditioning system, my sore feet, or the news that a good friend is moving away. Then each patient gets a turn to share his feelings. Most times we just *talk*, but we also welcome occasional moans or sighs as appropriate expressions of our feelings.

Although at first glance the focus of the session may seem negative, we all leave the session *positive* that our needs for self-expression were met.

Holly Bennett, RN, NE

Clock it to them

Intensive care units usually have no windows, so lights are on around the clock. Small wonder, then, that patients frequently don't know whether it's day or night. To help orient them, put a card indicating a.m. or p.m. next to the clock on the wall. This will help relieve a bit of the frustration patients feel in the often stressful atmosphere of the unit.

Marylou Hughes, ACSW, DPA

A time to reminisce

Reminisicing can be therapeutic for elderly patients. It develops their sense of self and stimulates their minds.

When students at the University of South Carolina, two nurses used a "timeline" to help elderly patients reminisce.

In their work with a group of 6 geriatric patients, they listed 5-year intervals starting with 1890 to 1895—the interval in which the oldest patient was born. They then asked the patients to list important events that occurred in each interval; medical and technological advances, and political and historical events. The patients listed the San Francisco earthquake, the sinking of the Titanic, and the Lindbergh kidnapping, for example.

They also volunteered dates of personal importance to them: when they were born, when they were married, when their first child was born.

The timeline was a great success. One patient, who rarely participated in any group activity, regularly attended the meetings to help complete the timeline. Many patients stayed after the meetings to discuss it.

Besides helping the patients review their lives and accomplishments, the timeline got them to look to the future.

After the timeline was completed, the nurses gave each patient a copy. The patients were pleased because the timeline highlighted important events in their lives. And the nurses were pleased because it helped the patients develop a sense of self.

Jean A. Proehl, RN, BSN

Remembering the past

An elderly woman in a nursing home felt ignored and unnoticed by the staff—that is, until a friend brought in a picture from the patient's past. We posted the picture, which showed the woman in her twenties wearing a bathing suit, on the wall of her room.

Now when staff members pass by, they often stop and ask about the young woman in the picture. The patient enjoys telling them about her past. And staff members are reminded that every patient is a real person with an interesting, exciting history.

Sally Blumenthal, RN

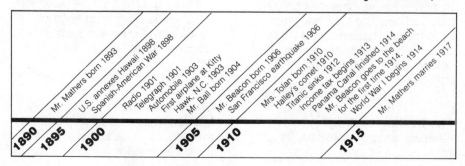

In-house art gallery

At the retirement home where I work, we're constantly looking for new and interesting activities for our residents. So ever since our local library began lending framed pictures to its cardholders, we've been borrowing two pictures a month and hanging them in the hall. The residents enjoy studying the art and following up their study with a lively discussion. They look forward to our new acquisitions each month.

Marilyn Moore, RN

Help for grieving adults

"People ask me how my mom's doing since dad died—but not how I'm doing. And I lost my father!"

That comment, and others like it, inspired a nurse and a social worker to form support groups for adults who've had a parent die recently. A clinical nurse specialist and thanatologist at St. Luke's Hospital, Milwaukee, and a social worker at Lutheran Social Services, Milwaukee, hold these group meetings to help adults understand, accept, and deal with the death of a parent.

The groups, each with about 10 participants, meet once a week for 6 consecutive weeks. At the 1½- to 2-hour sessions, participants talk about their feelings, their relationship with the surviving parent, and topics of special interest to them, such as sibling disagreements or a child's grief. They also watch and discuss a filmstrip on death and mourning, and receive handouts that explian stress, grief, and guilt.

Among the techniques used is one in which participants list five things they enjoy doing and five things they find stressful, then decide how often they did these things within the last month, week, and 24 hours. This exercise makes the grievers aware of what makes them feel good and helps them avoid what depresses them. Participants also learn breathing exercises, deep muscle relaxation, and other techniques they can use when they feel stressed.

At the final meeting, participants share wine and cheese and receive "gifts"—positive statements about themselves from the other group members. Many also exchange addresses and phone numbers for future contacts. Before they leave, the participants evaluate the sessions. Their responses have included: "The group helped bring me out of a prolonged state of shock and denial," "I feel I can cope now," and "I've learned that I'm not alone."

Virginia Bourne, RN, MSN
Judy Meier, MSW

Any messages?

Looking for a fun way to encourage your depressed or unmotivated patients? Try "balloon" writing.

Inflate a nonsterile rubber examining glove and secure the opening with a knot or rubber band. Use a felt-tipped pen to write a message on the glove, then tie or tape the glove to the patient's overhead bed frame, bulletin board, or other furniture. By combining wording such as "Happy Birthday," "Keep those feet moving," and "Cough, please" with diagrams, drawings, and smiling faces, you'll get your message across—even when you're not with the patient.

And when the patient's discharged, he can deflate his glove—*cum* balloon—and take it home with him.

Martha G. Oestreich, RN

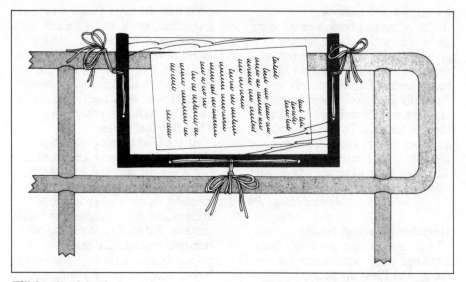

Fill in the blanks

If you have a patient who's paralyzed or immobilized and must spend a lot of time in a side-lying position to prevent decubiti, here's a way to help him. Make an inexpensive magazine or book holder to attach to the bed so the patient can read rather than just stare at the wall. The holder is ideal for one-page articles, poems, or letters.

First, get one of those report cover kits with clear plastic sheets and plastic slide locks. (They're available at most variety stores or drugstores.) Cut two of the plastic sheets about 3″ longer and 1″ wider than the book or magazine that will go into the holder. Next, staple the sheets together on three sides to make an envelope or pouch.

Then, cut the slide locks to fit the envelope's sides and bottom (miter the adjoining edges of the slide locks for a tighter fit). With a hot ice pick or small drill, make two holes in each slide lock. Lace a 4-ply yarn through the holes, leaving about 8″ on each side and on the bottom to loop around the top and bottom bed rails.

Finally, tie the holder to the bed rails, adjust it to the patient's eye level, and slip in the book or magazine. The holder won't hamper the bed rails' movement. Best of all, because the materials just slide in, you can vary the patient's "side-show"— and keep boredom at bay—with just a flip of your wrist.

Pat Baggerly, RN

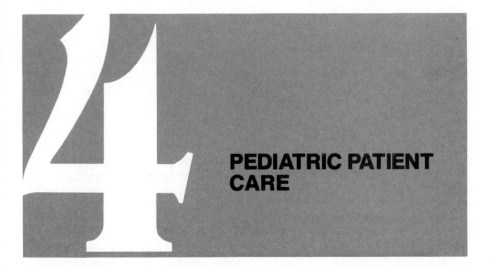

PEDIATRIC PATIENT CARE

FLUID AND NUTRITION

Keeping score
To encourage pediatric patients to take fluids after surgery, devise an attractive "scorecard."

Draw on a sheet of paper various

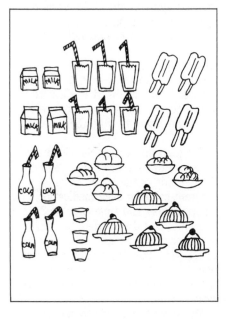

symbols representing fluids: soda bottles, Popsicles, ice cream, Jell-O, milk, and water. After the child takes the fluid, he colors the appropriate symbol on his scorecard.

Martha Clark, RN

Inventive incentive
A pediatric patient sometimes balks at drinking all the fluids his doctor orders. As an incentive, we give the child an animal picture (which we've cut from magazines and children's books) each time he drinks the prescribed amount of fluid. The child then pastes the picture on a poster board attached to his bed or bulletin board.

The child is proud when visitors and staff note how many animals he's accumulated on his poster. And the poster reminds everyone to encourage the child to drink more fluid.

Karen A. Bender, RN, BSN

Circuitous solution
Getting small children to force fluids can be a problem. Use plastic "crazy straws," which are constructed in

complicated shapes. The youngsters love watching the path of the juice when they sip. They take adequate fluids and won't let the straw out of sight.

Dianne Charron, RN

Small is better
Getting toddlers to increase their fluid intake can be a real problem, as you know. One solution is to offer small amounts of fluid in a 1-oz medicine cup. The cup doesn't intimidate the patient as much as a large drinking glass would, and the child will more readily sip a teaspoon or two of fluid.

By offering the cup frequently, you can substantially increase your patient's daily fluid intake. Also, since the cup is premeasured, keeping an accurate record is simple.

Urusuline Ferguson, RN

Down the spout
Getting bedridden patients to drink used to cause more fluid spilled than consumed, especially with tots who haven't quite mastered drinking through straws, or with postoperative patients who aren't allowed straws. Eliminate the mess by using special drinking cups—the kind that have a snap-on lid with a spout in it. They can be found in most grocery stores or drugstores. So, if a patient can raise his head, he can drink—unassisted and unafraid of spilling.

Diane Voellner, RN, MN

Feeding easy
Feeding a baby with a cleft palate can be discouraging for a new mother—even when using a commercial cleft palate nipple. But if you put a small slit through the hole of a regular nipple, the baby can feed easily.

Tell the mother to place the nipple into the baby's mouth with the slit in a vertical position. Make sure the nipple's angled so the baby's tongue and existing palate can compress it.

Although the baby can't form a vacuum to suck, he'll work at the nipple and cause the slit to open and close to produce a flow of milk.

Remind the mother to hold her baby in an upright position while feeding him. He'll also need to be burped more often than babies who suck normally.

This simple "nipple-slit" allows mothers and babies to enjoy feeding time together—a real boon for both.

Nancy Finnegan, RN

PLAY THERAPY

In a spin
How can you encourage a child who has just had surgery or who has a respiratory disease to do his breathing exercises? Give him a simple pinwheel toy that spins as the child blows on it. It's good for him, and fun, too.

Vicki Lutterell, RN, BSN

Charting = Child's play
Medication sheets are *not* just for nurses. I give modified medication sheets to my pediatric patients to encourage them to take their medications.

For each medication the child has to take, I draw a circle in a column on the left side of the sheet. (I use a different color for each medication.) I write the day and time each medication must be taken across the top of the paper and make columns for them. After the child takes a medication, I let him fill in the appropriate space in the column with that medication's color.

My patients are usually so eager to

fill in all the spaces on their sheets that they forget to fuss about taking their medications.

Jennifer Fransen, RN

Body painting

If you have a hard time putting calamine lotion on wiggling, squirming children, try my method. Get a small paintbrush and paint the child's skin with the lotion. Most children love the novelty of having their body painted, and they'll be sure to sit still during the procedure.

Kathie Dougherty, RN

Paging in the ED

To keep a frightened child occupied while he's waiting to be examined in the emergency department (ED), give him an "activity page" and a box of crayons. On one side of the page include drawings and descriptions of objects and people he'll see in the ED. On the other side include spaces in which to write his name, his doctor's and nurse's names, and the reason he came to the ED. Also offer a connect-the-dots drawing of a child with a broken leg and crutches.

Besides giving children something to do, these activity pages introduce them to the ED in a pleasant, non-threatening way. And parents think the activity pages are a better reward than candy.

Ginger Kropp, LPN

Gone fishing

Have you ever tried to apply an ice pack to a small child's hurt finger? Not an easy job, at best. Next time, instead of struggling, turn the ice treatment into a game.

Fill a plastic mug with ice and water, and challenge the child to get the ice out of the mug. While he's

fishing for the ice, the icy cold water will decrease swelling and pain. He'll forget about his sore finger, and you can dry his tears.

Cathy Parker, LPN

Bath-time fun

Feverish babies and children usually don't like tepid *sponge* baths. So if you find no obvious contraindications, ask the doctor if you can give the child a tepid *tub* bath instead.

Add some toys (disposable plastic items found on your unit) to the bathwater, and the child will probably play in the bath, without coaxing, for as long as necessary.

Jean R. Bear, LPN

Nutrition rummy

To encourage children to select from the four basic food groups and avoid junk foods, use a card game to teach them sound nutrition principles.

To play the game, you need 52 playing cards, color-coded according to food groups and divided as follows:
• 10 *milk-group* cards (black borders).
• 10 *cereal-group* cards (blue borders).
• 10 *fruit/vegetable-group* cards (green borders).
(Each of these groups has five cards labeled for one serving and five labeled for two servings.)
• 10 *meat-group* cards (red borders), all labeled for one serving
• 12 *junk-food* cards with one picture on each (such as popcorn, candy, cookies, and gum).

To make the playing cards, cut 3″×5″ cards into 2¼″×3½″ pieces. Then label each card, color in its border, and paste on an appropriate magazine picture.

Before the children start the game, make sure a "Guide to Good Eating" poster from a local dairy or nutrition

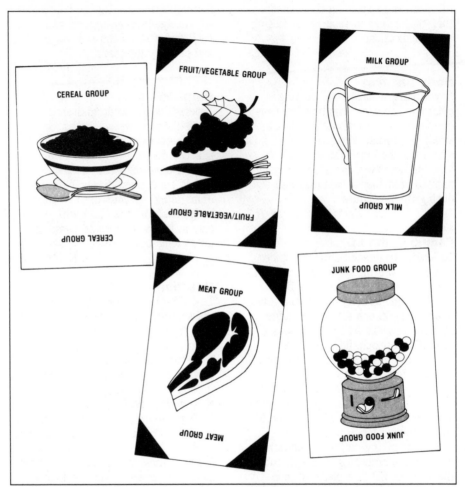

center is hanging close by. The poster will guide the children as they play, especially regarding the servings suggested for each food group. Once the game begins, it's played just like rummy.

Two to four players are dealt 11 cards each. The remaining cards are placed face down, except for the top card, which the dealer turns over to begin a discard pile. Each player then draws the top card from the face-down pile or the discard pile.

The player then discards one card,

so he doesn't have more than 11 cards after his turn. The first player to lay down 10 or 11 cards with the correct number of servings in each food group wins the game. For example, a winning hand might have two 1-serving and one 2-serving fruit/vegetable cards, one 1-serving and one 2-serving milk cards, four 1-serving cereal cards, and two 1-serving meat cards.

To test the game's effectiveness, give the children a nutrition quiz before the game. Then see if the children answered more questions correctly *after* playing.

Nancy Matheson, RN

Soaking procedure
In the busy emergency department where I work, I frequently have to soak a child's finger or hand wound. But just as frequently, I run out of basins for the soaking solution.

Then I use a clean plastic urine container instead. The container is transparent, so I play finger games with the child to encourage him to move his fingers or hand for a more thorough cleansing.

Mary Eggen, RN

Pinwheel play
A simple, old-fashioned pinwheel makes an excellent substitute for an incentive spirometer for pediatric patients. They love to blow on the pinwheel and watch the colors go round. They can even have contests to see who can blow the hardest. Besides helping the children comply with their respiratory therapy regimen, the pinwheel also promotes social interaction.

Nancy Jo Murray, RN, MS

Put up a happy face
To increase visual stimulation for infants who require restraint (such as those undergoing cleft lip repair), tape pictures of happy, smiling faces inside their cribs. Toothpaste advertisements in magazines are especially good, and the little ones seem to enjoy gazing at human faces.

Rita A. Fleming, RN

Injection question
Remembering to rotate injection sites can be difficult for young diabetic patients. Turn this problem into a game by cutting out a large, cardboard doll and marking the injection sites on the doll's arms, legs, and abdomen. On the back of the doll, draw a chart with the various sites on the left and the days of the week across the top. Every time a patient gives himself an injection, he checks off the site under the appropriate day. And you need only check the doll to see where the next injection should be given.

E. Weinstock, RN

Soaking solution
When burn wounds or infected cuts on an active toddler's hand or fingers need to be soaked several times a day, how do you gain his cooperation? Try placing brightly colored, nonfloating objects or large coins on the bottom of the soaking basin. Then challenge the toddler to reach into the warm solution and bring them out. He may have trouble grasping some of the objects or he might drop them before getting them out of the solution, but this will prolong the soaking time.

When he has all the objects out, ask him to place them back on the bottom again. Although this method takes longer to achieve the desired soaking time, it keeps the toddler interested.

Rose Alayne Wilkerson, RN

Picture pride
Give pediatric patients crayons and paper and ask them to draw self-portraits while they wait to see the doctor. When finished, they can hang their pictures on a picture board—a bulletin board on the waiting room wall.

This activity keeps young patients busy, and they're proud of their contributions to the waiting room's decor.

Toni Piller, RN

Everybody wins

If you do skin tests on children, make the testing less traumatic by using this guessing game.

First, divide the child's back into sections according to the different types of allergens (weeds, trees, and so on). Next, ask both the child and his parent to guess how many allergy extract drops you'll administer in each section.

Then, as you administer the drops, count them. If someone guesses the exact number, he gets two points. If neither parent nor child guesses correctly, the player with the closest guess gets one point. The player with the highest score wins. Repeat the game for each section of the child's back, until the allergy testing is complete.

The game lets the child relax between administrations and diverts his attention from the test. The few minutes you spend explaining the game beforehand save many minutes of fighting, crying, and struggling. So, really, everyone—child, parent, and you—wins.

Beverly Opitz, RN

Tales of distraction

Suturing a minor laceration or changing a dressing on a squirming child is always a challenge. Rather than use sedatives or restraints to keep him still, try to enlist the child's cooperation with story-telling and a reward.

If you rarely have a person available just to stand by and read a story, tape some children's favorites on cassettes. After you explain the procedure, the child chooses a story and

puts the proper cassette in the player. Then, instead of concentrating on his discomfort, the child becomes engrossed in the story.

When you finish the procedure, blow up a rubber glove, tie a knot at the cuff, draw a face on it with a felt-tipped marker, and give the child the "balloon." This reward is simple, inexpensive, and appealing.

Capt. Susan B. Shipley, RN

Puppet pal

Getting a young patient to sit still for 20 minutes while his hand soaks in povidone-iodine (Betadine) solution can be an ordeal. So turn the treatment into a game.

Soak some 4″ × 4″ bandages in a Betadine solution, apply them to the laceration, and then slip your patient's hand into an examination glove to keep the 4″ × 4″ bandages in place. Using a marking pencil, draw eyes, a nose, and a mouth on the glove, creating a hand puppet. After this your patient looks forward to his next treatment—and a new puppet pal.

Lynn Broesch, LVN

Exit ennui

Boredom and short attention spans are problems in pediatrics.

Use a "Game Crash Cart" filled with cards, crayons, books, tracing paper, puppets, and other toys liked by both boys and girls of all ages.

The gaily decorated cart creates an air of excitement and joy for bedridden patients. It's an orderly way of keeping many diversionary objects available for the children.

Joanne Serapilia, SN

Show and tell

Explaining a procedure before doing it

is just as important with children as it is with adults. But if a very young child can't understand a verbal explanation, try drawing a picture.

You needn't be a great artist—stick figures will serve the purpose very well. Show the child what will happen as you explain the procedure to him.

The picture also serves as a distraction while you're actually doing the procedure. The child can compare the real equipment with the picture you've drawn for him.

Sandra Dewulf, RN

Egg roles
Those plastic egg-shaped containers for panty hose can help your adolescent and pediatric patients beat the hospital blahs. For example, have the older children make small toys for the younger ones. They can put a wooden spool or similar object inside a container, glue the halves together, and decorate them with decals. Or adolescents can create attractive cradle mobiles by punching holes at both ends of a decorated egg, then stringing several together.

To add a seasonal touch to hospital trays, let patients transform the containers into candy-filled Easter eggs or bunnies, Thanksgiving turkeys, or Christmas Santas or elves. And, of course, with a little imagination, patients can make festive Christmas-tree ornaments from the containers.

You'll find that choosing new roles for these egg containers is fun for both the adolescents who hatch the projects and the youngsters who receive the results.

Mildred A. Feliz, RN

Disposamobile
Use a disposable face mask to make a mobile for a crib-bound infant in an intensive care or isolation unit.

Tie a favorite rattle, small toy, or even a colorful hospital bootee to two tie strings of a face mask. Secure the other two tie strings to the crossbars of the crib.

The "mobile" is sturdy enough to last several days, but you can change the toys more often to provide new stimuli for the infant.

Kathryn Wheat, RN

Bouncy mobile
Here's a way to make a colorful, inexpensive mobile to stimulate infants and bedridden youngsters. Punch eight holes in a paper or Styrofoam dinner plate, making a circular pattern. Cut a long piece of string into four 24" pieces; then thread each piece up through the bottom of the plate and down through the next hole.

Now you can be creative. Cut animal pictures from magazines, or make snowflakes or other shapes from colored paper, and tie your creations to the strings hanging from the plate. To suspend the mobile, just punch two more holes in the center of the plate, and thread a strong rubber band through the holes, tying it to a long string at the top. Then tape the string to the ceiling or hang it from the I.V. pole.

The rubber band makes the animals and snowflakes dance if the child pulls on the mobile, and gives the plate some bounce so it won't tear easily.

Sylvia Spearr, RN

Road bed
How can you keep the pediatric patient on complete bed rest occupied? After the novelty of new coloring

books wears off, the child longs for an action game. Some paper towels—plus imagination—make the perfect answer for a little boy who loves playing with model cars.

Laying eight to ten paper towels end to end, tape them together and draw a "road" down the middle. After cutting out the road, encourage the boy to add his own twists—for example, passing zones, curves, and so on. The young road designer will contentedly drive his toy cars up and down pillow mountains and through blanket tunnels for hours.

Sally Goodhart, LPN

Let's pretend
Trying to get my 2-year-old to take her medicine used to be a real battle. Now, we pretend to give some to one of her dolls. After watching her "sick" dolly take the medicine, my daughter happily takes her dose. The game works well with my young patients too—even when bad-tasting medicine is prescribed.

Patricia Trefethen, RN

MOBILITY

Getting punchy
A child in skeletal traction needs exercise and diversion. So make a personalized, personable punching bag for him. Here's how.

Fill a pillowcase with baby blankets or towels. Wrap a piece of 2" wide adhesive tape around the middle of the pillowcase and another piece around the opening of the case to close it. This makes a punching bag with a head (the part near the pillowcase's opening) and body.

Wrap more tape around the head of the bag so you can draw eyes, ears, nose, and mouth. Then hang the

bag from the overbed frame so it's within easy reach of the child.

Encourage the patient to nickname the punching bag or to personalize it with a mustache, hair, or hat drawn on the tape. Let him punch away whenever he needs to release pent-up energy or frustration.

When the patient is discharged, you can simply dismantle the bag and send it to the hospital laundry.

Karen A. Bender, RN, BSN

Get a grip on it
The barrel of a plastic syringe makes a nice hand-grasp exerciser for unresponsive children.

Remove the plunger from the syringe, cover the end of the barrel with tape, and place the barrel in the child's hand. It's narrow enough for the small hand and fingers to grasp, yet wide enough to prevent the child from clenching and embedding his fingernails into his palm. (A 3-ml syringe usually fits the grasp of children to age 2; a 10-ml syringe fits most older children.) But to avoid a contracture, remove the exerciser for 2 hours after every 2 hours of use.

Marian Swist, RN

Children only, please
Do you use oversized wheelchairs or large carts to transport children from the pediatrics unit to other areas of the hospital? This often adds to their fright in unfamiliar surroundings.

To make this experience as pleasant as possible, use a large red wagon that comfortably carries children up to the age of about 9. Since most children have a wagon at home, it gives them something to relate to and makes their trip a happier experience.

Barbara Berger, RN
Barbara Jurgelis, RN

Help for handicapped tots

To help a handicapped toddler learn to walk, make a set of sturdy, economical parallel bars from wooden dowels and ordinary kitchen chairs.

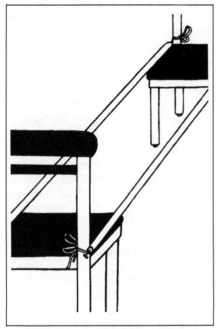

At a lumber company, buy two 8' dowels, 1" in diameter. Sand and varnish the dowels and attach a piece of clothesline rope to each end with a small nail. Then place the dowels over the seats of two kitchen chairs and tie the ends of the dowels to the chair backs. The height and width of the chair seats are just right for a toddler.

When the bars aren't in use, untie them and put them away.

Helen Hoke, RN

See and saw

To help children in Halo-Tibial traction watch TV or even see around the room, use a car clip-on mirror. Not only can it be swiveled in any direction but also it fits perfectly on the bars of the traction.

Cheryl Izenour, RN

PHYSICAL CARE

Disappearing ink

The footprinting and fingerprinting procedure in the delivery room leaves hard-to-remove ink stains on baby and mother. But with some gauze dabbed in a bit of baby oil, cleanup is easy. Just wipe the stains with the gauze and the ink will disappear—in a jiffy.

Jackie Angle, RN, BSN

Countering *Candida*

When a baby has thrush, lactose in his formula or his mother's milk can promote the growth of *Candida albicans.* To prevent such growth, advise the mother to rinse her baby's mouth with water after each feeding.

Beth L. Haug, RN

Upside-down shirt

Disposable diapers with plastic covers are great timesavers in an intensive care nursery. But they can create problems, too—such as chafed babies' bottoms. Exposing the affected areas to the air will speed healing, but the babies may get cold.

Solve the chafing problem and keep the babies' temperature stable by putting long-sleeved infant shirts on the babies when you expose them to air. Their legs go through the sleeves, and their bottoms stick through the neck openings—keeping everything covered except the affected areas. Mothers like the way their babies look, too.

Sue Leonard, RN

Padding the preemie

Occasionally, an unswaddled, over-zealous premature infant will rub his knees, elbows, toes, and even his chin against his bed linens, causing painful abrasions. To protect these delicate areas, apply small karaya pads to his skin.

When moistened, the pads adhere, making a soothing barrier against harsh linens. And removal is easy: the pads come off in one piece without pulling the skin.

Michele Dawson, RN, BS

An easy weigh

Standard baby scales are usually too small for large or handicapped young patients. Adult scales aren't much better; they're often imprecise (espe-

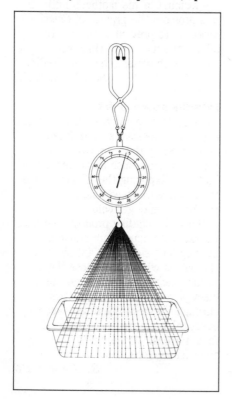

cially at lower weights) and are inadequate for handicapped children who can't stand on the base of the scale.

As pictured here, a "bathtub swing scale" can hang on a door frame with the clamp from a baby's jumping exerciser. Place a hanging scale (available from feed stores) on the clamp, and attach a fishnet hammock—which you can find in a boating or sporting goods store—to the bottom of the scale. Finally, place a plastic baby's bathtub in the hammock to assure smooth sailing during the weigh-in.

The scale is lighter, less expensive, and more easily dismantled and transported than the typical baby and adult scales.

Barbara Cheyney, RN, PHN

Tiny tongue blade

You may have trouble examining the mouth of a newborn—a tongue blade, even a junior one, is too big for the tiny patient's mouth.

Use the *handle* end of a cervical scraper as a tongue blade. Because it's only half the width of a conventional blade, it ends problems with oral examinations.

Gale B. Johnston, RN

Cast offs

"When is my cast coming off?" is a question pediatric patients ask repeatedly. But since many patients have only a vague concept of time, invent a visual aid to help them count the days: calendar cards.

Number a set of cards—one card for each day the child has to wear his cast—and hang them above his bed, like a mobile. The patient can remove one card each day, and see the numbers get smaller, or can count the remaining cards to see how many days are left.

As the number of cards decreases, the number of smiles increases!

Linda Wyszinski, RN

Cap it off
When children have a sutured laceration on the scalp with a dressing that needs to be kept clean, use a bathing cap. Choose one that's a size larger than needed, and it will keep the bandage clean and secure. The caps come in decorative colors so children can pretend they're airplane pilots with their rubberized headgear.

Ann Cunningham, RN

Cuddly caps
Make stocking caps for the babies in an intensive care nursery. Since the babies' greatest heat loss is from their heads, the caps help keep their temperatures stable, decreasing their caloric needs. Also, the caps seem to make parents less preoccupied with the monitoring equipment and more aware of their babies' normal aspects.

Dian Loomer, RN
Linda MacKenzie, RN

A hat trick
To keep a newborn baby's head warm (and prevent heat loss), make him a cap from an 8" piece of stockinette. Put a rubber band around one end of the stockinette to close it, roll up the other end 1" to make a cuff, and place the cap on the baby. You can also use the cap to keep a baby's head dry when he's in an oxygen hood.

Mary Kraft, RN, BSN

Quick-cooling gauze
Here's an easy way to bring down a child's elevated temperature.

First, remove the padding inside a 4" × 4" gauze pad, leaving the wide-gauge gauze. Soak this gauze in lukewarm water. Then, place the wide-gauge gauze over the child's abdomen, wrists, and ankles, and rewet the gauze every few minutes.

This technique brings a child's temperature down more rapidly than sponging or using heavy rags and cloths.

Cynthia Sundman, RN

Diaper lift
Ever care for a young child who had a hernia repair and circumcision? Pressure irritates his penis and he can't wear a diaper—at least not in the regular fashion.

So to keep him dry *and* comfortable, take an 8-oz paper cup and devise a penis cradle for him. After

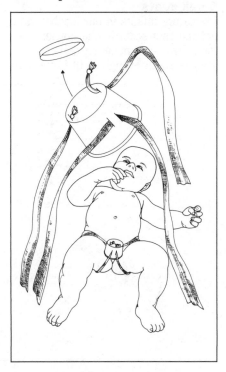

removing the cup bottom, slit the cup in four places: two slits in the front and one on either side. Then cut four long gauze pieces, thread one piece through each slit, and knot the ends inside the cup so they won't pull out.

Next, put the cup over the child's penis, with the cup front facing his buttocks. After bringing the two side gauze pieces around the child's waist and the front pieces up from under his buttocks, tie all four together at his back like a belt. Finally, put a diaper on the child *over the cup.*

By lifting the diaper up, the cup keeps pressure off the child's penis. Yet the diaper "does its duty" and helps keep the child's clothes and bed dry.

Jamie L. Hafer, LPN

Small seats

Premature infants in our incubators get the best seats in the house: toy infant seats made for dolls. They're small enough to fit in incuba-

tors and sturdy enough to hold the infants securely. We put the infants in the seats for feedings or just to change position.

Kathy Cohen, RN

How dry I am

Advise new mothers on how to promote umbilical cord healing and how to treat diaper rash. Getting plenty of air to the area being treated is an important part of the healing process, and a hand-held blow-dryer works perfectly. Set the dryer on "warm," and hold it 6 to 8″ from the skin for 5 minutes four times a day. Besides helping to heal the skin, the warm air may lull the babies into a quiet state.

Barb Prior, RN

Percussion discussion

For an effective, reusable infant chest percussion tool, tape a *plastic* medicine cup (a paper cup weakens after one or two uses) to the end of a tongue blade. Cushion the blow with a

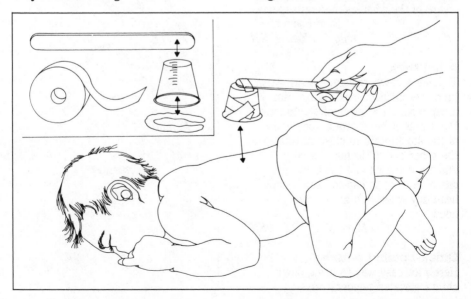

cotton ball taped to the edge of the cup.

Ordinary plastic nipples can also be used for infant chest percussion. They're safe, soft, and, with the base trimmed a bit, small enough to use on tiny and premature infants. They work especially well if you have to percuss between monitor leads on a tiny chest.

Mary Walker, RN

Let it slide

Filling the ice chamber on a Croupette may be a problem; the ice spills onto the bed or floor. Instead fill a brown paper bag with ice and place it with the open end down into the chamber. The ice easily empties from the bag into the chamber—without a mess.

Mary Beth Flickinger, RN

A better chair

Children with spasticity, partial paralysis, athetosis, or long-leg casts or braces have difficulty using a conventional toilet or potty chair. At Lenox Baker Children's Hospital in Chapel Hill, N.C., such children use a modified potty chair that resembles a cobbler's bench.

Designed by two nurses and the maintenance supervisor at the hospital, the chair has a broad base that makes it stable for children with poor coordination and balance. The narrow section of the seat extension prevents adduction or leg scissoring—problems often found in children with cerebral palsy. The extension itself supports the legs of children in long-leg casts or braces and prevents knee flexion. Arm supports and seat straps provide additional safety.

The wooden chair's polyurethane finish makes it easy to clean and eliminates chipping. Best of all, the chair lets the children assume a normal sitting position for excretion, rather than be limited to a bedpan or diaper.

Susan E. Parker, RN, MS

Superspenders

We recently cared for a 6-month-old baby who suffered burns on his torso. We applied dressings, then wrapped an Ace bandage over the dressings.

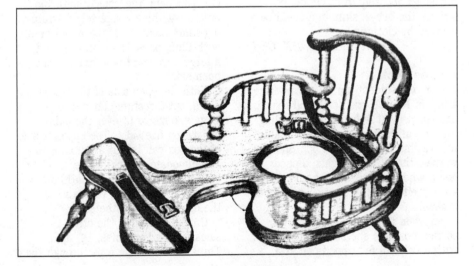

The baby was so active, though, that the bandage kept sliding down his torso.

To keep the dressings and bandage in place, we applied two Montgomery straps to the bandage on the child's chest and the two corresponding Montgomery straps to the bandage on the child's back. Then we tied each strap—suspender-style—at the baby's shoulder.

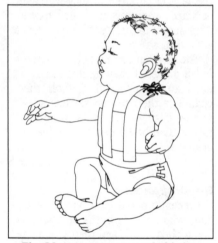

The Montgomery straps held the dressings securely in place, didn't irritate the baby's skin, and could be covered by clothing.

Frances Wartella, RN, CEN

A rope trick

One of our student nurses caring for a boy in Russell traction found that she spent most of her time reminding him to pull himself up in bed because his weights were on the floor. She worried that if the weights slipped down when no one was around, the pulling effect of the traction would be broken.

So when the weights were in the correct position, she marked the rope with a colorful felt-tipped pen at a point where the rope nearly touched the top of the foot of the bed. Then, when the patient could no longer see her mark on the rope over the foot of the bed, he knew it was time to pull himself up again.

This simple warning marker made the patient a little more self-reliant and freed the student nurse for other activities.

Sharon Zaucha, RN

Baby bands

If you're caring for an infant who has his legs in casts, here's a way to keep the top of the casts clean and odor-free. Put a terry cloth wrist band on each of the infant's legs above the cast. (Make sure, of course, that the band isn't too tight.) The band will absorb any urine or moisture and can be removed regularly for cleaning.

Patricia Belous, RN

Refraining from restraining

Problem: A pediatric patient who's had urologic surgery has orders to stay on his back and not to touch his surgical site or catheter. How can you help him comply with his orders—without completely restraining him? Solution: Make a bed cradle with Chux pads, traction rope, and a large cardboard box that has one open side.

With the open side of the box facing down, cut a rectangular opening—large enough to fit over the child's waist—on one side. (The opposite side of the box can be cut away later to accommodate the child's legs, if necessary.) Then cut a small hole in the top of the box so you can see the dressing and catheter.

On the bottom of the other two sides, punch two holes, 14″ apart. Thread the traction rope through the holes, and tie the ropes to the bed frame to keep the box securely in place. Then make a small notch near the bottom of one side of the box to extend the catheter tubing, so it won't become compressed.

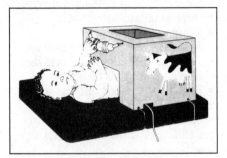

Finally, cover the box with the Chux pads and ask the patient's parents to help you draw pictures on it of the child's favorite things. You can also tie a rattle or small toy to the box within arm's reach of the patient.

Your bed cradle (which can be used with ankle restraints, if necessary) will restrain the patient while still allowing him some mobility. And it will help provide needed sensory stimulation, too.

Jan Leong, RN
Vickie Cegelski, SN

Perfect timing
Getting a child to void or drink at a certain time usually requires a little ingenuity. As an incentive, we use a kitchen timer.

For example, if a child must give a second-voided specimen in 20 minutes, or drink fluids every hour, we set the timer accordingly. While it's ticking away, the child mentally prepares himself for the task at hand. When the timer goes off, the child knows that he's "on," and usually performs with great enthusiasm.

Candy Pollack, RN

Tops on bottoms
I was recently given a challenging order in the special-care nursery: to expose to room air the red, sore buttocks of a 4½-lb premature infant without risking temperature loss. Since she was in an open crib, I was afraid that if I left her uncovered from the waist down, she'd get too cold. So instead, I put another undershirt on her—a bit differently, though. I put the baby's legs through the arms of this undershirt and left her buttocks exposed through the neck opening.

The baby's mother was amused when she visited and found undershirts on *both* ends of her little girl. But she was glad to learn that her baby was warm while her buttocks were healing.

Ellyn Presley, LPN, EMT

Diapers on duty
For the pediatric patient who has a sacral incision and must remain prone, here's a way to keep him and his incision free of stool and urine contamination.

I cut two 1″ × 2″ strips of Stomahesive and place one strip on each of the patient's hips. Then I attach the adhesive tabs of a disposable diaper to each Stomahesive strip and bring the diaper down between the patient's legs. This end of the diaper cups up below his buttocks and is left open to catch and absorb stools and urine.

When removing the soiled diaper, I gently press on the Stomahesive as I pull off the tabs so it stays in place. The strips do need to be replaced, though, every 2 or 3 days.

Jane Marner, LPN

Percussion protection
A nipple from a baby bottle makes a good chest percussor for an infant.

But before you begin, put a light blanket or diaper over the baby as a buffer, so the nipple won't irritate his skin.

Mary H. Coons, RN, MSN

How dry they are

A disposable diaper isn't always absorbent enough to keep a baby and his bed dry all through the night. That's why we place a sanitary napkin in the baby's diaper at bedtime. The napkin is soft, highly absorbent, and readily available from our supply department. Now we no longer have wet babies and beds in the morning.

Kimberly A. Stotts, RN, BSN

Easy-off dressing

We use nonadhering dressings (Xeroform petrolatum) for circumcision care in our newborn nursery. The dressing keeps the diaper from sticking to the baby's penis. But sometimes the dressing itself sticks to the baby and is difficult to remove without causing trauma or fresh oozing.

My solution is to apply petroleum jelly to some sterile gauze and place the gauze over the dressing. After about 20 minutes, I can remove the gauze and the dressing usually comes right off with it—with no difficulty. Then I apply a new dressing and repeat the procedure as needed.

Donna Henry, LPN

Throw in the towel

You're probably familiar with the use of warm, wet towels to bathe adult patients. Nurses at Huguley Memorial Hospital, Fort Worth, Tex., have adapted the towel bath for infants. They found that the towel bath not only saves time, it also conserves heat, an important consideration when caring for infants.

The nurses start the procedure by adjusting the room temperature to 75° F. (23.9° C.). Then they gather these supplies:
• ¼ ounce Septi-Soft (Vastal Laboratories, St. Louis), a liquid soap that cleans and softens the skin
• a quart of 110° F. (43.3° C.) water
• three standard bath towels
• a large plastic bag.

Next, they follow these directions:
• Pour the soap and water into the plastic bag; add two towels.
• Knead the solution into the towels and squeeze out the excess.
• Undress the infant, place him on his back, and cover him with a dry towel.
• Test the towel temperature with your elbow to make sure it's comfortable. (The temperature should read between 100° F. and 105° F. [37.8° C. and 40.5° C.] on a bath thermometer.)
• Remove the dry towel from the infant and replace it with a wet one.
• Gently massage through the towel, cleaning the infant from head to toe.
• Replace the wet towel with the dry towel and turn the infant on his stomach.
• Use the other wet towel to wash the infant from his head to his heels.

When Shirley J. Pinterich, RN, MS, and Reulita P. Vigilia, RN, MS, compared the towel baths and pan baths, they found that pan baths averaged 3.6 minutes; towel baths, 2.7 minutes. The greatest temperature loss with pan baths was 2.7° F.; with towel baths, 1.6° F.

Shirley J. Pinterich, RN, MS
Reulita P. Vigilia, RN, MS

COMFORT

Socks to swim in

To prevent children with spina bifida from scraping their feet against a swimming pool's side or bottom, put terry-cloth tennis socks on the children's feet before they go into the pool. This way they can splash to their hearts' content without scraping their feet. What's more, the socks don't interfere with the pool's filtering system.

Pat Hunter, RN

Take a breather, kid
My 5-year-old niece has unlimited confidence in my nursing abilities. When she recently suffered from an intestinal virus with frequent attacks of vomiting, my reputation was put to the test. Though I couldn't prevent the vomiting, I decided to put my knowledge of relaxation techniques to work. I taught her basic breathing exercises and imagery techniques (how to imagine relaxing, calm scenes). With her energy and attention diverted from "being sick," she felt better and more in control of the situation.

I learned how successful my teaching had been when she later suffered a minor injury and automatically started the breathing exercises on her own. And when she was sad because her grandmother was leaving, she said, "Tell me something happy to think about so I'll feel better. I already tried puppy dogs, rainbows, and flowers, but they're not working."

Pediatric nurses can try this when their patients undergo painful procedures.

Sr. Carol Taylor, RN, MSN

Throat soak
Children with sore throats don't always take their cough syrups and fluids as prescribed, so their recovery is prolonged.

To speed up the healing process, we offer them warm gelatin desserts to drink. Although they're not a substitute for cough syrups, they help promote comfort and recovery. They coat the throat, relieve soreness, provide necessary fluids, and—best of all—they come in many popular flavors.

Carol Wilt, RN, BSN

Relief in the round
After some of our patients get their allergy injections, their injection sites become red, swollen, and itchy. So we tell them to apply frozen teething rings to the injection site. The rings soothe as well as ice cubes, but they're easier to store and not as messy.

Rita Bleivik, RN, BSN

Give it a shot
Injections and pediatric patients: the two mix about as well as oil and water. So to make the procedure a little easier for you and less fearful for your patient, try this.

Ask the child to hold the bandage (one illustrated with comic characters or superheroes if possible) to give him some control and divert his attention away from the needle. Then say, "This will sting a little. If you think it hurts, I want you to say, 'It hurts; take it out, please.' But you have to say it *just* like that, and then I will take it out." Then give the injection. By the time your patient says, "It hurts; take it out, please," you'll have finished giving the injection.

Giving the patient some control and a diversion helps alleviate some of his fears and the pain of the injection.

Annette Hicks, RN, PNP

ComforTIEable
We recently cared for a 2-month-old

infant with a tracheostomy tube.
His tube wasn't the problem—his tube
tie was: it rolled into a string and
left an indentation on the infant's
chubby neck.

To make the tie more comfortable,
we put some foam-padded, adhesive-
backed tape around the back of the
baby's neck, with the foam side
against the baby's skin. Then we tied
the tie and folded the tape over the
tie onto itself. The padding kept
the tie from cutting into the baby's
neck, and it seemed to absorb moisture, too. In fact, it worked so well
we've begun using it on all patients
whose tracheostomy tube ties bother
them.

Donna Jenkins, RN, MEd

Painless pulse taking

We recently cared for a 12-year-old
patient with a supracondylar fracture
of the left humerus. Skeletal traction
was applied to his elbow, and his
wrist and forearm were placed in a
sheepskin sling.

Because his left radial pulse was
very faint, we had to monitor it with
a Doppler ultrasound stethoscope
every hour. Besides that, of course,
we had to check the color, temperature, and sensitivity of his arm.
All this checking, probing, touching,
and sliding the Doppler into the
sling caused the patient a lot of discomfort.

To alleviate some of this discomfort, we cut a small window opening
in the sling over the radial pulse.
We slipped the Doppler into the opening and took the patient's pulse
painlessly. And we made some of our
observations of his arm through
the window, too.

Margaret P. Carson, RN, BSN

With an eye to eye pads #1

When jaundiced newborns need phototherapy, we make eye pads for them.
First, we put a piece of polyurethane
dressing (for example, Op-Site, Bioclu-
sive, or Tegaderm), about 1½" long,
on each of the baby's temples. (See "A"
in illustration.) These pieces of dressing remain in place throughout the
phototherapy. Next, we cut an adult-
sized eye pad in half to fit over the
baby's eyes and tape these halves
together. We attach another piece of
tape (see "B" in illustration) to the
outer edge of each pad and attach the
pads to the dressings on the baby's
temples. (The tape only touches
the dressing—not the baby's skin.)
We turn the ends of the tape under for
easy grasping and removing.

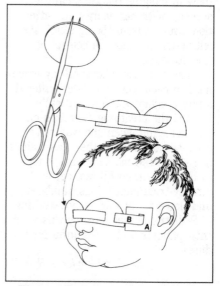

We can remove the pads easily to
change them, give eye care, and
provide visual stimulation without
applying and reapplying tape to the
baby's delicate skin.

Martha Andersen, RN

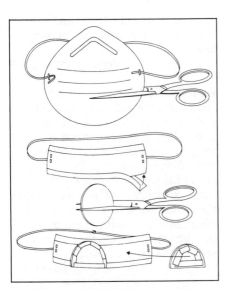

With an eye to eye pads #2

We make comfortable, *tapeless* eye pads for newborns. We cut a disposable face mask across the width— ½" above and below the elastic band—and cover the edges with paper tape to prevent fraying. Then we cut an adult-sized eye pad in half, lay the halves on the inside of the mask, and secure them to the mask with doubled paper tape. We also cover the edges of the eye pads with paper tape to keep them from fraying.

We adjust the elastic band to fit the baby's head by tying a knot in the band.

Roberta Poulton, RN

Band aid

Here's a way to ease some of the discomfort for children who must wear corrective leg braces. The leather frequently rubs against their lower legs and feet, irritating tender skin. But stretchable wrist sweatbands, available in most sporting goods stores, can serve as a cushion against this continual rubbing. The bands

are inexpensive, machine washable and dryable, and easy to put on. What's more, children love the many colors.

Sarah H. Benton, RN, CCRN

EMERGENCIES

Bright sights

Each patient room in our pediatric division has a large, brightly painted wooden animal propped against the wall. The puppies, frogs, bears, and other creatures delight our patients. But—more important—they make an easily accessible board to place beneath a child during a code.

Karen Pasley, RN

Milk *is* a natural

As you know, children are forever getting their teeth knocked out. But did you know that immediately replanting a tooth is the best way to preserve the tooth's life?

One course of action is to replace the tooth in its socket and ask the child to hold it in place until you get him to his dentist's office or the hospital emergency department (ED).

Another is to try a cold glass of milk—not to drink, though. Instead, place the tooth in the cold milk. Then get the child (and the glass of milk and tooth) to the ED or dentist's office as quickly as possible.

Milk's osmolality keeps the root cells from enlarging or shrinking. By immersing the tooth in milk, more than half its cells will be kept alive, even after 12 hours. If the tooth is left out in the air (on a table, for instance), most of its cells will die within 18 minutes.

So for healthy teeth, milk really *is* a natural.

Ronald Johnson, DDS

Rx for emergencies

Standard equipment on our ambulance includes a box of lollipops. Young children seem to accept our help more readily if we greet them with a lollipop in hand, rather than with unfamiliar, scary-looking emergency equipment.

Ann Hauser, BA, EMT-P

Cart smarts

We keep a small three-shelf pediatric emergency cart in the recovery room where I work. On the top shelf is a fishing tackle box containing pediatric doses of emergency drugs, pediatric endotracheal tubes and equipment, I.V. catheters, and monitor electrodes. The other shelves contain small arm boards, diapers, blood pressure cuffs, and gowns. Face masks and oxygen tubing are kept in a cloth bag hung on the side of the cart.

When a pediatric patient is brought to the recovery room, we place the cart next to his bed. Then, if an emergency arises, we'll be prepared.

Deborah Stout, RN

SUPPORTIVE MEASURES

Give 'em a band

On our pediatric surgical unit, our patients *and* their favorite toys (teddy bears, dolls, or other security blankets) get identification bands. This way, we can quickly reunite the children with their toys after surgery, saving our young patients unnecessary emotional upset.

Mary Lu Rang, RN, BSN

Puppet treats

Rather than give lollipops or candy to pediatric patients in our emergency department, we give them brightly colored hand puppets made by our volunteers. The children—and parents—love them. And they're harmless, too.

Maureen Anthony, RN

Familiarity breeds content

Here's how we add an extra touch to a child's routine hospital orientation. A few days before he's admitted, we give him a tour of the pediatric unit. Then we take a picture of him in one of the patient rooms. All the rooms are alike, so the child can take the picture home to show his friends where he'll be staying. Then when he's admitted, his assigned room will seem like a familiar place.

C. Duran, RN

A teaching toy

Our small hospital doesn't have many pediatric patients or the time or staff for patient-teaching classes. Just the same, we want to make sure the children understand hospital procedures and their treatments.

So whenever possible, we demonstrate procedures (starting an I.V., a dressing change, an examination) on a stuffed frog that each child gets on admission. When he sees that the frog made it through the procedure, he's confident that he will, too. Parents are grateful that their children are relaxed and understand the procedures. And the frog is a great conversation piece: the children enjoy explaining the frog's condition to visitors.

Laboratory personnel and respiratory therapists can also use this show-and-tell teaching aid when drawing blood or giving treatments.

Melinda Crawford, RN

Isolated assessment

Being in isolation is no fun, especially

for a child. To help me assess what he's thinking as well as how he's feeling, I do this.

Before entering the patient's room for the first time, I draw a nose and smile on my mask. Each time I enter the room thereafter, I ask him to do the honors. If the child draws a frown instead of a smile, I understand that all is not well and we talk about what's on his mind. This gives me a chance to stem any fears or misconceptions before they become big problems. And my just being there wards off loneliness for a while.

Marie M. Shanahan, RN

Starred charts

When pediatric patients take their prescribed medications for the day, help them see stars. Stars on their medication charts, that is.

To make a chart, take a sheet of paper, print the patient's name on it, and list his prescribed medications down the left side. Then print the days of the week across the top of the page and rule in the necessary columns. When the patient takes his medications, put an adhesive-backed star in that day's space.

Giving stars as a reward really encourages patients to take their medications. And to encourage at-home compliance, give the chart to the child's parents when he leaves the hospital.

Brian J. J. Cole, SN

Baby keepsake

Many infants in a neonatal unit need to have an I.V. tube inserted into a scalp vein at one time or another. Already worried about the newborn's illness, the parents become upset about having their baby's head shaved.

To allay the parents' anxieties (especially for the first shaving), tape the infant's shaved hair to a card listing his name, age, weight, and the date.

Besides letting them know that you understand their concern, the card is a nice baby keepsake for the parents.

Nancy Hogg, RN

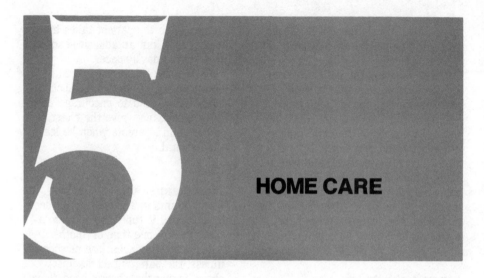

5

HOME CARE

ADMINISTERING SELF-MEDICATION

Home helpers
To help our home care patients keep track of their medication schedules, we use cardboard "sliding pill boxes." (They look like matchstick boxes with an inside compartment that slides in and out. Some pharmacies stock them for their patients.)

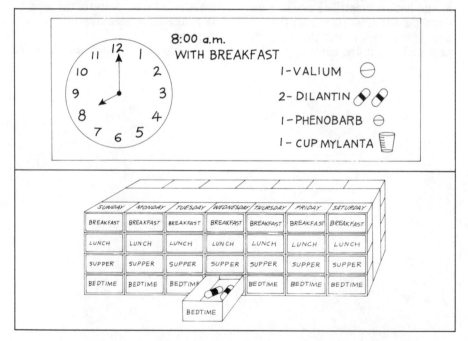

8:00 a.m.
WITH BREAKFAST

1 – VALIUM

2 – DILANTIN

1 – PHENOBARB

1 – CUP MYLANTA

	SUNDAY	MONDAY	TUESDAY	WEDNESDAY	THURSDAY	FRIDAY	SATURDAY
BREAKFAST	BREAKFAST	BREAKFAST	BREAKFAST	BREAKFAST	BREAKFAST	BREAKFAST	BREAKFAST
LUNCH	LUNCH	LUNCH	LUNCH	LUNCH	LUNCH	LUNCH	LUNCH
SUPPER	SUPPER	SUPPER	SUPPER	SUPPER	SUPPER	SUPPER	SUPPER
BEDTIME	BEDTIME	BEDTIME	BEDTIME	BEDTIME	BEDTIME	BEDTIME	BEDTIME

BEDTIME

We stack four boxes on top of one another and tape them together. Then we set seven of these taped stacks side by side and tape the seven stacks together. We label the top of each stack with a day of the week. The four boxes in each stack are labeled "breakfast," "lunch," "supper," and "bedtime."

When we visit the patient each week, we fill the boxes with medications for the upcoming week. At the next visit, we can tell by simply checking the boxes whether the patient's missed any medications.

Becky Weber, RN

On schedule

Nurses new to our oncology unit frequently are overwhelmed by the number of chemotherapy drugs they must know about, the variety of possible combinations of drugs, and the many potential adverse reactions. Besides all this, they must learn how to give the drugs in appropriate sequence. So we've devised a treatment schedule to help them keep this information straight.

We transcribe the chemotherapy orders from the doctor's order sheet to the treatment schedule. Then we put a check mark at the time each drug is to be given. (We use pencil because the schedule may be changed.) We write a new schedule for each patient every day.

The treatment schedule gives a 24-hour overview of the treatment plan; shows exactly when chemotherapy drugs, antiemetics, and sedatives are to be administered; and provides a good follow-up plan and reference after the course of treatment is completed.

Edith Kellnhauser, RN, BA

Eggsactly the right dose

A big problem for a patient who's discharged with a lot of medications is how to adjust his hospital medication schedule to his at-home schedule. To help him, I review *both* schedules with the patient before he's discharged.

First, we discuss the patient's normal routine at home, for example, when he wakes, eats, sleeps, and so on. With this routine in mind, we list the times it would be convenient and appropriate for him to take his medications. To make it easier, we try to group medications by scheduling the b.i.d. medications for the same time as two of the q.i.d. medications.

Using an egg carton, we mark one of these times in front of one of the depressions in the front row. Then we mark another medication time in front of the next depression, and so on until all of the medication times have been marked on the egg carton. We place the medication containers in the second row.

Each night at home, the patient sets up his next day's medications in the egg carton. Taking one container at a time from the second row, he removes the medications and places them in the appropriately marked time depressions in the first row.

The next day, he just takes his medications at the times marked on the carton. He doesn't have to worry about double or missed doses.

Tell your patient to keep the egg carton out of the sunlight. And if you're worried about the medications' exposure to room air and moisture, check with the patient's doctor or pharmacist before setting up the system.

Anna Juskiw, RN, BS

Shoe box/pill box

If a blind patient is taking a variety of medications, all in pill form, and wants to take them by himself, use this system: Using letters cut from sandpaper, label seven envelopes with the days of the week. Place the pills in small zip-lock plastic bags labeled with sandpaper numbers, according to the time the pills are to be taken. Then, place the bags inside the envelopes, and file the envelopes in a shoe box within the patient's reach.

At the beginning of each day, the patient simply pulls the first envelope from the box, "reads" the numbers on the plastic bags with his fingers, and takes his pills at the designated hours.

This system not only gives the patient a feeling of independence, but it also gives you an accurate way to tell whether he's taken all of his pills.

Barbara Boles, RN

Bottle clip

A simple, inexpensive broom clip holder helps a one-handed diabetic patient prepare his insulin independently.

The clip, available in most hardware stores, holds a standard-size insulin bottle securely and can be mounted on any convenient surface with a single screw. An easy-to-reach kitchen cabinet shelf usually works well. (Of course, the clip shouldn't interfere with the cabinet door closing.)

June B. Jackson, OTR

Right side up—and down

Do your patients on twice-daily medications have trouble remembering whether they've taken their morning or evening dose? Here's a way to help them keep track.

Tell them to mark the top of the medication container "a.m." and the bottom "p.m." Then, as soon as they've taken the medication, they can turn the container to show the time for the next dose. Later, if they've forgotten whether they took their medicine that morning, they can simply look at the container. If it shows "p.m.," they know they took the morning dose.

Wilhemina K. Patterson, RN

Bottle opener

Opening a medication bottle with a child-proof cap can be difficult (if not impossible) for a patient who has the use of only one hand. But some Velcro can help.

Tell your patient to apply an adhesive-backed piece of Velcro to a counter or other flat surface and another piece of Velcro to the bottom of the bottle. Place the bottle on top of the Velcro on the counter, press down on the bottle cap, and turn the cap. To prevent spilling the medication, remind your patient to leave the loosened cap in place when he lifts the bottle off the counter.

Doris Kozlowski, GN

Caps off

If you're caring for arthritic or elderly patients who skip medications because they can't remove child-proof caps from medicine bottles, these tips may help.

Many child-proof caps have two parts: an inner part that screws onto the bottle and a revolving outer part that provides the safety feature. Dig out the inner part, discard the outer, then use the inner part to cap the bottle. The patient will now be able to open the bottle easily.

Better yet, you can avoid this

whole problem by suggesting that your patients request regular caps for the bottles the next time they get their prescriptions filled.

Of course, if children are present in the home, you'll want to disregard these tips.

Lorraine Castellino, RN

A feeling for healing
A pharmacist came up with this idea to help a blind patient identify the different medications he had to take at home every day. He devised a code using letters and simple symbols to represent the medications and times they were to be taken.

For example, a triangle (three sides) represents t.i.d.; a square (four sides), q.i.d.; and a letter of the alphabet, the name of the medication. He cut these letters and symbols out of carpet tape and attached them to the appropriate bottles. The patient could "read" these labels, using his sense of touch.

Sylvia T. Joseph, RN

FOSTERING INDEPENDENCE

Homemade hanger
Home care patients who use wheelchairs or walkers to get around may also have catheter or urinary drainage bags. Finding a place to hang the bags when the patients want to move around may be a problem. Use this idea:

With wire cutters, clip the bottom rung from a wire clothes hanger. Spread the two sides straight out and bend both ends down 1½". Attach the wire, hook side down, to the walker or wheelchair with a pair of radiator clamps. Hang the catheter or drainage bag on the hook.

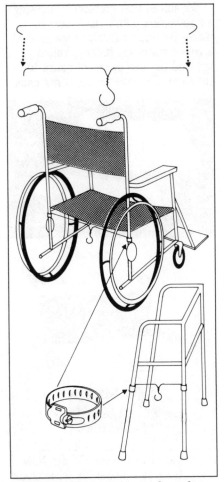

This wire hanger is sturdy and ensures good drainage with no backflow.

Agnes Moore, RN, BSN

A rehab roll
In the rehabilitation hospital where I work, we encourage patients with total hip replacements to propel their own wheelchairs. Most patients have had trouble with this, however, because they're too busy trying to keep the abduction pillow between their knees.

We solved that problem by making an abduction pillow that stays in place. We wrap adhesive tape around a rolled towel (so it stays rolled up) and tie long pieces of gauze to the tape. Then we tie the other ends

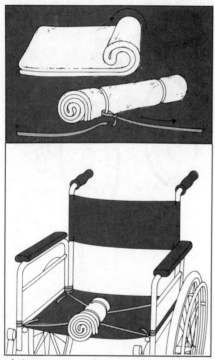

of the gauze to the wheelchair. Now the patient can propel his wheelchair and not worry that the towel will slide out from between his knees.

Victoria A. Schnaufer, LGPN

A pencil pusher
In the large nursing home where I work, some wheelchair patients couldn't reach the elevator's eighth-floor button. So I suggested they carry a new, unsharpened pencil with them and use the rubber eraser to press the button.

The pencil adds almost 4″ to their reach and gives them a new feeling of independence. Now they don't have to wait until someone has time to take them to their eighth-floor rooms or activities—they just reach up and go themselves.

Catherine Barnshaw, LPN

Improved walker
Help a patient with a walker become more independent and surefooted by buying a bicycle basket and attaching it to the front of his walker. He can then go to stores by himself and carry his packages home in the basket. And he'll become much steadier, thanks to the increased practice and exercise.

Suzanne Devine, RN

Carry-all pockets
After breaking her hip, my mother needed a walker to get around. But she couldn't carry anything in her hands when she walked.

She solved the problem by wearing an apron with pockets. She could walk from room to room taking along whatever she needed (books, pens, pencils, snacks, and so on) right in the pockets.

Devon Leguillette, RN

Cane and stable
My grandmother has stiff legs, and when she gets up from bed or from a chair, she's wobbly.

So before rising, she grasps the bottom of her cane, places one foot into the cane handle's crook, and then uses the cane to pull her leg up and down several times. After exercising both legs this way, her circulation's better, her legs aren't so stiff, and she feels more stable when standing.

Maybe some of your patients could take a lesson from grandmother—

and learn to use their canes to limber their legs.

M. Ellen Campobasso, LPN

Stuck-up cane

A friend who has multiple sclerosis and uses a cane passed along this tip to me. Whenever he'd lean his cane against a wall or counter to free both his hands, the cane would invariably drop to the floor. Retrieving it was always a struggle.

To solve this problem, he attached a small piece of Velcro to the handle of his cane and attached matching pieces to his belt, workbench, filing cabinet, kitchen counter, and wherever else he usually propped his cane. Now whenever he has to use both hands, he "hangs" his cane on the Velcro, and it stays upright until he needs it again.

Ann T. Nandrea, RN

Care for the casted

Because the patient can't carry anything while he's in a body cast and on crutches, suggest that he wear a carpenter's apron with lots of pockets. That way, he can carry almost anything he needs.

Mary S. Duff, RN, CCRN

Cane catcher

Crutches and canes can fall easily and are difficult to retrieve. For example, if you let go of a cane momentarily to try to prop it somewhere while you're sitting, it's sure to fall to the ground.

Solve this problem by buying a leather dog leash and cutting it down to just a few inches. Then have a shoe repairman stitch the shortened leash around the top of the cane and nail it in place. Slip the patient's arm through the collar, using it just as he'd use a wristlet on a ski pole.

Agnes Mohnar, RN

Working on the rails

I recently cared for a patient in his home who spent most of the time in bed. Whenever he tried to raise himself, he'd have trouble holding onto the slippery bed rails.

To help, I bought two 3' pieces of formed foam rubber from a hardware store (they're usually wrapped around hot water pipes for insulation). I wrapped the pieces around the bed rails and taped them in place.

The foam rubber rail pads are inexpensive. They've been in place for more than 4 months and still look fine. Best of all, they do the job: they give the patient a sure grip whenever he wants to lift himself in bed.

Ethel Hamilton, LPN

A pull sheet

One of my elderly home care patients is a big man who's too debilitated to pull himself up in bed. His wife, a small woman, isn't strong enough to pull him up either. With a little ingenuity and teamwork, though, they discovered a way to move him.

They twisted a flat bed sheet into a rope and placed it across the bed, under the patient's shoulders. They brought the ends of the sheet under his armpits, over his shoulders, and over the head of the bed. Then the wife gripped each end and, with the patient pushing with his feet, she pulled him up in bed.

Pam Barton, RN

Opening doors deftly

Have you ever realized that opening a refrigerator door can be a problem for some patients? For instance, a patient with a fractured vertebra can't open his refrigerator door because the pulling effort causes spinal pain. To help him, suggest he use a smooth, wooden mixing paddle. Tell him to insert the edge of the paddle very gently, near the door handle, between the rubber and the refrigerator. This releases the suction, and the door will open easily.

Or try this for a patient who has rheumatoid arthritis in both hands and can't grasp the handle to open the refrigerator door. Loop an 18" piece of rope around the refrigerator handle and tie the ends together. The patient can slip the rope over his arm to pull the door open.

Louise Wiedmer, RN, MS

Brush up on fun
Some elderly patients in nursing homes and those who have arthritis or paralysis may be missing out on some fun because they can't hold playing cards or magazines. To help them participate in such activities, give them a scrub brush. With the bristle end up, the brush can hold cards, pictures, and even light magazines.

Linda Jeronovitz, RN

A gripping story
When you want to check a patient's grip, don't offer him your whole hand; offer only two *ringless* fingers, such as your index and middle fingers. With just these two fingers you can determine the strength and equality of your patient's grip. And you needn't worry that a strong grip could press your ring into your other fingers, causing cuts, bruises, or fractures.

Patricia A. Diehl, RN

Portable pouches
Since many homebound patients use

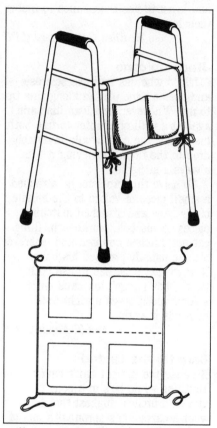

walkers to help them move around, use this device that enables them to carry along such items as tissues, snacks, books, and so forth. Make apronlike carriers from vinyl that fold over the front bar of the walker. These carriers can have four pouches—two in front and two in back—and four strings to anchor them to the front legs of the walker. Besides being handy, these carriers give patients a greater sense of independence.

Joanne Dorbury, RN

Bed 'n' board ('n' bag 'n' books)
Bedridden patients sometimes need

the head of their bed raised for comfort. With a hospital bed, this is no problem. To raise a regular bed, though, you might suggest they try one of the following:

• Wedge a beanbag chair between the mattress and box spring. The chair will raise the head of the bed about 30 degrees. (Before doing this, though, the patient should check with the mattress manufacturer to make sure that bending it at this angle won't damage it.)

• Put a few boards or books under the legs at the head of the bed.

• Slant a wide board (or a few boards) from the middle of the bed to the top of the headboard. Then tie the boards to the headboard and bed to keep them in place, and pad the boards with sheets, blankets, and pillows.

Whatever method the patient chooses, he'll have the comfort of a hospital bed without the expense.

Ann McCormick, RN, CCRN

No more bath blues

If a rheumatoid arthritis patient can't bathe himself, use a special bath sponge and heavy wire coat hanger. Stretch the top and bottom of the hanger. At the bottom, shape a triangle, stitch a folded sponge around it, and then fold a washcloth around the sponge. Adjust the hook at the top for the patient's best grip and bend the handle to suit his washing needs. If his elbows or wrists are too stiff to use the device, he could bend the handle into another position.

And how can a patient with stiff fingers squeeze out the sponge and cloth? Place the sponge against the side of the basin and press his hand flat against the sponge.

Louise Wiedmer, RN

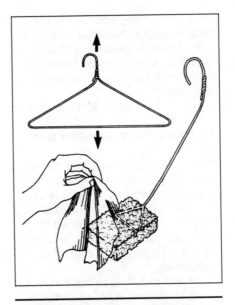

IMPROVISING EQUIPMENT AND SUPPLIES

Workable walkway

Here's an economical way to help hip surgery patients, stroke patients, and others practice walking in their own homes. Arrange six or eight sturdy chairs, such as dining room chairs, side-by-side in two rows so their backs form a pathway. The patient can practice walking with the same support he would get from parallel bars.

Teresa Rose, RN

Improvised foot cradle

If ever you need a foot cradle and find that they've all "disappeared," improvise.

Get a cardboard carton from the hospital stockroom and remove the top. If you want to protect the feet, simply cut an opening on one side of the box and place the box over the feet. If you want to protect another part of the body, cut openings on two facing sides and place the box over the area where protection is needed.

Such improvisation is especially helpful for invalids in the home who cannot afford to rent or buy costly equipment.

Nancy M. Crombie, LPN

An improvised over-the-bed table

To make an improvised over-the-bed table, select a strong cardboard box large enough to hold a bed tray at a comfortable height for the patient. If the box is too tall, cut it down to size. Then cut out enough room for the patient's legs to fit comfortably underneath.

The box can then be used as is. Or it can be covered with a colorful self-adhesive paper for easy wiping after use. Young patients enjoy decorating this piece of "furniture."

Linda N. Gunby, RN

Overboard

An ironing board makes a useful overbed table for home care patients. The board's adjustable, sturdy, and large enough to hold many of the patient's belongings.

Nancy Westerbuhr, RN, PHN

Expedient extract

Liquids and tablets for deodorizing ostomy appliances are sometimes expensive and ineffective. Vanilla extract is an effective and inexpensive alternative. Instruct patients to saturate a small wad of tissue with vanilla extract and place it in the bottom of the appliance. They can repeat this procedure as often as necessary—every time they empty the appliance, if they desire.

Diane Deegan-McCrann, RN, ET

Undercover table

Even lightweight bed covers can rest uncomfortably on the feet of patients who've had orthopedic surgery. To beat this problem after they're discharged from the hospital, tell them to try this:

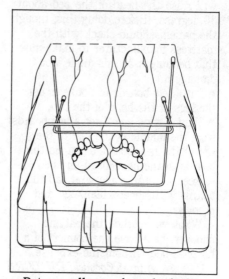

Put a small, open-legged television table under the top covers, with the tabletop facing the foot of the bed. This keeps the covers off the patient's feet, while allowing enough room for a pillow to elevate the feet. Also, the tabletop bottom makes an excellent footrest.

Note: If the patient doesn't have a table, an empty cardboard box works just as nicely.

Lynne Davies, RN

Postpartum pads

If your postpartum patient is nursing her baby, she may appreciate this tip.

Instead of commercial bra pads, try using beltless sanitary minipads. Simply cut a minipad in half, peel the backing off both halves, and affix one half to each side of the bra.

The minipad halves are highly absorbent and have a stay-dry lining that helps prevent irritated nipples and leaking. Besides, they're much cheaper—less than half the cost of most commercial bra pads.

Susan Lea, RN

Handled with care
When a patient is nauseated and vomits heavily, an emesis basin may be inadequate or unavailable. Instead, give him an empty plastic gallon milk carton (with the top cut off and the rim taped for padding). The patient can easily pick it up by its handle, giving him better control and less spillage.

Marion Dolan, RN

Home care chair
When your surgical patient is discharged, suggest that he use an adjustable lawn chair at home in lieu of a hospital bed. The patient can raise or lower the chair's back and foot sections, and he can pad the chair with cushions or pillows for extra comfort. Also, the chair is light enough to be moved from room to room as needed.

Pam Bloch, RN

RESOLVING ELIMINATION DILEMMAS

Nighttime convenience
One of my home care patients has nurses assigned to her in the day and evening but not at night. Urinary frequency is a problem because she can't get out of bed to go to the bathroom without someone helping her. So before the evening nurse leaves, she puts a bedpan on top of a bucket near the patient's bed. During the night, the patient can reach over, get the bedpan, use it, and empty it into the bucket. She can reuse the bedpan as often as necessary without worrying about spilling.

Pauline Lamia, RN

A filter tip
Here's a tip for your patients who must strain their urine for renal calculi or gravel. A cone-shaped filter for an automatic coffee maker makes a handy urine strainer. The filters are small-pored and can be easily handled and disposed of. Also, if the patient passes any blood that's not readily visible, a pink or red stain will appear on the white filter paper.

Arline M. Brice, SN

Skin saver
If diarrhea is irritating your patient's skin, suggest that he use a peri bottle (the kind given to new mothers for perineal care during the postpartum period). Tell him to clean his perineum with fluid from the bottle instead of wiping with tissues.

To use the bottle, he simply fills it with warm water (and some soap, if desired) and directs the water over the anus and perineum. Then he can blot the skin dry.

Caution: Tell the patient to store the bottle with the cap off, to discourage bacterial growth between uses.

Barbara J. Smith, SN

Colostomy cleanup
Here's a tip for your patient with a colostomy: Suggest he spray the inside of his colostomy bag with a cooking oil spray (such as Pam) before applying the bag. His stools won't stick to the bag and cleanup will be easier.

Teresa Ryan, RN

SOLVING INTAKE PROBLEMS

To a tee
Surgical patients discharged with a long-term or permanent feeding tube, which must be clamped between feedings to prevent backflow, sometimes lose the clamp and are unable to find a replacement. A readily available substitute that fits perfectly into the end of a nasogastric tube is a plastic or wooden golf tee.

D. Peters, RN

Self-serve solution
For a thirsty patient who can't pour his own juice or water, try rigging up this self-dispenser.

Put a 2-qt container of fluid on the overbed table at a higher elevation than the patient. Then attach two pieces of I.V. extension tubing together to make a long tube, clamp the tube, place one end in the container, and give the other end to the patient. Teach the patient how to unclamp and clamp the tubing, so he gets a feel for regulating the flow and doesn't choke on too much fluid. Then let him drink whenever he wants.

Mark Adam Smith, Corpsman, USN

Measure for measure
Here's a way to help a homebound patient on fluid restrictions keep track of his daily intake. Mark a pitcher, bucket, or some other household container at the level showing his total daily allowance of fluids. Then tell him whenever he drinks some fluid, he should pour an identical amount of water into the marked container. This way, he can see at a glance how his intake compares to his total allowance.

Lindsay Lake, BSN

IMPROVING PHYSICAL CARE

Piercing the infection
Tell your patient with pierced ears she can prevent earlobe infections by simply applying some antibiotic ointment to the earring post before inserting it into the lobe. Of course, check first to be sure she's not allergic to the ointment.

Mary Stringer, RN

Leg writing
When I discovered that my postoperative patients who'd had cesarean sections weren't doing their leg rotations and flexions in bed, I came up with another exercise routine. I asked them to pretend each leg is a pencil. They're to lift their "pencils" (one leg at a time) and print their newborn's *full* name in the air. No shortcuts with nicknames are allowed.

Now my patients are more compliant and even do their exercises more frequently.

Rita A. Bednarczyk, LPN

Cast care #1
Here's a way to help a patient protect the bottom of the foot of his leg cast from becoming broken, scraped, or dirty: Place a piece of used carpet or a carpet square over the bottom of the cast. Slash or cut out a "V" at the back so the carpet fits around the heel when you bring it up toward the ankle. Hold the carpet in place with a large sock or slipper sock. Extending the carpet out beyond the toes a little will also provide some protection against bumped or stubbed toes—a welcome protection, since the toes tend to become somewhat extra sensitive to jostling.

Judy Hutchins, RN

Coded clothes

An elderly, blind woman who lives alone recently told me how she coordinates the colors in her wardrobe: she uses safety pins to code the clothing by color. For instance, one pin placed on a garment in a vertical position indicates that the garment is white. Two vertical pins indicate that the garment is blue. Pins placed horizontally indicate other colors.

The coding system helps the woman retain her independence because it allows her to dress properly without assistance.

Sr. Carol Taylor, RN, MSN

Cast care #2

Here's a tip to pass on to patients wearing arm casts.

If the cast snags clothing and furniture, make a cast cover from an old nylon stocking. Cut the stocking's toe off and cut a hole in the heel. Then pull the stocking over the bulky plaster, poking the patient's thumb through the hole in the heel. Trim the stocking to about 1½″ longer than the cast and tuck this end of the stocking under the cast's edge.

Cyrena Gilman, RN

Kitchen cream

Since diabetic patients need to take special care of their feet, tell them they probably have an effective, inexpensive cream right in their own kitchen that'll help soften their dry, calloused skin. It's solid vegetable shortening.

Tell the diabetic patient to put a dab of shortening in the palm of his hand after bathing. Then have him add a few drops of water and mix with the shortening until he gets a nice cream that rubs in well and doesn't leave a greasy covering. Using this treatment once or twice a day will bring dramatic results. What's more, the "cream" can be used on elbows, hands, knees—wherever rough skin is a problem.

Joyce A. McCarthy, RN

Zippy tip

A patient who has a leg prosthesis usually has to remove his pants to get his prosthesis on or off. To eliminate this bother, suggest that he put a zipper on the inside seam of his pant leg (so the zipper opens at the *bottom* of the pant leg). Likewise, a patient who has an arm prosthesis can put a zipper in the sleeve of his shirt. This will make putting on and taking off the prosthesis a lot easier...a real zip.

Fidelita Lim-Levy, RN, CS, MSN

Diminutive dressing

Here's a suggestion for postoperative patients who need just a small dressing or protective cover for their incision when they're discharged. Apply a sanitary pad with an adhesive strip to the undergarment covering the incision. The pad protects the incision, is more economical than a sterile dressing, and has no adhesive touching the skin to irritate the sensitive surgical site (the adhesive strip is attached to the garment).

Carol I. Lewis, RN

Double-duty crutch

Pass this tip along to the patient who has a leg cast and must keep the leg elevated whenever possible. Tell him to use one of his crutches to prop up the leg.

After the patient sits down, he should adjust the crutch to the shortest position, then place it between his chair and thigh, with the handgrip pointing away from him. He can place his casted leg over the crutch so his ankle is supported by the handgrip and his foot rests below it.

Because the crutch goes wherever the patient goes, he'll always be able to keep his leg elevated and still while sitting.

Linda M. Schultz, RN, BSN

Reflections on wounds

After being hospitalized for abdominal surgery, I was sent home with instructions to clean and redress the wound. To accomplish this, I improvised the following method.

I put a disposable underpad on my bed and arranged all the necessary supplies nearby. Then I lay down on the bed with two pillows under my shoulders and head, knees flexed, and a hand mirror propped against them. This way I could see the wound and use both hands for the cleaning and dressing change.

Donna M. Babao, RN, MA

PERFORMING EMERGENCY SELF-CARE

Finger splinting good

In an emergency, a hollow roller-type hair curler or the top half of the clamp-on curler will make a sturdy finger splint or protector for an injured finger.

Kathleen Cruzic

Dental assistant

Here's a tip to pass on to postoperative dental patients. If bleeding occurs at home, and the patient has no gauze on hand, he can use a tampon instead. Tell him to just cut the tampon in half, place one half at the bleeding site and bite down. This

will stanch the bleeding and save a phone call to the dentist.

Lynne Cole, RN

Emergency tapes

Before a patient with a laryngectomy is discharged, pass on this helpful—sometimes lifesaving—hint: Ask a relative or friend to tape-record several "emergency" phone messages that can be played over the phone to the fire company, police department, ambulance service, or doctor.

The messages might say: "My name is *(patient's name)*, I live at *(his address)*. I'm a laryngectomy patient and need a *(doctor's, ambulance's, or whatever)* assistance at *(repeat address)*. Please notify *(name of friend or relative)* at *(phone number)*."

Tell patients to mark all tapes clearly (only one message should be recorded on each side of a tape) and to keep the tapes and emergency phone numbers by their phones.

The messages allow patients who live alone or are alone for long periods of time to be independent and confident that they can get help if needed.

Suzanne S. Stephens, RN

TRAVEL TIPS

Quick fix for stoma leaks

Stoma patients may worry about what to do if their pouches or sites leak. So show them how to prepare an emergency kit. The contents are a pair of underpants, a stoma bag, a small facecloth or premoistened towelettes, and a small, plastic bottle of deodorant.

Men can put all this in a shaving kit; women in a makeup kit. Then the kit can be placed in a glove compartment or desk drawer, where it'll be readily available yet not arouse anyone's curiosity.

Jean Bourgelais, RN, ET

A bathing beauty

A patient who'd had a mastectomy told me how she solved a problem on her recent vacation. She wanted to wear her breast prosthesis under her bathing suit, but she didn't want to get it wet when she swam.

So she bought a natural sponge, trimmed it to the shape of her breast, and inserted it in her bathing suit. She wore her inexpensive sponge prosthesis with confidence, both on the beach and in the water. In fact, she told me, when the sponge got wet, it filled with water, giving her a quite natural appearance.

Heather Wright, RN, PHN, BSN

Homemade first aid

If any of your patients are planning camping trips, you'll do them a service by reminding them to take along a first-aid kit. And it needn't be expensive—they can make it themselves.

Here's what they should do. Take any sturdy container, such as a workman's lunch bucket, and fill it with the following: an antiseptic for killing germs that cause infection; calamine lotion for soothing bites and itches; sterile cotton or cotton-tipped applicators for applying medications; 4" × 4" gauze pads for large cuts, blisters, or compresses; a 2" roll of gauze for bandaging a wound; adhesive tape; an Ace bandage for easing pain and swelling of sprains during the trip to the doctor; a pair of scissors; a thermometer; tweezers for removing splinters; ammonia capsules for reviving someone who has fainted; and a reputable first-aid guidebook.

Also suggest that they include a list of emergency numbers in their kit, such as the phone numbers of their family doctor, an alternate doctor, and a relative or neighbor; their hospitalization policy number; and medication prescription numbers.

When they arrive at their vacation site, they can look up the phone numbers of the nearest hospital, a 24-hour or local pharmacy, the police and fire departments, ambulance service, and poison control center and add these to their list of emergency numbers.

Catherine O'Boyle, RN

In the can

A diabetic patient can carry an insulin bottle and two alcohol wipes in a 35-mm film can. The can allows a patient to take his insulin with him wherever he goes, without worrying about leakage or breakage.

Sue Ingram, RN

PEDIATRIC MEASURES

Medi-minder

An infant with cardiac problems requiring at-home drug therapy obviously must depend on his parents to follow through.

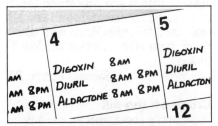

To simplify compliance, give parents a monthly open-block calendar. In each daily block, ask them to list the infant's prescribed drugs and their administration times. After administering each dose, the parents should check off the time administered.

Be sure to advise parents to fill out only a week's worth of blocks at a time, because their doctors might add to or discontinue the regimen. Also suggest that they not list doses, because these, too, could be changed. Instead, supply a small card listing the dosage for each drug, which can be kept with the drugs for handy reference.

The calendar really helps parents organize and keep track of their infant's multiple prescriptions. As a result, it's a real spur to parent compliance—and to infant good health.

Anne L. McKinnon, RN, BSN

The kit's a hit

A "Mother's Sick Child Care Kit" will save you from dashing to the grocery store for clear liquids and diversional activities when your children are sick. Use a brightly colored tote bag and fill it with packages of gelatin, powdered fruit drinks, crackers, tissues, a can of soft drink, a thermometer, children's aspirin, some crayons, and a coloring book.

Give these kits as gifts (they can be modified for children of different ages) to friends and patients so they'll be prepared the next time one of their children comes down with the flu or some other common childhood illness.

Shannon Patton, RN

Cross off the pill

Don't worry about whether parents give their children's medications properly. Instead, create a visual aid for parents—a cross-off-the-pill chart. Each chart should have 10 boxes— one for each day of the antibiotic

course. Inside each box, write "1, 2, 3, 4" to designate the number of pills to be taken each day. Have the patient simply cross off a number after each pill he takes. On the flip side of the chart, list general instructions for taking antibiotics.

Now, patients can hang up their charts in a prominent place, remind their parents when they need a pill, and cross off the numbers themselves.

Phyllis Yetka, RN

Easier postural drainage

When parents have to perform daily postural drainage and percussion on a young child with cystic fibrosis, suggest they get a beanbag chair for their home.

Using this chair, they can easily place a child in several comfortable positions. As a bonus, the smaller chairs are often decorated with cartoons and bright colors, which children like.

Sharon Bean, LPN

Splish splash

As you know, when a pediatric patient has had a bilateral myringotomy with tube placement, keeping water out of his ears is a must. But with active youngsters at bath time, this is almost impossible. So suggest to his parents that they cover his ears with a terry cloth sweatband. They can simply stretch it from around the nape of his neck, over his ears, and up to his forehead. The patient can splash to his heart's content and his ears will stay dry.

Lois Dunwoody, RN

Edible ice bag

If you're a pediatric or public health nurse, here's a tip you can pass on to parents of small children.

The next time Junior bumps his head (or leg or arm), don't waste time finding a towel and filling a plastic bag with ice cubes. Instead, just reach for a bag of frozen vegetables from your freezer and apply it to the injured area.

Suggestion: If by chance you've grabbed Junior's favorite vegetable, promise to let it thaw and serve it to him for dinner.

M. Lorraine Stewart, RN

Dressings in stock(ings)

Home care patients can keep leg dressings in place without using a lot of tape by putting a pair of old, clean panty hose on over the dressing. If men balk at the idea, remind them they can wear trousers, shoes, and socks over the panty hose.

Debra Fearing, LPN

Soaking sets

When your home care patient has to soak his hand or foot in a prescribed (but nonsterile) soaking solution, suggest this method.

Pour the solution into a clean plastic bag and have the patient put his hand or foot into the bag. Fasten the bag (not too tightly) with a rubber band. Place the bag in a bucket of warm water.

The water not only warms the solution but also causes it to rise in the bag to the level of the water in the bucket. This way, the patient will use less solution to cover his hand or foot for each soak, and will save money.

Erma Shea, RN, BSN

Nursing aid

Engorged breasts or flat, inverted, or sore nipples sometimes present problems to mothers who want to breast-feed their babies. A less expensive (and readily available) alternative to a breast shield is a regular bottle nipple.

Just bore a slightly bigger hole into the nipple's end with a pair of sterile scissors and remove the rim. The mother can place this nipple over her own, and the baby will grasp it easily.

Diane Theisen, RN

Face saver

One of my home health care patients has arthritis, and when I wash her hair in the shower, she can't tilt her head back to keep the water and shampoo from getting into her eyes and ears. To help her, I cut a big circle out of the top of a plastic shower cap. I put the cap on her head, pulling her hair through the cut-out circle. The elastic rim is now above her eyes and ears, so I simply flip down the remaining plastic to protect her face.

Now she doesn't have to move her head at all, and she doesn't get any water or shampoo in her eyes or ears either.

Ruth Sagehorn, RN

Cube feedings

Many nursing mothers like to express extra milk and freeze it for later feedings when they have to be away from their babies. But some of this mother's milk is wasted when the baby can't finish a full bottle.

To save this precious commodity, tell the mother to pour her expressed milk into an ice cube tray and cover the tray tightly with a plastic bag. She can keep adding her milk to the tray (chilling it first so it won't defrost the cubes) until the tray is filled, then empty the cubes into another plastic bag.

When the mother has to be away from her baby, she can thaw as many cubes as needed (each cube is about 1 oz of milk). Since the mother can usually estimate how much the baby will drink, waste is minimal this way.

Daryl Seifert, RN

Nursing reminder

A nursing mother should alternate breasts for each time she begins to breast-feed her baby. To help her remember which breast to use for the start of her baby's next feeding, suggest she put a small safety pin on the cup of her bra. After each feeding, she should move the pin to the other side to remind her to start with the other breast next time.

Bonnie Handerhan, RN, BSN

A tip with teeth in it

As a school nurse, I see a lot of children who have loose baby teeth. Sometimes a tooth is so loose I have to pull it out so the child won't swallow it. To ease the child's fear and pain, I apply a small amount of benzocaine on the gum around the tooth. The benzocaine numbs the area so I can pull the tooth quickly and easily.

Tonya Rhodes, RN, BSN

Kids in casts

When my 5-year-old son came home from the hospital in a body cast, I wanted to make him as comfortable as possible while allowing him mobility. To do this, I put pads on his elbows so his skin wouldn't become irritated when he pushed himself up. I also got a mechanic's creeper so he could propel himself on flat surfaces. And to boost his morale, I made some pants and shorts from brightly colored material and sewed Velcro at the side seams and crotch for ease in putting them on and taking them off. We had fun together, inventing these and other ideas.

Lois Smith, RN

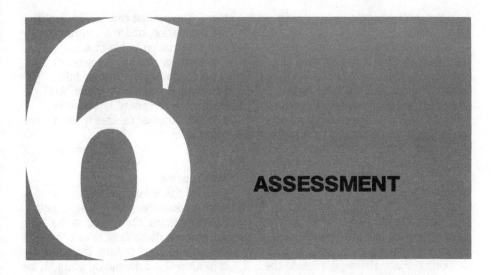

6

ASSESSMENT

OBTAINING A HISTORY

Nursing history helper
To help you remember all the pertinent information you need to take a complete, systematic nursing history, use a pocket-sized card as a guide. Here's how to make one.

First, list the categories you wish to include. For example:
- vital statistics
- patient's understanding of illness
- indication of expectations
- social and cultural history
- significant data.

Then type these subjects, with questions or specific items to ask the patient about, on both sides of a 5" × 7" card. Take the card to your hospital's print shop or a local printer and have it reduced in size (to about 3" × 5") and laminated to withstand the wear and tear of daily use.

The card is handy, easy to use, and lasts for years.

F. Kate Davis, RN

Quick assessment
When you need to make a patient assessment in a hurry and still obtain a maximum amount of information, try the 3-step SPADE technique.

First, determine the patient's status (or progress) in relation to his admitting diagnosis.

Next, assess his general status with SPADE: S—sleep, P—pain, A—activity, D—diet, E—elimination.

Finally, determine his most important request for assistance: "What's the most important thing you'd like to have help with today?"

This abbreviated assessment will help you in reviewing medical orders with doctors and in planning and implementing nursing care.

E. Jane Mezzanotte, RN, MSN

Drug identification
Nurse: *"What drugs are you taking?"*
Patient: *"A little white pill."*

Sound familiar? Some suggestions from the clinical nurse coordinator of pediatric neurology at the Medical College of Georgia, Augusta, can help you help patients identify their medications.

One suggestion is to make a drug display board. Gather old copies of the *Physicians' Desk Reference* (PDR) and cut out pictures of the drugs most frequently prescribed for your patients. If you're a neurology nurse, for example, you'd cut out pictures of Dilantin, Phenobarbital, and so on. Tape the pictures on a piece of cardboard and write the drug name beneath each.

If you don't have old copies of the PDR, ask the doctor to write a prescription for one pill of each medication your patients are likely to be taking. Place these pills inside the compartments of a fishing-lure box or a plastic box designed to hold nails and screws. Again, label each drug. (Be sure to store this container safely.)

Identifying liquid medications is more difficult. This suggestion may help: gather clear plastic bottles from the pharmacy and put 1 oz of the appropriate medication in each. Label the bottles and secure them side by side in a Styrofoam or balsa-wood base.

Once you have your drug display, show it to your patients and ask them to point to the drugs they're taking. Chances are they'll recognize their medications, or at least narrow the choice to a small group.

Diane G. Batts, RN

Medication board

Many of the patients we see in the emergency department don't know the names of medications they're taking. To help us get this information, we made a medication board. We glued samples of the most common pills and capsules on the board and labeled

them. The patient can easily identify his medication, and we can record this information in his chart.

A word of caution: As soon as possible, double-check your information with the patient's doctor. And make sure the board is stored in a locked room or cabinet when it's not being used.

Maureen Dew, RN

Medicards

Some of the elderly patients who come to our emergency department can't remember the names of the many medications they take or when they're supposed to take them. To help keep this information straight, we give them pocket-sized medication cards. The cards have spaces in which to write the names of their medications, how often to take them, and the reason for taking them. The cards also have spaces to record allergies, last tetanus inoculation, and family doctor's name.

We encourage the patient and a family member to carry the cards in their wallets. We also suggest that the patient have his card updated whenever he visits his doctor. Then the next time the patient is questioned about his medications, he'll have the answer—right in his pocket.

Nancy Davidson, RN

INFORMATION THROUGH EXAMINATION

Neurovascular check chart

Orthopedic nurses have to check neurovascular signs on postoperative and postcast-application patients every 2, 3, or 4 hours; yet nurses' notes provide space for recording them only once.

To resolve the dilemma, devise a

neurovascular checklist on a data sheet, which you'll keep at each patient's bedside. The sheet lists the patient's name and room number and the orders for checking neurovascular signs—e.g., right leg, q2h × 48 hr. Then list the signs (sensation, temperature, motion, color, edema) in chart form with blanks to be filled in every 2 hours or according to orders. This checklist becomes part of the patient's permanent chart. Although you could use your nurses' notes in this way, the separate chart is easier and allows a more accurate assessment of the patient's neurovascular status.

Laverne M. Hamill, RN

Heel assessment

When a patient's leg is in traction or in a cast, you know you should inspect his heel constantly for signs of skin breakdown. But if you can't raise his leg high enough to inspect the heel thoroughly, just raise it slightly and slide a flat mirror under the heel. The reflection will tell the story.

Esther Mulheron, RN

Picture story

Even careful documentation of a patient's skin condition doesn't always tell the story as clearly as possible. That's a good reason to include a "Rule of Nines" form—minus the numbers—with your written notes in your nursing care plan.

Indicate all skin abnormalities on the anatomical form by marking the appropriate areas with red ink. Also write a brief description of the abnormality, including size, appearance, type of wound, and so forth. This gives a picture that's truly worth a thousand words.

Pat Elswick, RN

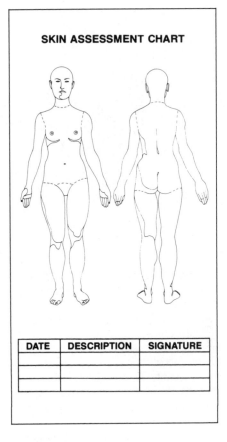

DATE	DESCRIPTION	SIGNATURE

Neuro kit

On our neurosurgical unit, we were frequently asked to gather items for assessing cranial nerve function, so we made up an assessment kit.

The kit is a plastic basket with a handle (similar to an I.V. tray) containing cotton, safety pins, pennies, keys, peppermint, reflex hammer, tuning fork, pencil, tongue blade, blocks, and an ophthalmoscope. For added convenience, we mark each item with the name of the cranial nerve function it tests. The easy-to-tote kit saves us time when a neurosurgical test is called for.

Barbara Martin, RN

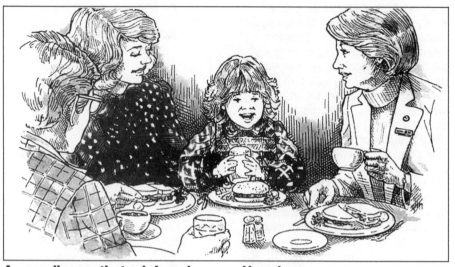

A new diagnostic tool: Lunch

When a child comes to the University of Illinois Hospital Affective Disorders Clinic for a 1-day evaluation, he and his parents are treated to lunch by a nursing staff member. But this "family luncheon" is more than just a social event. Conceived by doctors and carried out by the psychiatric clinical nurse specialist, it's also a diagnostic tool.

The informal luncheon is held in the hospital cafeteria or, if the weather's nice, in the hospital courtyard. While giving the child and parents a chance to meet with a member of the nursing staff away from the unit, the luncheon also lets the nurse see firsthand how the family interacts.

The result? The family feels more comfortable with the staff, who in turn gain greater insight into the child's problems.

After the luncheon, an assessment form documents the findings which are shared with other staff members.

Janet York, RN, MSN

Hear here

If you suspect a patient has a fractured femur, hip, or pelvis, here's a way to immediately confirm or refute your suspicions.

Place your stethoscope on the patient's symphysis pubis and percuss each patella with your finger or a pen. On the side of the fracture, you'll hear a sound lower in volume and pitch than you'll hear on the unaffected side. (The reason is simple: the break in the bone interferes with the sound's conduction and decreases its frequency.)

Likewise, you can detect a fractured humerus, clavicle, or scapula by placing your stethoscope on the patient's sternum and percussing both funny bones (that is, the backs of the elbows where the ulnar nerve rests against a prominence of the humerus).

This technique is especially helpful for nurses who work in nursing homes or on geriatric units and need to assess a patient immediately after a fall.

Dasha Pisarik Ziegler, RN, BSN

Lung assessment

I've found a good way to demonstrate the sound of rales to new staff nurses. I pour a carbonated soft drink into a paper cup and tell the nurses to listen to the soft drink while it fizzes. They'll hear a good imitation of rales.

Joe Niemczura, RN, MS

Flower power

Have you ever had to assess the lung sounds of 2- and 3-year-old patients? Often they don't understand what to do when you tell them to take a deep breath. Or they may be too frightened to cooperate.

To get them to breathe deeply, give them a brightly colored plastic flower and ask them to smell it. Since they're familiar with flowers, they're not frightened. In fact, most children will smell it several times if necessary.

Besides eliminating the child's fears, you'll make the examination easier for yourself, too.

Joan Turner, RN, BSN

A flash point

I work the night shift at a nursing home. When doing rounds, I can't always tell whether the patient in the dark room is breathing unless I turn on the light or shine a flashlight on his chest—and this almost always wakes the patient. But I found that if I point the flashlight at my uniform, the reflected light lets me see the patient's chest without waking him.

Carrie Plotz, LPN

Telltale tape

Once you've inserted an endotracheal tube, you can't easily tell if it's staying in place or if it's slipping out of position. To see at a glance whether or not the tube has moved, put a small piece of adhesive tape around the tube so that one end of the tape touches the patient's lip or naris. Then if the tube moves out of position, you'll know because it will have pulled the tape from the patient's lip or naris.

Jacqueline Zabresky, RN

If the tube fits

The patient has just been intubated and will be hooked up to a ventilator. After auscultating his chest, you suspect the tube is too long and may be in the right main-stem bronchi. But how do you know for sure?

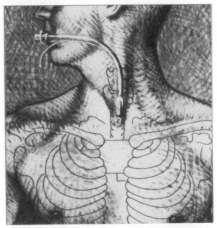

Besides the usual method of observing for symmetrical chest expansion and auscultating for lung sounds, use this method developed by doctors at Henry Ford Hospital in Detroit. Hold an endotracheal tube (the same length as the one inserted) beside the patient's neck. If the tube's the proper length, it shouldn't exceed the distance from the patient's lower incisor teeth to a point midway between the thyroid cartilage and the angle of Louis. In most cases, the 20- to 23-cm mark on the endotracheal tube will be at the corner of the patient's mouth. (The doctors say 21 cm is almost always a good length for average-sized adults.)

Annals of Emergency Medicine,
February 1982

Postpartum pointers

To assess a postpartum patient who's had a vaginal delivery, remember this: *For Every Lady Be Vigilant.* It'll remind you to check her:
*F*undus
*E*pisiotomy site
*L*ochia
*B*reasts
*V*oiding.

Donald M. Grubb, RN, MSN, ARNP

Exemplary exam

Before examining a patient's breasts, I warm a bottle of skin lotion in a basin of warm water. I apply some of the lotion to my hands. The lotion warms and softens my hands, which helps take the chill and friction out of the examination.

Kathleen Kerrigan, RN, BSN

Schooltime sights

One of my duties as a school nurse is to test the vision of preschool children. Two problems in doing this are: (1) getting the child to stand at the correct distance from the eye chart; and (2) having him cover one eye without spreading his fingers and peeking.

To solve the first problem, I cut small feet patterns out of colored construction paper and tape them to the floor where the child should stand. He'll usually take great care to stand right on the paper feet during the vision test. To solve the second problem, I give the child a construction paper fish, which he holds by

the tail so the fish's body covers his eye. No peeking now.

After the test, the child can take the fish home.

Betty Hedlund, RN, BSN

OBTAINING ACCURATE MEASUREMENTS

Marking mls

A lot of patients on the geriatric unit where I work are restricted to 2,000 ml of fluid/day. We know these patients receive a total of 1,050 ml on their meal trays each day, but keeping track of the other 950 ml used to be a challenge.

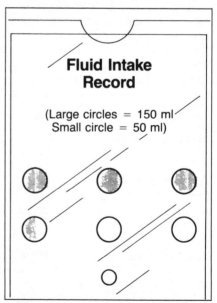

What helps us meet this challenge is a small white card with six large circles drawn on it, each representing 150 ml of fluid (the usual amount in a plastic cup). One small circle represents the remaining 50 ml of fluid. Like a wallet-sized photo, the card's enclosed in a clear, plastic cover.

We ask each patient to carry the

card and a grease pencil with him in his pocket. Then, when the patient gets a drink, the staff member who gives it to him colors one of the circles on the card with the grease pencil. If the patient receives only a small drink (with medication, for example), only half of the circle is colored.

Every night we collect all the cards, calculate how many ml of fluid each patient has had for the day, and record that amount on his I&O sheet. Then we erase the cards with an alcohol wipe and return them to the patients.

The cards help us keep more accurate I&O records. And, perhaps because patients feel more in control, the cards also help them comply with their fluid restriction orders.

Karen A. Jacob, RN, BS

A spillproof cup
Do you have a patient who's unable to drink from a cup without spilling? Then this tip is just for him.

Punch a hole in the top of a sterile specimen cup, fill the cup with fluid, and put a straw through the hole. To disguise the cup, insert it into a regular paper cup and secure it with tape.

The cup's screw-on lid will prevent spills. And the measurement markings on the side of the cup will allow you to accurately assess the patient's intake.

Judi Williams, RN, BSN

Picture this
A quick and easy way to measure intake is with a picture chart. Use a paper tray (such as those used to serve meals to patients in isolation) as the background. Cut in half the various sizes of paper or plastic cups,

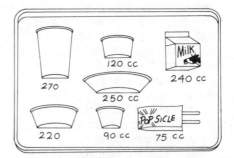

bowls, cartons, and so forth, and glue them to the tray. Then print the amount of fluids each holds underneath—for example, a carton of milk is 240 ml. Keep this chart on display at the nurses' station. This aid helps you measure intake at a glance when you pick up trays after meals.

Sarah Pettus, BSN

Length wise
To measure the length of a squirming baby when you don't have a measuring board or someone to help hold the measuring tape or the baby, use examination table paper. Lay the baby on the paper, hold him still with one hand, and mark the paper at the top of his head and at his heel. Be sure his leg is extended. Then remove the baby and measure the length between the two marks.

Janette Hoffman, RN, BSN

More than hems
A 6" hem gauge does more than just measure hems; it also helps measure the size of lacerations or contusions and the amount of bleeding or drainage on surgical dressings and casts.

Carry the gauge with you throughout the day—it takes up no more room in your pocket than a pen or bandage scissors.

Diane Klaiber, RN

Body measurements

When you need to measure something (such as a skin lesion) quickly, and your measuring tape isn't handy, here's a good substitute.

At your leisure, measure some of your own accessible body parts—such as the nail bed of your little finger—with a metric ruler and memorize these measurements.

This measuring equipment is easy to remember, water resistant, portable, never gets lost—and is always *right at hand.*

Douglas C. Korrow, RN

DISK-advantage

As a home health nurse, I frequently need more equipment than I like to carry with me. For instance, when measuring the size of lesions or decubitus ulcers, I find the tip of my finger not exact enough but rulers too bulky *and* breakable.

My solution is to carry a measurement disk made for reading the results of intradermal skin tests. It's accurate and easy to carry. If the disks aren't available at the home health agency, I can get a supply simply by writing to the drug companies that manufacture the skin tests.

Jill Dailer, RN, BSN

In large measure

Tape measures sometimes aren't long enough to measure large abdomens, so use twill tape instead. Wrap the twill tape around the patient's abdomen, mark the tape with a pen or pencil, then measure it against the patient's own tape measure. After determining the patient's girth, throw the twill tape away to prevent cross-contamination.

Marie Fait, LPN

Pupil paper

Determining a patient's pupil size is an important part of neurologic checks. But in recording the size, terminology may not be specific. For instance, a pupil that appears "moderate" in size to one person, may appear "dilated" to someone else.

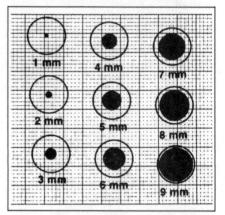

To estimate and record pupil size more accurately, make a chart of pupil sizes on EKG paper. A pinpoint pupil is 1 mm—the size of one small square. A moderately sized pupil is 5 mm—the size of a large square. A fully dilated pupil is 8 or 9 mm. Keep the pupil-size chart at the nurses' station for quick reference.

Frances Marshall, RN

Eliminating guesswork

When you phone a doctor to report a patient's bleeding, do you have trouble describing how much? Many nurses do. Estimating isn't easy. Terms such as "bleeding heavily" could mean anywhere from 10 ml/hour to five or ten times that much.

To avoid this problem, use a visual aid.

Take three perineal pads. Onto the first, place 10 ml of blood from a syringe; onto the second, 30 ml; and onto the third, 60 ml. Then lay the three pads side by side, with cards underneath telling the amounts. Take a color photograph. Enlarge it to $8'' \times 10''$, and place copies on each unit as a ready reference.

Helen Gracey, RN
Michael Bruser, MD, CRCS(C)

Cushion the noise

If you ever have to take a patient's blood pressure in an ambulance, air-ambulance plane, or some other noisy place, remember this tip. Put a pillow under the patient's antecubital area first. The pillow seems to cut out the distracting noise and allows you to get an accurate blood pressure reading.

Stephen M. Keller, EMT

A counterpoint

As you know, a patient with arterial peripheral vascular disease usually experiences leg pain that intensifies with walking. What you don't know is exactly how far the patient can walk without such pain. Vague descriptions such as "only a short distance," "not too far," or "from my house to the street corner" don't allow you to judge the severity of his disease.

For a more accurate assessment, have him count the number of steps he takes before he feels pain. This gives you objective data that you can use to measure the patient's progress.

Barbara Engram, RN, MSN

Get it straight

When you need to measure urine output with a urine meter, be sure to get it straight—the urine meter, that is. If the meter's tilted, the urine in the meter could overflow into the collection bag, making the measurement inaccurate. So take a

moment to be sure the meter is hanging straight. It'll save minutes later.

T. Jesaitis, SN

Bedpan lining

When careful stool measurements are ordered for a patient with gross rectal bleeding, try collecting specimens this way. First, rinse a bedpan with water. Next, press a large plastic bag into the contours of the pan, so the bag's edges form a collar over the edge of the pan. (The moisture in the pan keeps the bag in place.)

After the patient has passed the stool, lift the bag out of the pan and place it in the measuring container. Neither blood nor stool clings to either the bedpan or the container. This increases accuracy while eliminating cleanup.

To reduce odor, twist and tie the bag. You can save the specimen in a tied bag without telltale odors or much change in color.

Ruth P. Whitney, RN

Watch the weight

Are you ever asked to keep accurate records of sputum output for patients who require postural drainage with percussion? If so, you know that transferring a sputum specimen into a graduated cylinder not only gives you inaccurate measurements but also is aesthetically unpleasant.

Weighing rather than measuring specimens is more accurate, more convenient, and more aesthetically pleasing. Use previously weighed plastic drinking cups with lids to collect the specimens. Then, with specimen inside, again weigh the cup on a gram scale. Determine the weight of the sputum by figuring the

difference between the two weighings.
Cups with the same lot number
are consistent in weight.

D. Joan Trapani, RN

Collections on the move
If you're transporting a patient who
has a nasogastric tube and you need
to collect drainage from the tube
while you're moving him, try this.
Secure a disposable plastic glove
to the end of the tube with a rubber
band or piece of tape. The glove will
collect the drainage, and later, you
can easily empty the drainage from
the glove into a cup for measuring.

Kimberly A. Stotts, RN, BSN

Small measure
As you know, a young child on intermittent nasogastric suctioning usually
has only minimal drainage. So getting
an accurate measure of the amount
can be a problem.

To solve this, we channel the
drainage into a plastic container for a
35-ml syringe. As the illustration

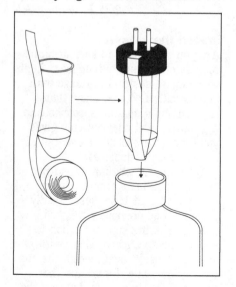

shows, the container is taped to the
inside stopper of the patient's suction
bottle. By using only one thickness
of tape to secure the container, we
can easily fit the bottle stopper
in place.

After each suctioning, we simply
remove the bottle stopper and empty
the drainage into a small measuring
device. Then we take the reading
and chart the amount accordingly.

Mary Loeffler, RN

Plain drain
Used I.V. bottles are a boon for measuring gravity drainage from Levin
tubes and the like. Be sure to wash
the bottle first and remove the metal
part of the cap. Leave the rubber
stopper in the bottle and attach it to
the patient's drainage tube.

The markings on the bottle will
show you the amount of drainage, so
you won't have to empty the bottle
to measure it. To keep track of the
amount over a period of time, mark
the bottle with tape each time you
measure.

If the patient's drainage tube is too
short, you can use I.V. tubing to
lengthen it. If drainage is too thick
for I.V. tubing, use the regular drainage tube but attach it to a Foley
catheter bag rather than an I.V. bottle.

R. Hager, LPN

Ideas that stick
Another type of sticker makes it easy
for you to keep track of the amount
of drainage in your patient's Hemovac.
The sticker, which you place on top
of the vacuum unit, should have room
to record the patient's output for
each shift over several days. It could
look like this:

OUTPUT STICKER

Date:	Date:
7-3:	7-3:
3-11:	3-11:
11-7:	11-7:
Date:	Date:
7-3:	7-3:
3-11:	3-11:
11-7:	11-7:

You record the amount of drainage on the appropriate line whenever you empty the container. Anyone who wants to know the patient's total drainage output can simply look at the sticker rather than having to search through the patient's chart.

Elizabeth Ward, RN

Penrose drainage
To collect wound drainage from a Penrose drain, place an ostomy appliance over the drain, taking care not to irritate the suture line. The drainage will accumulate in the appliance away from the patient's skin. This not only prevents skin breakdown and decreases dressing changes, but it also allows you to evaluate the color, consistency, and amount of drainage in the appliance.

Lana Sue Zinkon, RN

Check the chart
Do you ever find that another nurse describes a wound drainage as moderate, when you'd consider it small? Or do you have trouble visualizing the size of an inflamed area that someone else describes as 4 cm?

One way to take the guesswork out of such situations is to have everyone use a standard chart for reference. The chart used in labor and delivery to measure cervical dilatation is ideal. Simply display the chart where it's accessible to the entire unit staff and have them refer to the chart for assessment of wound drainage or measurement of any area up to 10 cm in size.

The use of such a chart makes charting simpler and more consistent and saves time in shift reports.

Mary S. Hall, RN

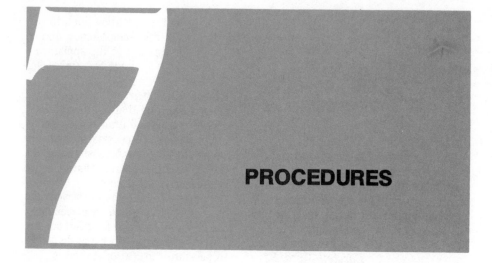

7 PROCEDURES

PERFORMING MOUTH CARE

No-mess mouth care

Giving mouth care to a patient who must lie flat in bed isn't easy—especially the rinsing and spitting. But here's a way to avoid the mess.

After the patient's teeth are brushed, offer him mouthwash or water through a straw. Then, have him use the same straw to expel the mouthwash or water into an emesis basin.

Although using a straw may be a bit awkward at first, patients usually master it quickly and become proficient in the ins *and* outs of rinsing and spitting with straws.

Kathy Scheeve, SN

Foam in the mouth

To remove blood from a patient's mouth, try a solution of half peroxide and half ginger ale. Just dip a toothbrush, mouth swab, or gauze into the solution, brush or wipe the patient's mouth, and let the blood foam away. Follow with a plain water rinse.

This method works especially well on unconscious patients. And most conscious patients find it a pleasant mouth rinse.

Janice Heistand, RN, CCRN

Using dental floss

If your patient has trouble using dental floss to perform his own oral hygiene, you can help him this way.

Tie one end of some floss to the end of a tongue blade and the other end of the floss to the end of *another* tongue blade. (Or make pinholes through the ends of two tongue blades, then thread one end of the floss through one pinhole and the other end of the floss through the other pinhole. Knot the ends of the floss to prevent them from slipping through the pinholes.) Then hold one tongue blade in each hand, pull the floss taut, and floss your patient's teeth.

Marie A. Frasca, RN

Irrigation project

When patients have advanced oral cancer, their lesions give off foul-smelling secretions. To reduce odors and keep patients clean and comfortable, irrigate their lesions regularly.

A primary concern is to reach every oral cavity. So apply solution from a catheter-tip syringe or a disposable enema bag with tubing, rather than simply rinsing from a cup.

For each irrigation, use at least 1 qt of either half-strength hydrogen peroxide and astringent mouthwash or sodium bicarbonate and warm water in a mild solution, followed by clean tap water. Whichever solution you use, try to irrigate regularly— once every 4 hours that the patient's awake.

These methods work especially well when patients' lesions open to the outside of the face or neck. Then the solution comes through these openings to clean the lesions without damaging surrounding tissue.

Nancy Delano, RN

What a difference a tray makes

Reuse disposable dressing trays as oral hygiene trays; they have three compartments to store all the equipment you need to give patients good mouth care.

In one compartment, put 2" × 2" pieces of gauze; in another, pour your oral cleansing solution; and in the last compartment, store cotton swabs, tongue blades, petrolatum, and plastic Kelly forceps. (These forceps are small enough to reach into tiny areas and strong enough to grip the gauze firmly while you're cleaning the patient's mouth.)

The trays help keep supplies together, making mouth care much easier and neater.

Debbie Niemi, RN

Natural cleanser

Many times we clean a patient's

mouth by swabbing it with papaya juice, a sponge, and a Toothette. Papaya juice, available at most health food stores, is a natural enzyme that removes most debris without injuring the patient's mouth. And no harm is done if the patient swallows some of the mouth "cleanser." Afterward, we irrigate the patient's mouth with water.

Mary T. Knapp, RN

PROVIDING E.E.N.T. CARE

Lens lifter

Ever have to remove contact lenses from multiple trauma patients? The quickest and most painless way to do this is to use the suction tip of a glass eyedropper. By depressing the suction tip and gently applying it directly over the lens, you can lift the lens off the cornea quite easily.

Marleen Kaechele, RN

Eyewash

Patients with eye traumas need copious eye irrigations. An easy and efficient way to give them is to attach I.V. tubing (without the needle) to 1 liter of normal saline solution, then use the tubing to direct the saline solution into the patient's eye. If necessary, you can regulate the stream by using the flow clamp.

Barbara Sosaya, RN, BSN

Eye-opener

Need to improvise an eyecup if one isn't readily available? Use a sterile spoon—either teaspoon or tablespoon size. Fill the spoon with the eyewash solution. As the patient bends his head forward, place the spoon over the eye with the point resting on the inner corner of the eye. Then tell the patient to tip his head backward, open his eyelid, and wash the eye.

Your patient can use this improvisation at home or even away, as on a camping trip, for example.

La Donna Kolman, RN

Icy fingers
When the weight of a regular ice pack on the eyelid is too painful for a patient, make an "icy finger" ice pack instead.

Fill finger cots with water, tie them shut, and freeze them. Place two ice-filled cots inside a piece of 2" stockinette and pin or tape two pieces of twill tape to the stockinette—one at each end. Place the stockinette over the patient's eye and tie the twill tape at the top of the patient's head.

This icy finger pack is lighter than regular ice packs and stays in place itself so the patient can freely use both hands. We keep a supply of them in the freezer for fast and easy replacement.

Barbara Simonds, RN

An eye piece
Problem: A patient comes to the emergency department complaining of eye pain and photophobia. He won't let you put an eye patch on him because he's afraid it will put pressure on his eye.

Solution: Cut the bottom from a clean plastic cup, tape the rough

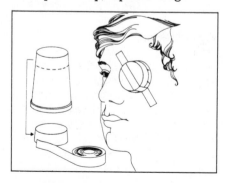

edges, place the cup over the eye, and secure it with a piece of tape. The cup protects the eye without actually touching it.

Sydney Anne Gambill, RN

Irrigating ears
For ear irrigation, home dental hygiene equipment (the kind with the pulsating stream of water) works better than a syringe ever did. Here's how to use it.

First, make sure the patient's tympanic membrane isn't perforated. Then fill the machine's container with tepid water. Position the patient over a sink or have him hold a basin under his ear. Next, straighten his external ear canal—with children, gently pull the auricle straight back; with adults, pull it back and down.

Then turn the machine on to the lowest pressure setting and aim the water stream directly at the tympanic membrane. If the wax is hard, increase the pressure until the wax begins to break up, then decrease the pressure to finish irrigating the ear. Afterward, tell the patient that if he still feels water in his ear, it will eventually run out.

Finally, sterilize the equipment with a cold sterilizing solution.

Terry Schumacher, RN

Wrap, tape, and irrigate
To absorb leakage and keep the patient's shirt dry while you're irrigating his ear, try this: Wrap the long edge of a disposable diaper around the patient's neck—absorbent side up—and fasten it with the tape tab. Curve up the outer edge to catch any solution the diaper doesn't absorb.

You can use whatever size diaper fits your patient's neck.

Jackie Pederson, RN

*Ear*igation
Next time you irrigate a child's ear, try this. Use a 20-ml syringe with an I.V. plastic cannula (such as Cathalon 4) instead of the traditional irrigating syringe. This smaller syringe is softer, more pliable, and less frightening to your patient.

W.A.C. MacDonald, MB, ChB

Ending epistaxis
It's awkward enough for a nurse to apply pressure to a patient's bleeding nose, let alone having the patient do it himself.

From your inhalation therapy department, borrow a nose clip—the ones used during IPPB treatments and pulmonary function studies.

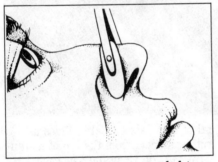

These exert the pressure needed to stop the bleeding.

Margaret A. Powers, RN

CLEANING EQUIPMENT

A suction tip
If you use a tonsil suction tip for mouth care, here's how to keep it clean between uses. Tape the cover of a 60-ml syringe to the back of the headboard. Then, after using the suction tip, place it in the syringe cover to keep it from falling onto the patient's bed or the floor.

When you change the tonsil suction tip, change the syringe cover, too.

Paula Chelewski, RN

Handy dryer
Ever have a problem drying empty hot water bottles and ice bags? A simple help is a wire coat hanger. Hang a hot water bottle upside down by placing the hanger hook through the hole in the bottom of the hot water bottle.

To dry ice bags, pull down on the bottom of the coat hanger, then bend elongated hanger in half. Slip the ice cap over the end of the bent portion of the hanger.

Marilyn A. Metker, RN

A feeding tube flush
Small-diameter enteral feeding tubes often get clogged from the feeding formula residue. To prevent this residue buildup, we flush the tubes every 4 hours (and each time the feeding is interrupted or discontinued) with 5/8 oz of cranberry juice, followed by 3/8 oz of water.

The acidic cranberry juice breaks up the formula's residue, and the water rinses away the juice, preventing sugar from crystallizing in the tube.

Dee Adinaro, RN, MSN

A bubble bath
A simple, effective way to clean used glass suction bottles before they're sterilized is to fill the bottle with hot water and drop in an effervescent denture-cleansing tablet. In a short time, all tenacious material is dissolved and ready to be rinsed out.

Judith Webb, RN

Deodorizing drops
Want to eliminate odors from your patients' urinals, bedpans, commodes, and suction bottles? Just pour a few drops of mouthwash in them. The unpleasant smells will disappear.

Janet D. Stolarz, LPN

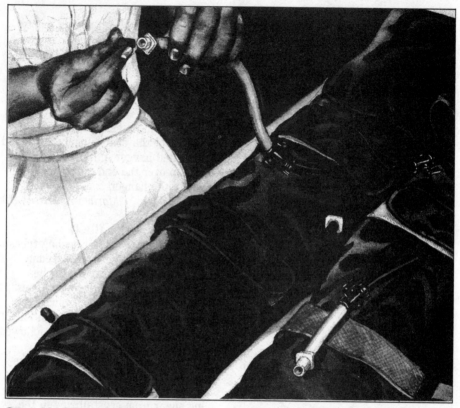

Stop MAST contamination

Blood-soiled medical antishock trousers (MAST) must be carefully washed to prevent blood-transmitted diseases. The *MAST Manual* suggests using a washing machine with medium-temperature water and household detergents. It also suggests closing the inflation/deflation valves before washing.

But what if a valve's left open, or opens inadvertently during the wash cycle? The contaminated wash water enters the chambers and is difficult to remove.

To prevent this problem, follow the procedure used at Community Hospital of San Gabriel, Calif.: Place a rubber stopper from the top of a standard red top vacutainer in each valve. The stopper seals the valve so water can't enter the chambers.

Annals of Emergency Medicine,
June 1984

Cleaning with cola

When a feeding tube becomes clogged with formula, unclog it with diet cola. Get a doctor's order first, then flush the feeding tube with 1 oz of cola. Clamp the tube for 15 minutes. The cola will dissolve the formula and unclog the tube.

Nina S. Ehle, RN

PREPARING HOT/COLD THERAPY

Hole in one

Have you ever tried to fill a disposable ice bag—and found you just don't have enough hands? Here's an easy way to do it. Punch out the bottom of a paper cup, fit it in the neck of the ice bag, and use it as a funnel. The ice slides right in.

Warning: Don't leave the cup near your supply of paper cups—you might help yourself to a "bottomless" cup of coffee!

Noreen Cechocki, RN

Ice in easy

Unless you have three hands, filling an ice bag can be a messy procedure. Try this ice-bag filler that's inexpensive, washable, long lasting, and—best of all—does the job without the mess.

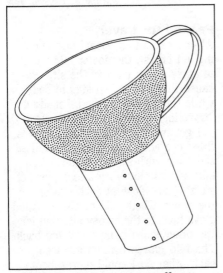

Have the maintenance staff cut and rivet a piece of metal into the shape of a *bottomless* 6-oz paper cup.

Then have them solder the top of the cup to the bottom of a wide-mouthed metal funnel—the kind used for home canning.

The funnel fits into an ice bag and has a handle for convenient hanging on a hook near the ice machine.

Phyllis Boone, RN

Frugal funnels

Have you ever tried to make an ice bag out of a hot water bottle by stuffing crushed ice into it? Wet and messy, wasn't it? Here's a tidier way. Simply cut the top from an empty half-gallon plastic bleach bottle. Turn it upside down and you have a wide-mouth funnel. Insert the neck of the funnel into the neck of the hot water bottle. The ice will slide in easily, with no mess.

Brother James Martin, LPN

Or, to aid in filling ice bags, caps, and collars, cut the large end off a plastic urine specimen bottle and insert it into the neck of the ice bag to make a funnel. You can fill the bag easily without spillage.

Hollis Roberts, RN
Cynthia Harrison, RN

Alcohol on ice

To make a moldable ice bag, fill one finger of an examination glove with 70% alcohol and the rest of the glove with water. Gently shake the glove to mix its contents. Then tie the glove's wrist in a knot to seal it.

Place the glove in the freezer—in a short time you'll have an ice bag of slush that molds to almost any shape and stays colder longer than regular ice bags.

Kathleen Hendrixson, RN

Cool aid

Fill #5 pleated paper cups (the dispenser type) with water, and place in the freezer. When needed, you just remove, fold down the rim extending above the ice, whirl a cloth around the ice end to absorb droplets of water, and apply to the injured part. The paper cup makes it comfortable to hold and easy to move over the injured part, reducing the possibility of ice trauma.

Anne Saloka, RN

Ice sealing
To improvise an ice pack, try using the kitchen appliance that seals a meal into a plastic bag. Fill a large-size bag with ice and seal it. Apply this pack to the affected area. The ice will melt, but the pack remains cool. And no leakage.

Place the bag of water in the freezer and you have an ice pack ready for the next injury. You can make a few in various sizes and keep them in the freezer at the hospital for your patients.

Sherri Sener, RN, BSN

Ice bags that fit
Need a good ice pack for hard-to-cover areas such as your patient's knee, cast, or forehead? Use the plastic bag that holds the supplies issued to each patient on admission.

Fill one fourth to one third of the bag with ice and secure it with a heavy rubber band. Then turn the remaining portion of the bag inside out—over the ice-filled part—and pull the drawstring or fasten with another rubber band. You'll have an ice pack that's double thick, moldable, and usually just the right fit.

Daveen McClure, RN

Cold eggs
Do you need many sizes and shapes of instant ice packs? For handy, disposable ice cube trays, use old plastic egg cartons. Separate these trays into individual cubes, each in its own egg-shaped container. Then if someone has a lacerated lip or tongue, he can hold the cube to his mouth without freezing his fingers or dripping water on the floor.

Rosalind Goldman, RN, SNP

Refreezable cold packs
Fill plastic ziplock freezer bags half full with water, remove excess air, and freeze them. They're inexpensive, stay cold longer than the chemical packs, and are available in a variety of sizes for convenience.

Marguerite Quinn, RN

Warming hot packs
Use a slow-cooker crock pot to heat hot packs. Set it to the desired temperature, and you'll have moist hot packs readily available.

Joanne E. Gerson, RN

Packed for travel
After I had an excisional biopsy on my left breast, the doctor told me to apply an ice pack to the site. Because I didn't want to stay in bed while the ice was applied, I made a "traveling ice pack."

I got two disposable rubber gloves, filled one with tepid water, and filled the other with ice and water. I tied both gloves shut with a long piece of gauze—one glove at each end of the gauze. Then I placed the ice-filled glove next to the biopsy site and let the other glove hang down my back. The two gloves counterbalanced each other so I could move about freely and still keep the ice pack in place.

Nancy Deveney, RN

POSITIONING PATIENTS

Get the picture?

Here's an aid to repositioning paraplegic and brain-injured patients
without having to ask for assistance.
Use printed diagrams showing a
body in various positions to indicate
where padding should go. After the
admitting nurse checks the patient's
bone structure and examines him
for paralysis and decubiti, she draws
arrows on the diagram to show
pressure points that should be padded.
She also briefly describes what kind
of padding is needed (*small pad, large
pillow*, and so forth). Then, referring
to the diagram, an aide can safely
and comfortably reposition patients
without the nurse's help.

Jean Sorrell, RN

Pillow prop

When you're positioning a patient on
his side in bed and you prop a pillow
behind his back, does the pillow
slip away? If so, untuck the drawsheet
and place the pillow *under* the drawsheet. Then tuck the sheet back

under the mattress. The pillow won't
slip, and the patient will stay on
his side.

Betty Ann Ulmer, RN

Trash bag transfer

A large plastic trash bag will help
you transfer a helpless patient from
his bed to a stretcher. Just place
the unfolded bag between the drawsheet and top sheet of the patient's
bed, positioning it between the patient's shoulders and buttocks.

Because the plastic bag reduces
friction between the sheets, you can
grasp the drawsheet firmly and move
the patient from his bed onto the
stretcher with ease.

Dorothy J. Lasalle, RN

One-step transfer

Here's how to weigh and transfer a
semicomatose, obese patient to a new
bed. Use a bed scale for the weighing.
Then, with the patient still on the
scale and two more nurses stationed
at his head and feet, push the bed
out from under the patient and slide
the new bed—all made up—underneath in its place. Then move him off

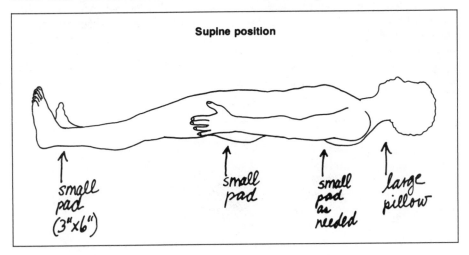

Supine position

small
pad
(3"x6")

small
pad

small
pad
as
needed

large
pillow

the scale and onto the new bed.

The whole procedure takes about 5 minutes and is easy on your back and your patient's delicate skin.

C. Debra Strutman, RN

Lean on water
If a patient's confined to a wheelchair and develops pressure sores from leaning against the armrest for support, reduce the pressure this way. Partially fill a small hot water bottle with water and place it on the armrest. It makes a handy cushion that's just the right size.

Ann H. Phillips, RN

Wheelchair fare
Need an easy way to reposition a patient in a wheelchair? Try a towel.

Fold the towel in half lengthwise and place it on the chair's seat so that it extends slightly over the front and back edges. When the patient slides forward, stand behind the wheelchair, lock the wheels, and pull the back edge of the towel. The patient will be pulled back on the seat and you won't strain your back.

If too much of the towel hangs out in back so it drags on the floor, you can bring the end up and over the backrest, placing it behind the patient's shoulders.

Ramona Dekrey, RN, BSN

A gravitational pull
When you have to move a patient up in bed, put gravity to work for you. Flatten the head and raise the foot of his bed, then slide him up toward the head. Put the bed back in the original position.

Caution: Don't move the patient this way if his legs shouldn't be elevated for some reason.

Martha G. Oestreich, RN

Keeping patients in place
If you've ever given decubitus care to a restless or uncooperative patient, you know how difficult it can be. A student in the BSN program at Creighton University, Omaha, devised a sling to position such patients for decubitus care.

To make the sling, she folds a drawsheet lengthwise twice so it is one fourth its original width. She places the drawsheet sideways across the bed, positioning it beneath the patient's buttocks, and tucks one end under the mattress. Then she places the patient on his side near the edge of the bed and pulls the drawsheet taut over his hip, keeping the ulcerated area uncovered. After wrapping the other end of the sheet around the top of the side rail, she tucks it under the mattress to secure it.

Then she places pillows behind the

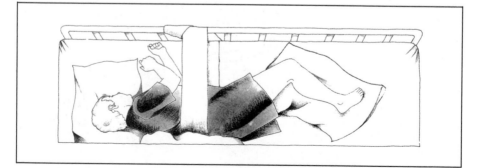

patient's trunk and between his knees to keep his body properly aligned.

The student nurse has used the sling on many restless patients and finds it keeps them on their side every time.

Elizabeth Shonquist, SN

Straight legs
When a patient has an arterial line in his femoral artery or a temporary pacemaker in his femoral vein, we try to keep his leg straight so he won't disturb the line. Restraining his leg would do the trick, but we've found an even better alternative: a knee immobilizer.

The immobilizer can be applied loosely for comfort, yet will still keep his leg straight and his line undisturbed.

Lynn Versaw, RN

Abduction instruction
Next time you need an abduction pillow and can't find one, try making one yourself. Place a drawsheet under the patient from his upper thigh to midcalf and a firm pillow (or two soft pillows) between his legs. Then drape a second drawsheet over the pillow and tuck the ends under the patient's legs. Bring the first sheet up and around the patient's legs and fasten the ends of it together with large safety pins. There you have it: an abduction pillow that's easy to put together—and it *stays* together as well.

Margaret A. Artaserse, RN

About turns
When a lot of patients need to be repositioned every 2 hours or so to prevent decubitus ulcers, how do you keep track of who's been turned

when? One way is to set up a system in which all the patients are placed in the same position at the same time. For instance, at 12, all patients are placed on their backs. At 2, they're turned to face the door. At 4, they're turned to face the window. At 6, they're placed on their backs again, and so on.

As a reminder to those doing the positioning, post a drawing of a clock over each patient's bed. At 12 and 6, write "back"; at 2 and 8, write "door"; at 4 and 10, write "window." Then when making rounds, you can easily see whether patients have been turned on schedule.

Connie Smith, LPN

High tops
Footdrop in comatose, paralyzed, or bedridden patients can be prevented by using footboards, but working with them is awkward and cumbersome. After trying a number of preventive methods, I found that high-topped canvas basketball sneakers seem to work best.

First put a pair of socks on the patient, then snugly lace up the sneakers. To keep the feet aired and dry, keep the sneakers on 4 hours, then off 4 hours.

It's also much easier to turn and position the patient wearing sneakers rather than work with boards and bolsters.

Carol Schreiber, RN

Head support
Here's a way to provide head support for debilitated patients so they can sit in an armchair or wheelchair.

First, position the patient comfortably and safely, with his body in proper alignment. Next, wrap a 2" to 3" felt collar twice around his neck.

Then, apply a well-padded cotton halter under the patient's chin, padding the sides of the halter with cotton strips or bandages, to protect the patient's face. Attach the other ends of the cotton strips or bandages to an I.V. pole placed behind the patient. Using this method, the patient can still swivel his head to see what's going on around him.

This technique strengthens the neck muscles and boosts the patient's morale as well as his head.

Lucy Dalicandro, RN

Drape a drawsheet

To drape a patient in the lithotomy position, fold a drawsheet in half lengthwise, then fold it in half the other way. The sheet is now folded in quarters.

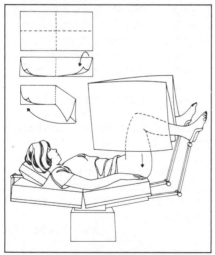

Hold the sheet where all the folds meet, and place it at the patient's waist. Drape each of the two long folds over each of her legs. The drape resembles the front half of a pair of pants—and covers the patient effectively.

Sandra J. Shafer, RN

MAKING OCCUPIED BEDS

A sheet feat

Changing the drawsheet on the bed of an immobilized patient is not only a difficult task for you, it's an uncomfortable experience for your patient as well.

To make the procedure a little easier on everyone, do it this way. Untuck the old drawsheet and attach one side edge of the new drawsheet to one side edge of the old one with three safety pins. If possible, have the patient lift himself with an overbed trapeze. Then pull the old drawsheet across the bed. The new drawsheet will follow and replace the old one—wrinkle-free—underneath the patient. Just remove the pins, tuck in the new drawsheet, and you're finished.

Pat Wheeler, RN

A bed roll

Recently, I cared for a bedridden patient who was on a ventilator, had lower GI bleeding, and could tolerate being turned on his side for only a few moments at a time. As you can imagine, changing his bed wasn't easy—for him or me—until I came up with this technique.

I took all the new bed linens (except for the top sheet) to an unoccupied bed; I made up this bed but didn't tuck in any of the sheets. Then I went to one side of the bed, picked up the edge of the bottom sheet, and rolled it to the center of the bed, making sure I caught the drawsheet and pads in the roll. I repeated this procedure on the other side of the bed. (Now I had two long, cigar-shaped rolls in the center of the bed.) After I folded the bottom third of the two rolls up toward the head of the bed and the top third down toward the foot, I had a complete, compact bottom linen change.

I placed this linen change on a chair near the patient's bed, cleaned the patient, and untucked his soiled linen. I moved the patient to one side of his bed and quickly pushed the soiled linen toward the center of the bed. I placed the new linen on the bed near the center, unfolded the ends (so it looked like two cigars again), and rolled out the roll nearest me.

After turning the patient to his other side, I pulled the soiled linen off the bed and unrolled the other linen roll. Then I helped the patient move onto his back.

At a more leisurely pace, I tucked in the bottom sheet and drawsheet, added the top sheet, and changed the pillowcase. In no time, and with minimal discomfort for the patient, the bed was changed.

Margery Emge, RN, MSN, CCRN

On a roll
Changing a bed with the patient in it means a lot of tugging, rolling, confusion, and—for some patients—pain. But you can save yourself and your patient some trouble and discomfort by partially *premaking* his bed on an empty bed, if one's available.

Layer the bed linens (including Chux, lift sheets, and drawsheets) on the empty bed just as if you were going to make it—but don't tuck the linen in. Starting at one side, roll the linen into a tube. Place the linen tube alongside the patient's bed. Then, roll the patient to the far side of the bed, push the dirty linen toward the patient, and roll the new

linen tube out onto his bed. All the layers of new linens will be in place on one side of the bed, and you can tuck them in. Roll the patient back and finish pulling off the old linen and tucking in the new linen.

If your patient is in balance-suspension traction, you may find it easier to roll the linen from the top of the bed to the bottom instead of from side to side.

Gail Chark, RN

Padded pull sheet
When you're making the bed of a bedridden patient who needs a disposable under pad, prepare his bed as you normally would—with one exception. Instead of placing the pad on top of the pull sheet directly under the patient, sandwich it between the pull-sheet layers.

This technique will mean fewer soiled bottom sheets, thereby saving you time and cutting your hospital's linen consumption. It'll also add to your patient's comfort, because paper from the pad won't cling to his skin.

Janet Markey, RN

MANAGING ELIMINATION AND DRAINAGE

The sole answer
My patients include some women with spinal cord injuries who have indwelling (Foley) catheters. Changing the catheter is difficult because I have no one to help position the patient, so I can't get a clear view of her urethra. To solve this problem, I carry a pair of tennis or crepe-soled shoes with my equipment.

I position the patient on her back and put the shoes on her feet. I then place her feet close to her buttocks and let her legs open. The rubbery soles of the shoes keep her feet from slipping, and I can see what I'm doing. This makes catheterization quicker, and easier on the patient, too.

C. Bess Farrell, RN, BSN

A viewpoint on catheterization
One of the biggest problems in catheterizing a woman patient without assistance is getting a good view of her perineal area. So try placing a bedpan or fracture pan upside down on the bed with a pad over it. Then position the patient's buttocks on the pan. You'll be able to see the area more clearly, and catheter insertion will be easier.

Cathie Holtzinger, RN

Cath care comfort
Here's a tip for catheterizing a female patient who has a fractured hip or who finds the dorsal recumbent position uncomfortable.

Turn the patient on her left side in the Sims' position, with right knee and thigh drawn up, if possible. Place a sterile drape over her buttocks, covering the rectal area. Then separate the labia and proceed to catheterize her.

Elderly patients especially find this position more comfortable than the traditional position.

Sonja Feist, RN, MS

Constriction site
When a male patient who has a constricted urinary meatus needs to be catheterized, you have a problem. The plastic catheter in the catheterization kit is too large and a small, red rubber catheter is too soft and flexible. So I use a small plastic, sterile disposable suction catheter instead (with the doctor's order, of course). This catheter is firm and

passes through a constricted meatus when a softer or larger one won't.

Betty J. Glenn, RN, BRE

In control again
Pass this hint to a patient who's having trouble voiding after his urinary catheter is removed. Tell him to blow bubbles through a straw into a glass half-filled with water. The water sounds should help the patient void easily again.

Florence Mackinnon, NA

No cath? No problem
When you have a male patient who's incontinent but can't use an indwelling urinary catheter, try a newborn-size disposable diaper instead.

Just gently wrap the diaper around the patient's entire penis, secure the tape tab, and fold over or tape the open end shut.

The disposable diapers are more comfortable and safer than conventional incontinent pants and pins, and they look better under trousers than bulky rubber pants. Also, after the patient has voided, you can weigh the diaper for an accurate intake and output measurement. And before applying a fresh diaper, all you (or he) need do is clean the genital area.

Judith B. Schwandt, RN

Diaper's on, pressure's off
Here's a technique we've devised for toddlers who've had hypospadias surgery. Although they usually have a suprapubic or perineal catheter, they still need to wear a diaper for bowel movements. But to protect the penile operative site or dressing from pressure by the diaper, we make the following modification.

We cut an "X" shape in the front half of a regular disposable diaper.

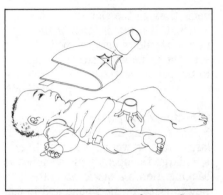

Then we cut the bottom from a Styrofoam cup and insert the cup through the "X" until the rim is flush with the inside of the diaper. We tape the cup in place on the outside of the diaper.

Now the diaper can be fastened securely around the baby's waist without putting pressure on the penile dressing. And we can easily check the dressing by looking through the bottom of the cup.

Lois S. Chin, RN

Pantastic idea

The next time a patient who's in a chair or wheelchair needs a bedpan, try reversing the position of the pan. The reversed pan supports the patient's thighs without digging into them, as it does in its regular position. Also, there's less chance of spillage with the pan in the reverse position.

Loretta A. Debus, RN

Urine-free cast

To prevent urine contamination of a hip-spica cast, cover its crotch area with a polyethylene drape. The drape's hypoallergenic adhesive sticks to the cast and won't irritate the patient's skin.

Ann Cunningham, RN

Tender-touch terry

Here are some ways to make a urinal more comfortable for a man:

To protect the patient's scrotum and penis from irritation, place a terry-cloth wristband on the opening of the urinal. And to prevent irritation of the patient's inner thighs, slip a terry-cloth headband around the middle of the urinal.

A money-saving hint: Rather than buying the bands, make them. Sew a 2″ × 3″ piece of stretch terry cloth together to make the wristband. And sew a 2″ × 4″ piece of terry cloth together to make the headband.

The bands can be easily removed for laundering whenever necessary.

Dale S. Lohmann, RN, MSN

No-friction fracture pan

Before giving a fracture pan to a patient, apply some body lotion to the pan rim. The lotion will decrease the friction—and the pain—of using the pan.

Deborah Wood, RN
Helen Kelsey, RN

Bedpan comfort

When you take a patient off a plastic bedpan, does his skin stick to the seat? If so, try sprinkling some powder on the rim of the bedpan before he uses it. And a light dusting of powder on a patient's legs before applying antiembolism stockings helps the stockings go on easier.

Nila C. E. Sadek, RN

No overflow woes

When a fracture pan overflows, changing the bed linens can be painful for your patient. But you can easily prevent such overflow by siphoning urine away from the fracture pan. Here's how.

Get some straight tubing, a 30-ml syringe, and a urine collector. Place one end of the tubing into the fracture pan, the other end onto the syringe's needle. Position your patient on the pan and place the urine collector at a lower level.

As the patient starts to void, pull the syringe's plunger back. This will create suction and start a flow of urine. Remove the syringe from the tubing, and quickly place the tubing into the collector.

Besides reducing your patient's discomfort, this technique will reduce your hospital's linen usage. You can also use the technique when giving perineal care.

Linda Hooker, RN

Bedpan ease
If using a bedpan is too awkward for your patients in traction, try this.

Put a stadium chair (the kind with only a seat and backrest—no legs) on the patient's bed. Place the bedpan on the chair. The patient can help transfer himself on and off the bedpan by using a trapeze.

The chair supports the patient's back, making the bedpan routine more comfortable and less awkward. (Of course, this method works only for patients who can sit up or bend at the hip.)

Cecelia Moore, RN

Avoiding problems
If you care for incontinent male patients—some comatose, others paralyzed from the waist down—here's how to keep both bed and patient dry without risking urinary tract infection from catheterization.

Cut a 2″ slot in a bed liner and place it (absorbent side down) over the patient's pubis. Slip the patient's

penis through the slot and position a urinal. If urine dribbles or the urinal overflows onto the polyethylene side, the urine won't soak through to the patient or the bed.

Ralph Vogel, RN

Plastic-wrap pattern
Before applying an ostomy pouch to a large draining wound, you may have to enlarge the opening in the adhesive backing. Here's a quick, accurate way to measure the wound and to cut an opening that'll fit around the wound without touching it.

Place a piece of plastic wrap over the wound. On the plastic, outline the wound with a broad felt-tipped marking pen. Mark the patient's top, left, and right sides.

Next, cut out the plastic-wrap pattern and place it with the marked side down over the opening in the pouch's backing. This way you don't reverse the pattern. Center the pattern as much as possible over the opening.

Trace the pattern on the paper covering the backing. Then cut the pattern out of paper *and* backing, and remove this section. Now, when you affix the backing to the patient's skin, the opening will accurately fit around the wound.

Lynda L. Brubacher, RN, ET

Ostomy aid
Patients with reusable ostomy equipment may have trouble removing the double-face adhesive disk from the faceplate when they want to clean their appliances. Here's a tip to make removal easier:

Tell the patient to apply Skin Prep protective dressing (the brush-on, spray-on, or wipe-on kind) to the faceplate and allow the dressing to dry for 1 or 2 minutes. Make sure the faceplate is covered evenly. (If he's using the spray, tell him to spread the dressing with his finger after spraying.) The patient can then apply the adhesive disk to the faceplate and proceed as usual.

The Skin Prep gives the faceplate a clean coating that makes the disk easy to remove. It helps to keep faceplates in good condition longer, too.

Patricia A. Nigro, RN, ET

Bedside matters
Do your patients use a bedside commode? To save steps, tie a roll of toilet tissue to one side of the commode with a strip of gauze bandage. On the same side, tie a small plastic bag containing soft pieces of cloth for cleaning patients. Tie another plastic bag for soiled cloths on the other side.

This arrangement not only saves time, but also separates the soiled cloths from the rest of the linen for laundry workers.

Connie Davis, RN

Tissue, tissue, everywhere...
Do you dislike having toilet tissue sitting everywhere and anywhere in a patient's room? And no matter where it is, it's always out of reach when needed.

The solution? Have your maintenance department install toilet tissue holders on an arm of each bedside commode. Then the tissue will always be where it's needed. And even though it's still visible, the tissue's new location seems more appropriate than the windowsill, or the bedside stand, or the dresser top, or....

Sandra Holdt, RN

Bring on the bran
No one—neither patient nor nurse—

enjoys a laxative or an enema. Yet, for long-term bedridden patients on a solid food diet, establishing bowel habits presents problems.

Here's a solution to some of those problems—unprocessed bran. With patients who are immobile for long periods and who have no dietary restrictions, sprinkle 1 to 2 teaspoons of bran on their food or in their fruit juice for each meal daily. Then leave the bran container at their bedside so they can regulate the amount to suit their own needs, perhaps decreasing it to twice daily. Patients using bran have no cramping, as they do after a laxative, and they don't have discomfort. And, oh, the nursing hours saved by the decreased need for enemas!

Myra B. Alexander, RN

Catheter keeper
If you change catheters on homebound patients, you need to keep several types and sizes of catheters on hand. So use a convenient carrying pouch. Here's how to make it:

Take a piece of canvas (or duck cloth) 72" × 45" that has bound edges along its length and cut edges along its width. Fold the canvas in half so the cut edges touch. Sew the cut edges together.

Now fold the canvas in half so the bound edges touch. You've folded the canvas in quarters, so your "pouch" is four pieces thick.

With the bound edges on top, sew a seam down each side. Then stitch seams 5" apart through all four thicknesses, from top to bottom. Your pouch should have 21 slots, in rows of seven across and columns of three deep.

Now take a felt-tipped marker and number the first row across according to catheter sizes. Then you can use one column (three slots) for different

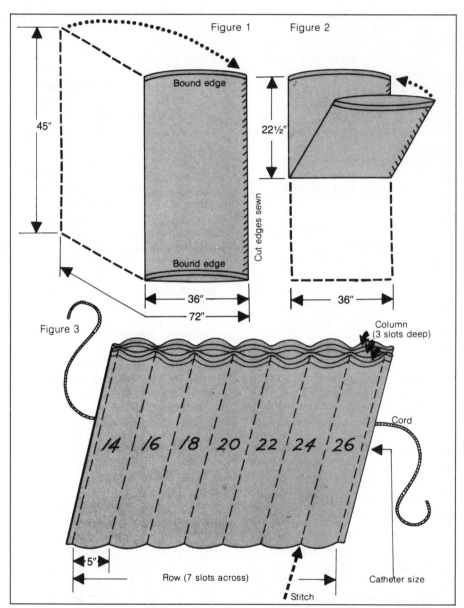

Figure 1   Figure 2

Bound edge

45″

22½″

Cut edges sewn

Bound edge

36″

72″

36″

Figure 3

Column
(3 slots deep)

Cord

14   16   18   20   22   24   26

5″

Row (7 slots across)

Catheter size

Stitch

types of same-sized catheters. For example, in the size-16 column, you can put packages of Teflon catheters in the first slot, plain catheters in the second slot, and silicone catheters in the third slot.

By keeping your catheters in slots, you can easily tell if you're running low. The pouch also keeps the catheter packages from tearing open, which could contaminate the catheters.

If you want to roll up and tie the pouch, sew a 12" piece of cord on each side.

Pam Stilger, RN

Heat-a-fleet

Before giving a Fleet (or similar) enema, place the unit in a microwave oven on a low setting for about 20 seconds. This will warm the liquid and make the enema much easier to administer.

Jane M. Johnson, RN
E.J. Richey, NA

From the mouths of babes

If your elderly or paraplegic patients have trouble retaining enemas because they lack muscle control, try cutting the tip off a baby bottle nipple and inserting the enema tube through the nipple. When the tube is inserted in the patient, the nipple rim surrounds

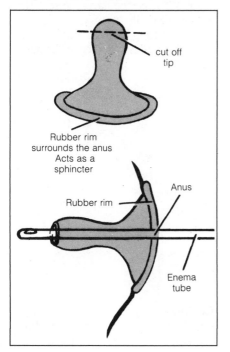

cut off tip

Rubber rim surrounds the anus Acts as a sphincter

Rubber rim

Anus

Enema tube

the anus and acts as a sphincter.

Ramona Chisholm, RN

In the bag

If you have a patient with an enema retention problem, position him on his left side at the edge of the bed. (Make sure the side rail is up; you can work through the bars.) Tape an extra-strength plastic bag to the left side of the mattress. Position the patient's buttocks so they rest on the bag's open end, and place the bottom of the bag in a wastebasket.

Run the enema slowly, allowing waste to drain into the bag. After a short time, turn the patient onto his back to use a bedpan.

This simple method of giving an enema means less mess for you and more comfort for your patient.

R.E. Jacobson, RN

Enema tactics

Have a problem using disposable enemas for elderly patients because of lax rectal sphincters or large hemorrhoids? To get the fluid well into the rectum, slide an ordinary rectal tube onto the tip of the disposable container before using it.

E. Rogers

Relaxing routine

Ever have difficulty inserting a rectal tube for an enema when the patient's apprehensive? First explain the procedure to the patient, then place a warm, wet cloth against his anal sphincter for a few minutes. This helps the patient relax his sphincter muscle, permitting easy insertion of the well-lubricated tube.

Renee Berke, RN

Warming enema packets

To warm an enema packet, we place

the packet in the coffeepot and run water through the coffee maker. The heated water runs onto the packet, warming it to just the right temperature.

Maisie Hubbard, RN, MSN

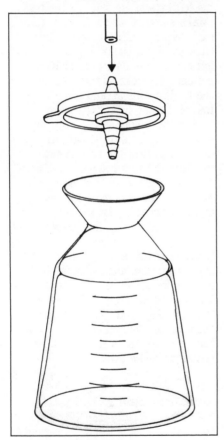

Look, no leaks

Here's a way to keep a patient's tube from leaking when it's draining by gravity. Use a plastic collection container with a cap. Make a hole in the cap and thread the tube through the hole. Then attach a plastic barrel connector to the end of the tube. With the wide part of the barrel connector holding the tube in the con-

tainer, no drainage will leak onto the floor, the bed, or the patient.

Maria L. D'Amato, RN, BSN

Soft tube

If you're having trouble passing a Salem sump tube because it's too large for your patient's nares, try running *warm* water over the last 5" to 6" of the tube. The water softens the tube, minimizing trauma and discomfort to your patient. Also, water left clinging to the tube helps advance it.

Deborah Lamb Mechanick, RN

Patent idea

Copious GI bleeding may clog a nasogastric tube despite hourly irrigations. To keep the tube patent, use this technique on the half hour.

Sandwich the tube between two tongue blades, placed lengthwise about 15" from the nares. Fasten the blades with silk tape—just tight enough to keep them in place. Then, press the blades together to dislodge clots.

Joy Murray, RN

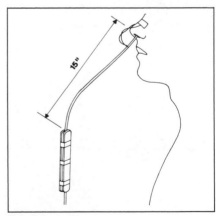

Draining dry

Ever care for a patient who'd had a ventricular drainage catheter re-

moved? The catheter site on his forehead continues to drain cerebrospinal
fluid, requiring dressing changes
every 1 to 2 hours.

So improvise a drainage system.
Put a sterile, disposable pediatric
urine collector over the catheter site
and connect the collector's drainage
tube to an empty, sterile I.V. bag.

This device not only eliminates a
possible source of infection—the
wet dressings—but it also serves as
a sterile, closed drainage system
to measure the cerebrospinal fluid.

Vivian E. Lyons, RN

A routine change
When a Gomco suction machine isn't
suctioning well—or at all—don't
reposition the patient or his nasogastric tube until you've checked the
collection bottle.

If the bottle has more than 1,000
ml of drainage, the machine doesn't
work efficiently. So routinely change
the bottle when the contents reach
this point, and you may not have
to disturb the patient.

Kimberly Anton, LPN

Tent the tube
Drainage that leaks out *around* abdominal sump or gastrostomy tubes
causes wet bedclothes and skin
irritation.

To prevent this, use a "tented"
tube-and-pouch device, which calls for
the following procedures:

Obtain a skin barrier (such as
karaya gum or Stomahesive), a drain-
able ostomy pouch with an adhesive
backing, and reinforcing tape. In
the centers of the barrier and the
pouch adhesive, cut openings no more
than ¼" larger than the opening in
the patient's abdomen.

Now turn the pouch around. Place

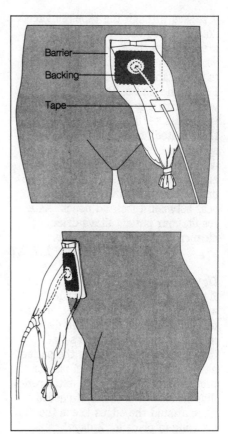

a piece of tape about 1" lower than
the bottom edge of the adhesive
on the pouch's other side. Then cut a
hole, slightly smaller than the tube
diameter, through the tape and pouch.

To apply the barrier, first clean
and dry the patient's skin. Then disconnect the suction momentarily,
slip the barrier over the tube, and
affix the barrier to the patient.

Next, thread the tube through the
hole in the pouch adhesive, then
out through the tape-reinforced hole
on the pouch's other side. Affix the
pouch back securely to the skin
barrier.

Now return to the pouch front and
wrap tape around the tube where

it passes through the tape-reinforced hole. Be sure the tape covers the area *between* the tube and pouch hole where drainage could leak. Continue to wrap tape about 4″ up the tube. Fasten the end of the pouch as you would with any drain.

Besides sealing the tube opening, this "tented" tube-in-pouch device serves as a splint to reduce tension on the tube. It also allows you to empty and rinse the pouch from the end, without disturbing the taped seal between tube and pouch. As a result, your patient stays drier, cleaner, and more comfortable.

Carleen D. Parlato, RN, ET

Dry dressing
If your patient has constant leakage around the cystostomy tubes, use half of a toddler-sized disposable diaper as a dressing. The diaper's liner draws wetness away from the patient's skin, and its outer layer of plastic protects his clothing. Put extra padding inside the dressing if needed. Tape around the edges keeps the dressing in place for 2 days.

Joann Tervenski, RN, BS

Bagging a drainage dilemma
Ever have difficulty managing the drainage from a ureterostomy incision? Then bag it. Apply an ostomy bag, that is.

An associate professor of nursing at Bucks County Community College (Newtown, Pa.) applied a colostomy bag to a patient's ureterostomy incision after his incision began to heal. To achieve a leak-free closure, she moved the drain from the incision away from any body fold before she applied the bag.

The bag saved nursing time because nurses no longer had to apply gauze dressings to soak up urine that

drained from the incision. And the patient appreciated the accuracy of measuring the amount of urine that leaked through the incision. When the amount he voided far exceeded that collected in the bag, he knew his incision was almost healed.

Judith E. Meissner, RN, MSN

Odor control
To control odor in your patient's colostomy bag, put a few drops of lemon-scented dishwashing liquid in the bag. The lemon scent masks the odor, and the liquid lubricates the bag so the stool slides to the bottom. Cleaning the bag is easier, too, since the soap is already in it.

Gale Nunn, RN

No more odor
If you notice a strong, unpleasant odor emanating from a urine drainage bag at a patient's bedside, try this. Add 10 ml of hydrogen peroxide to the bag every time you empty it. The hydrogen peroxide prevents bacteria from forming in the bag; hence, no odor. It also prevents bag discoloration and urine turbidity.

Jo Ann M. Camasso, RN, CNA, BSN

COLLECTING SPECIMENS

Throw in the towel
To get a 24-hour urine specimen from a newborn baby girl, place a rolled-up towel between the baby's knees and ankles, attaching it to her legs with 2″ paper tape. When her legs are separated (as if she had a hip-spica cast), the urine bag can be taped on securely, and she can't kick it out of place. Also, the baby can easily be turned from her back to her stomach.

Joan M. Moore, RN, MN

Collecting urine specimens

Here's how to collect a 24-hour urine specimen from an infant without using a catheter.

First, cleanse the infant's perineal area and let it dry completely. Then attach a 3" or 4" square piece of Stomahesive to a 24-hour collection bag. Cut a center hole in the Stomahesive and contour the edges to fit the baby's perineal area.

Next, remove the backing from the Stomahesive and moisten the Stomahesive with water to attach it to the baby's perineal area. The baby's body heat helps seal the adhesive, so hold the bag in place for a few seconds. (And for better adhesion, if the baby is a boy, place his penis *and* scrotum inside the bag.) For additional security, put nonallergenic tape around the edges.

Check the bag frequently and empty it into a jar.

Or, if you don't want to use adhesive tape on an infant, try this:

Make two small vertical slits in the Stomahesive—one on each side of the center hole—but don't remove the paper backing. Insert a piece of twill or trach tape through each slit. Then place the bag on the baby and tie it in place around his waist— just tight enough to be secure.

Bev Petrites, RN

Miniature urinal

How many times have you used a urine collection bag on a premature male infant, only to have the bag slip off the infant's penis?

Here's a more effective urine collector: a capped syringe, with the needle and plunger removed.

After inserting the infant's penis through the syringe's open end, place a strip of hypoallergenic tape over the closed end. Then, tape the syringe to the infant's lower abdomen or groin.

With this miniature urinal, you don't lose any of the infant's urine sample. So you get enough urine for testing, and you can measure intake and output accurately. Also, you can see the penis through the clear, plastic syringe, to check for pressure.

Nancy J. Urich, RN, BS

Specimen regimen

I work in a pediatrician's office where we do some of our own laboratory work, including urinalysis. We've found that urine collection bags don't work well on infants. Either they don't stay in place, or, if they're not secured properly on the infant's body, stool contaminates the specimen.

So we've devised another way to collect a sterile urine specimen. One person holds the child under both arms perpendicular to the examination table. Another person cleans the child's genital area with sterile wipes and holds a sterile urine container under the child. The wiping stimulates urination and within a minute or so, we have our specimen.

This method of getting a clean-catch urine specimen has become standard practice in our office now.

Pat Soukup, RN

A collector's item

Need to get a urine specimen from an infant or toddler? Apply a pediatric urine collection bag. But if you put a diaper over the bag, you risk squeezing the bag and causing the baby discomfort as well as having urine leak out. A safer, more comfortable alternative is this.

Make a large X-shaped slash in the

diaper at the front of the crotch, place the collection bag and diaper on the baby, and gently pull the bag out through the X-shaped opening. This way, there's no pressure on the bag, and you can readily see when the baby has voided.

Rose Marie Utley, RN, CPNP

What a catch
To get a clean-catch urine specimen from an incontinent man, we first cleanse his penis with povidone-iodine solution and apply an external collection device (such as a Texas catheter). Then we cut a slit in the plastic lid of a sterile specimen cup. We insert the drainage end of the catheter through the cap and into the cup.

This way, we get the specimen without increasing the risk of a urinary tract infection.

Donna Sabatelli, RN
Lurlene Williams, NA

A good catch
Most of the residents at the extended care facility where I work have trouble providing a clean-catch midstream urine specimen because they can't start and stop voiding easily. So I've found a way to obtain the urine specimen that's easier for them.

After cleansing the resident's genital area, I spread a disposable pad under the commode and remove its collection container. Then I seat the resident on the commode, and I squat behind it.

I hold the collection container under the commode to catch the resident's urine when he begins to void. Then I lower the container and hold a specimen cup under the commode to catch the midstream specimen. (I've also found that placing the container on the pad under the commode and

holding the specimen cup above it works just as well.)

This way, the resident doesn't have to worry about when to stop and when to start voiding, and I get a good specimen on the first try.

Sandra Werkheiser, RN

Preventive maintenance
When catheterizing a patient, here's how to prevent the sterile field from folding back on itself after you've carefully spread it out.

Roll two pieces of tape into rings with the sticky side out. Unpackage—but don't unfold—the sterile field, and place it between the patient's legs. Put one piece of tape on what will be the underside corner of the field that you'll be opening toward you. Pull open the field, and secure the taped corner on the thigh (for a man) or sheet (for a woman). With the other tape ring, do the same on the corner that opens away from you.

This little bit of tape is a great preventive maintenance tool—especially when the patient won't or can't remain still.

Warren G. Patitz, RN

Stool collection
To obtain stool specimens for guaiac tests from patients with bathroom privileges, give them filter paper instead of toilet paper and a stool cup to hold the paper when used. Most patients find this an easier and less offensive method of collecting stool.

Lillian Plodquist, LPN

A specimen problem
Recently, my mother underwent some diagnostic tests that involved collecting stool specimens at home, then sending them to the laboratory for

analysis. When she complained about the difficulty and unpleasantness of collecting the specimens, I thought of a way to make it easier for her.

I suggested she drape a piece of plastic wrap over the toilet bowl (with the lid up), keeping the plastic above the water. Then I suggested she tape the sides of the plastic to the outside of the bowl. The stool would fall onto the plastic wrap, which she could easily lift off the toilet to get the specimen. The remainder of the stool could be flushed away and the wrap placed in a bag for disposal.

Brenda Owens, RN

Fancy footwork

Have you ever had to do repeated heel sticks on a crying infant to get enough blood for a specimen? If so, hold the baby's feet in warm water for 5 to 10 minutes. (Better still, let the baby's parent do the soak.) Then, with just one stick, you should be able to draw an adequate specimen.

Johnnie Titus, RN, BSN

Preheated veins

I frequently need to collect blood specimens from our home care patients, but many of them have poor veins for venipunctures. To save the time and discomfort of repeated needle sticks, I call the patient's home about 20 minutes before I'm scheduled to visit there. I tell the patient or a family member to apply a warm compress over the patient's inner arm at the elbow (the antecubital area): first, apply a warm, wet cloth; cover it with a dry cloth and wrap plastic wrap around the arm; and leave this compress in place until I arrive.

When I remove the compress, the patient's veins are more visible and easy to dilate, so the venipuncture is usually successful—the first time around.

P. Stilger, RN

Blood lines

When a patient's admitted to our emergency department, we frequently have to start an I.V. line right away and draw blood for laboratory studies. To avoid inserting two needles into the patient for the blood specimen, I draw the blood when I insert the I.V.

Before securing the line or running the fluid, I draw about 15 to 20 ml of blood from the I.V. line's hub with a sterile syringe. I place the blood in collection tubes immediately. Then I secure the line and start administering the fluid. This way, the patient's blood specimens are ready for testing without my inflicting more pain on the patient.

Lynn Suprock, RN

Sample procedure

If you need to draw a blood sample from a patient who has an I.V. line, you can avoid a venipuncture by following this procedure:
1. Use a hemostat to clamp the I.V. line above the injection port for 1 minute.
2. Apply a tourniquet.
3. Insert the needle of a vacutainer into the injection port and apply a 10-ml vacuum tube.
4. Collect the first 2 ml of blood, then remove and discard the tube.
5. Attach a new tube and collect the pure venous blood that now flows.

If the blood flow is impaired, simply tap the vein at the tip of the I.V. catheter to break the seal between the catheter and vein.

Samples obtained this way can be

used for complete blood counts, coagulation studies, cross matching, and most serum chemical determinations. The procedure should not be used to draw blood for glucose or potassium levels if the infusate contains 5% or greater glucose or more than 10 mmol per liter of potassium.

Doctors at Pennsylvania Hospital, Philadelphia, who devised the procedure, say it gives good quality specimens without the need for a venipuncture.

The New England Journal of Medicine,
Dec. 5, 1985

Specimen bag

To collect a urine specimen from an incontinent male patient, I use a pediatric urine collection bag. I make the hole slightly larger and place the bag over the patient's penis. As soon as I see enough urine for the specimen, I remove the bag.

Caryn Jones, RN

Go with the flow

Next time you're taking a blood sample from a patient and the flow stops, loosen the tourniquet momentarily. If the tourniquet is too tight, it may impede arterial blood flow. Releasing pressure this way usually starts the blood flowing again.

Bertha L. Clarke, RN, CEN, BSN

Geriatricks

Collecting a urine specimen from an elderly woman patient when you can't get an order for an indwelling or straight catheter can be difficult. So try using a pediatric urine bag. Tape the bag over the patient's perineum. It holds about 50 to 60 ml of urine—sufficient for most tests.

Debora J. Burke, RN

SECURING TUBES AND DRAINAGE SETS

All strapped in

Use Montgomery straps to secure indwelling (Foley) catheters. First, cut a 4" × 4" section from a Montgomery strap. Then into the section's center, cut two parallel ¼" slits 1" apart. After weaving the string supplied with the strap through the slits, apply the strap's sticky side to the patient and tie the string around the catheter.

This simple device can all but eliminate the need to reposition Foley catheters. So you'll save yourself time and your patients considerable discomfort.

Jacqueline Kasulanis, RN

Waistbanded bag

For an ambulatory patient who has an indwelling urinary catheter, I recommend this alternative to strapping a collection bag to the patient's leg. Sew a large pocket to the inside of the patient's pant leg or skirt. Place the bag in the pocket, so the weight of the bag is on the garment's waistband—not on the patient's leg.

Velma Foley, RN

Comfy caths #1

To secure an indwelling (Foley) catheter to a patient's leg without using tape, wrap a long piece of Kling bandage around the patient's thigh. Be sure it's tight enough to stay up but loose enough to avoid constriction. Tape the bandage to itself and loop a rubber band around the catheter. Insert an open safety pin into the loop and attach the pin to the bandage.

The catheter will stay put, and you

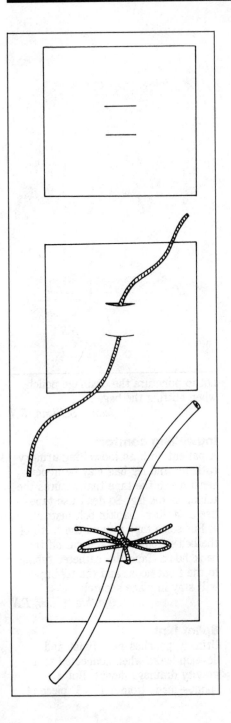

don't have to change tape, which may cause the patient discomfort.
Vicki Rios, RN

Comfy caths #2
Another way to secure an indwelling (Foley) catheter without tape is to tie a long piece of umbilical tape or gauze to the balloon port of the catheter. Then tie the rest of the tape around the patient's thigh. With the catheter secured this way, the patient can move about freely without the discomfort of sticky tape on his skin.
Kimberly Stotts, RN, BSN

Tapeless tubing tricks
Problem: To stabilize a patient's indwelling (Foley) catheter, you tape the tubing to his thigh—but the tape irritates his skin. Solution: Try using a long piece of gauze instead.

Wrap the gauze once around the patient's thigh. Lay the tubing over the gauze, then wrap the rest of the gauze around the thigh over the tubing and tape the gauze to itself. Now the tubing is sandwiched between two layers of gauze. To be doubly sure the tubing is secure, tape it to the gauze.
Carol M. Croston, RN

Cath comfort #1
Another way to stabilize catheter tubing without tape is to use transparent polyurethane dressing. Just apply a $4'' \times 6''$ piece of the dressing over the tubing where you'd usually apply the tape. The dressing holds the tubing securely and stays intact longer than tape. It also allows you to see the patient's skin under the dressing and helps heal inflamed areas.
Bonnie Thomas, RN

Pajama game

An irrational patient will sometimes risk traumatic injury by pulling on an indwelling urinary catheter.

Discourage this by putting a pajama bottom on the patient and running the tubing down the inside of the pajama leg. Usually, this is so successful that conventional restraints aren't necessary.

E. Rexine Stott, RN

Substitute straps

One of my elderly home care patients had an indwelling (Foley) catheter with a leg bag. The straps on the bag dug into his skin, causing irritation. In looking for substitute straps for the bag, I noticed the strap on a Depend adult disposable undergarment. This strap is wide and stretchy, and it has two buttons on each end. I wrapped the strap around the patient's leg and attached the leg bag to the buttons. The strap stays in place and doesn't harm the patient's skin.

Margaret Guilfoyle, RN

A Foley fix

If a patient with an indwelling (Foley) catheter complains that his leg drainage bag bunches up, make two simple alterations. First, cut four extra slits—two at the top of the bag and two at the bottom, each about 1" from one of the existing slits.

Next, thread the bag's top strap through the top four slits and sew the strap to the bag at the two threading points. Thread and sew the bottom strap the same way. Now, the bag stays securely attached to the strap and doesn't ride up.

Note: When passing this tip on to your patients, warn them to be careful

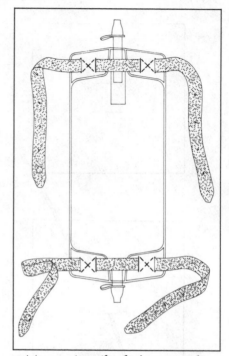

not to puncture the drainage pouch when slitting the bag.

Jeanne Sullivan, RN

Indwelling comfort

A patient with an indwelling urinary catheter and leg bag may be hypersensitive to the tape that secures the tubing to his leg. So don't use tape—use a sanitary napkin belt instead.

Put some tape around the teeth of the belt's front hook and cut off the back hook. Tape the catheter tubing to the front hook, and the tubing will stay in place securely.

Cynthia Walker, RN

Splint hint

Urinary pouches may twist and develop leaks when connected to a gravity drainage device. But a splint—made from a 1" × 3" piece of stiff plastic, cardboard, or tongue blade—can help prevent this.

Just tape the splint across the pouch's lower edge, about 1″ above the outlet. The splint will help maintain the bag's shape, keep it from twisting, and give the ostomate peace of mind knowing his bag won't leak.

Joyce Downing, RN, ET

Cath comfort #2

If the rubber strap on a leg bag digs into the patient's skin, try this. Before applying the bag, wrap a washcloth or Chux pad (with the plastic side away from the patient's skin) around his leg. Then strap the bag onto his leg. The cloth or pad serves as a cushion between the patient's leg and the strap.

Donna Anderson, RN

Drainage bag dilemma

Placing a urinary drainage bag in the correct position when a patient is in a wheelchair can be difficult. Either the bag is hung so high it's above the patient's bladder, or so low it's dragging on the floor.

Solve this problem by inserting a grommet (a metal eyelet) through the vinyl backing of the wheelchair—at the center bottom of the chair back—and placing a small "S" hook through the hole in the grommet. Then hang the drainage bag from the hook. This method keeps the bag below the patient's bladder, but away from the floor.

Dianne E. Dunne, RN

Floss works

When you need to secure a nasogastric tube but can't find any thread, use waxed dental floss. It's strong, and its convenient container keeps the

floss clean while providing a handy cutting edge.

Mary E. Anderson, RN, MS

Better adherence and appearance

I use Op-Site for taping nasogastric tubes.

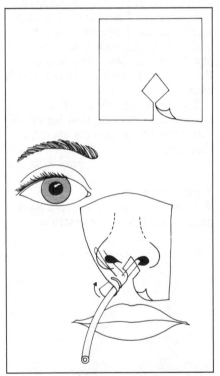

I fold a small piece of Op-Site about ¾″ from the bottom and cut a triangle into the fold. (When I unfold the Op-Site, I have a diamond-shaped hole.) I put the tube through the hole, then cut from the bottom edge of the Op-Site to the hole. I peel off the backing and apply the Op-Site to the patient's nose, with the green edge just below the bridge of his nose, and carefully cut off the green edge. Then I wrap the two bottom halves of the Op-Site around the tube.

The Op-Site keeps the tube in place as securely as tape—but without the irritation and unsightliness.

Lynda L. Lindsay, LPN

Secured with strips

Instead of using tape to hold a nasogastric tube in place, I use tincture of benzoin and Steri-Strips. I apply a small amount of benzoin across the bridge of the patient's nose. When it's dry, I wrap the Steri-Strip around the tube and place it over the patient's nose.

The strips not only adhere to the tube securely but also look better than tape, so the patients appreciate them, too.

Fran Ellis, RN

Tube twist

Whenever you need to clamp a nasogastric tube briefly (for instance,

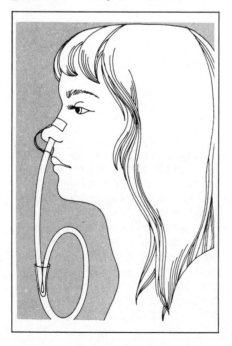

to ambulate the patient, between feedings, and so forth), use the tube itself as the clamp. Just fold the tubing 6″ from the end and insert this folded portion into the opening.

This handy maneuver saves time spent looking for clamps and doesn't strain the tubing with the added weight of a normal clamp.

Debra Schmaltz, RN, BS

Lightweight clamp

Use umbilical cord clamps on nasogastric and "G" tubes. You'll find them lighter and easier to fasten and unfasten than the Hoffman and other heavy clamps.

Jo Goldman, RN

Bag it

The drainage collection devices used after surgery can irritate your patient's skin when they're taped on and changed often. To avoid the discomfort of tape, take a 6″ piece of stockinette, seal one end to form a bag, and insert the collection device. Then attach the bag to the patient's dressing, or else make a gauze belt to hold the bag in place.

Because the bag stays in place without tape, you can change the collection devices whenever necessary and not worry about hurting your patient.

Louise Sweeten, RN

Tape a tube

Here's a way to keep gastrostomy tubes from slipping in or out of the abdomen.

First, cut two 4″ lengths of 1″ wide adhesive (or nonallergenic) tape. Then make two 3″ slits in each piece of tape, leaving about 1″ on one end unslit to make a tab. Both pieces of tape should have three strips and

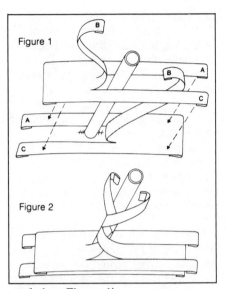

Figure 1

Figure 2

a tab (see Figure 1).

Place one piece of tape on the patient's skin on one side of the gastrostomy tube—with strips A and C secured to the patient's skin around the other side of the tube. Don't allow strip B to adhere to the patient's skin. Place the other piece of tape (in the opposite direction) on the other side of the tube the same way. This piece of tape will overlap the first piece. To secure the tube and prevent sliding, wrap both B strips around the tube in opposite directions (see Figure 2).

If you turn the tab ends and the ends of strips A and C under onto themselves, you won't have to pick at the tape on the patient's skin to remove it.

Sharon E. Feick, RN

Op-Site for ET tube
To secure a patient's endotracheal tube—without putting tape on his skin—try using Op-Site.

First, prepare the patient's skin with tincture of benzoin. Then apply

Op-Site to the area where the tape will be applied. Now tape the tube to the Op-Site instead of to the patient's skin.

Op-Site adheres well, is less irritating than tape because it permits airflow to prevent skin breakdown, and is transparent so you can easily assess the skin.

Patricia Fuchs, SN, CRTT, RRT

The tie that's kind
Obviously, taping a nasal endotracheal tube (ETT) to a burn patient's face is bound to cause additional skin irritation. So instead of taping the ETT on, tie it on as follows:

Cut both ends off a #14 French (or larger) suction catheter. Then cut the catheter into two pieces—each as long as the distance from your patient's nose to his ear (see illustration).

Next, thread umbilical tape (long enough to tie around the patient's head) through both catheter pieces. To simplify threading, use an 18G needle to push the tape through both catheters' lumens.

Wet the outside of the ETT with benzoin to make it sticky. Loop the tape—the part *between* the two catheter pieces—around the ETT. Then

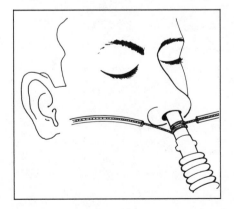

secure the ETT by tying the tape ends behind the patient's head.

This kind of tie will stay clean longer than tape. Best of all, it won't rub or pull your patient's delicate skin.

Adriana Sullenger, RN

Easy-off tape
To secure an endotracheal tube without getting tape stuck in your patient's hair, do this:

Cut a piece of 1" tape about 24" long. Cut another piece about 9" long. With the sticky sides facing each other, center the shorter piece over the longer piece and press the pieces together.

Now place the tape under the patient's head (double-thick section at the back of his head) and bring the ends around the tube, securing it in place.

This technique holds the tube in place, and you won't pull the patient's hair when you take the tape off.

Betty Horvath, RN

Unknotting a tying problem
How do you secure a tracheostomy cannula? The usual way is to knot a string to each flange on the cannula, then knot both strings together be-

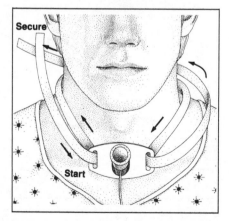

hind the patient's neck.

But this method can cause problems. For instance, the knot behind the patient's neck can cause skin breakdown. The knots on the flanges can pull the cannula to one side when the patient moves his neck, causing tissue damage, coughing, and ventilation leaks.

To avoid these and other problems, a nurse in San Antonio, Tex., uses a single string that's long enough to go behind the patient's neck twice. He describes how the string's attached:

First, slip one end through the front side of the flange opening. Then, pass the string behind the patient's neck and through the back side of the opposite flange opening.

Next, pass the string again behind the patient's neck and tie the two ends together. Knot the ends on the side of the patient's neck and make sure the string isn't too tight over the carotid arteries.

Besides being easy to apply, the single long string is easy to remove. Simply untie the knot or cut through the string, then slip the string back through the flange openings.

It helps to get the long string from a tracheostomy kit manufacturer or using extra-wide, sterile umbilical tape.

Edward L. Russel, RN, BSN

Self-taught timesaver
When you apply a condom catheter by first applying the double-sided adhesive tape, do you end up with a sticky mess? I did, until I tried doing it this way.

First, I place the condom sheath on the end of the patient's penis. Then, as I apply the adhesive tape to the shaft of the penis, I roll the sheath down over the tape. The catheter is secure, and the whole procedure is a lot neater.

Phoebe Hershenow, RN, BSN

APPLYING DRESSINGS, BANDAGES, AND COMPRESSES

One-handed bandage
Here's how to make a one-handed elastic bandage:

Sew a loop on one end of the bandage. Have the patient slip the loop over his foot as if he were putting on a sock, then wrap the remainder of the bandage around his leg. Not only does this decrease edema but also makes the patient more independent.

Joyce Meyers, RN

Wrap and roll
Applying an elastic bandage to a patient's leg can be a one-person job if you do it this way: Use an unwrapped roll of toilet paper as a footrest for the patient. This will lift the patient's leg far enough off the bed so you can easily wrap the leg without needing someone else to hold it.

Jean Kindle, RN

A net worth of comfort
If you're caring for a patient who has a wound on his hips or buttocks, here's a way to hold the dressing in place without tape. Use a large-sized, tubular, stretchy, net material. Just cut the length of material you need, then pull it over the patient's feet and up over his hips. This will hold the patient's dressing securely in place—without irritating his skin.

Danalee Nelson, RN

Well-dressed thigh
If you have difficulty keeping a bulky dressing in place on a patient's thigh

or groin, try using the panty section of a pair of panty hose.

First, cut off the legs and crotch. Then, slip the remaining panty section over the bulky dressing, with the elastic waistband toward the patient's foot. The panty section will hold the dressing in place without constricting circulation. It can be washed and reused several times before being discarded.

J. Swenton, RN

Circumcision wrap
To make a simple, inexpensive dressing for an adult circumcision, unfold a standard $4'' \times 4''$ gauze pad to $4'' \times 8''$. Then fold lengthwise to $2'' \times 8''$. Coat one side with petrolatum, leaving the ends uncoated. Place the coated side along the suture line on the ventral side of the penis and wrap around, crossing the gauze on the dorsal side and taping the ends to the groin.

The tape supports the weight of the dressing, and the patient can void without soiling it.

Tom Megow, SN

Patchwork
In the doctor's office where I work, minor surgical procedures are performed routinely. Applying dressings to irregularly shaped or hard-to-reach wounds (such as those behind the ear or over the coccyx) is always a challenge. I've found that small, flexible oval eye patches can be applied easily and securely to these wounds.

Kathy Smernoff, LVN

No fallout here
Bulky dressings on large or draining abdominal wounds sometimes slip off when patients get out of bed. To avoid this problem, apply Montgomery

straps in the conventional manner, that is, two straps affixed vertically along the wound. Then place a third, smaller, Montgomery strap horizontally below the other straps and lace it through the vertical straps' lower holes. The horizontal strap keeps the dressings in place so the patient can move about confidently.

Constance J. Gramzow, RN, BSN

Dressed for success

Need an easy-to-use, nonirritating dressing for a healing lower abdominal incision? How about an unscented sanitary minipad—the type with adhesive backing?

Just pull the backing off and affix the napkin to the inside of the patient's underwear, opposite the incision site. The soft, absorbent napkin has it all over regular dressings: it won't irritate the patient's skin as a taped-on dressing could, and it's easier to change, too.

Rachel Rosen-Thal, RN, BSN

Ouchless taping

Here's how to keep Montgomery straps in place without taping the straps to the patient's skin. Cut a piece of Stomahesive, a little larger than the tape, and apply the adhesive side to the patient's skin (preferably, to a flat surface). Then tape the Montgomery straps to the Stomahesive.

Using this method, you can remove the tape from the shiny side of the Stomahesive several times to change dressings without traumatizing the patient's skin.

Lynda Brubacher, RN, ET

Straps: Banded together

Next time you have to apply Montgomery straps to a patient's incisional

area, don't bother with safety pins or twill tape. Instead, reach for some rubber bands and paper clips.

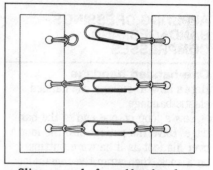

Slip one end of a rubber band through one of the strap's holes, then through the other end of the rubber band to secure it to the strap. Slip another rubber band through the opposite hole and secure it the same way. Then join the two rubber bands with a paper clip, as illustrated. Do the same with the rest of the holes in the strap.

The rubber bands allow the strap to expand as the patient moves. And since the paper clips lie flat, they won't dig into the patient's skin as a safety pin might if it popped open.

Barbara E. A. Naunchek, RN

A toe hold

If a patient needs a warm compress on his toe, use a disposable glove to keep the compress in place and his bed dry. After applying the compress, slip the glove over the patient's toes and lower part of his foot. The glove keeps the compress from getting the bed wet and holds the warmth in longer.

Pam Miller, LPN

Warm and dry

When a pediatric patient needs to

hold a warm soak against his arm or leg, I put the wet dressing for the soak in place and wrap a disposable diaper (absorbent side against the dressing) snugly around it. Then I secure the diaper and dressing with the diaper's adhesive tabs.

The diaper conforms to any shape, shields against wetness, retains the warmth, and allows the child to move freely. I can even draw funny faces on the outside of the diaper with a felt-tipped marker.

Anne Marie Berger, RN

Keeping a cool head
After oral surgery, most of our patients are too sleepy to hold regular ice packs on their jaws bilaterally, as ordered. So we help them this way: We tie a knot in the middle of a long piece of stockinette. Then we fill two examination gloves with ice and knot each glove at the wrist. We put the gloves in the stockinette—one on each side of the knot in the middle. Finally, we wrap the stockinette around the patient's head with the knot under his chin and the ends tied loosely on top of his head.

This stockinette ice bag stays put without being held in place. We can easily change the ice as necessary.

Sue Dillon, RN

Cool pad
Here's a method of applying ice to a patient's perineum after an episiotomy.

First, cut a sanitary pad in half—the short way—and soak the halves in water until saturated. Then take each half and fashion it into a 1" diameter roll. Next, cover the roll with a 5" × 5" square of plastic kitchen wrap and put it into the freezer.

When the roll's frozen, place one or two Tucks pads on the patient's

perineum, put the frozen roll over the Tucks pads, and hold both roll and pad(s) in place with another whole sanitary pad.

Denise Houle, RN

Postop pointers
A pediatric patient who came to our unit after eye surgery had postoperative orders for ice packs on both eyes, 30 minutes on and 30 minutes off, for 6 hours. When we tried to comply with the orders, the patient balked at the discomfort. Then we discovered a suitable alternative.

We soaked several cotton balls in water, froze them, and substituted them for the ice packs. We had to change them frequently, but the patient didn't mind because they were softer, smaller, and not as heavy as regular ice packs.

Nancy McStay, RN

Stay-put ice packs #1
When a baby gets an injection in his thigh muscles, here's how to prevent swelling. Cover a small ice bag with a cloth and slip it into the leg of his footed pajamas. No further securing is necessary; the pajamas are snug enough to hold the ice bag in place.

Linda Barker, RN

Stay-put ice packs #2
Another way to secure an ice pack is with stockinette. Cut a 6" to 8" length of stockinette (length depends on the size of the area you'll be covering). Place the covered ice pack on the patient's arm or leg and pull the stockinette over the pack. Tape the stockinette to itself and the ice pack is secure, leaving the patient's hands free for other activities.

An important reminder: Don't leave the ice pack in place any longer than hospital policy allows. And remember to periodically check the patient's skin.

Diane Clark, RN

Partial soaks

Soaks are sometimes prescribed for the patient with a plantar wart on the ball of the foot. When using an irritating substance such as dilute formalin solution for soaking, you'll want to minimize damage by limiting the area of surrounding healthy tissue in contact with solution.

Have the patient get a paint pan— the kind used when applying paint with a roller. Have him pour just enough solution into the deep end of the pan to cover the ball of the foot while the heel rests comfortably on the slanted pan bottom, high and dry. The technique works just as well for soaking the heel while keeping the toes dry: just turn the pan around and put the heel in the deep end.

Barbara McVan, RN

Dressing for success

If you've been looking for a way to secure a dressing without tape or other fasteners, your search is over. After applying a dressing, try the following technique.

First, wrap a gauze bandage around the dressing. Then slit the end of the bandage lengthwise about 8″ and twist the two ends together several times. Wrap one of the ends around the bandage, then tie the two ends together. (Don't tie the knot over the wound.) To make sure the bandage doesn't produce a tourniquetlike effect, check circulatory, motor, and neurologic functions below the bandage.

Linda Kerbs, PT

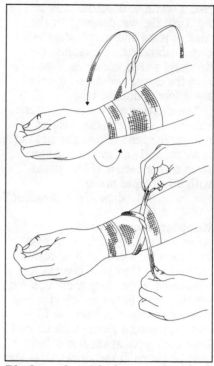

Binders that bind

One of my patients who'd had perianal surgery had to have bulky packings and dressings, saturated with povidone-iodine, applied every shift. The doctor ordered a T-binder to anchor the dressings.

Our hospital didn't stock cloth T-binders—only disposables. Once these binders became damp from the dressings, they fell away and the dressings followed.

My solution was to cover the outside of the disposable binder with waterproof adhesive tape. The dressings didn't soak through the binder and, what's more, everything stayed in place. The patient was more comfortable, and I was relieved that I didn't have to change the dressings so frequently.

Terrilynn M. Quillen, RN

CARING FOR THE SKIN AND WOUNDS

Socks under splints
A patient with arthritis or carpal tunnel syndrome who must wear a wrist splint may suffer skin irritation or breakdown under the splint. But you can prevent this with a pair of cotton knee socks.

Cut off the toe and make a hole in the heel of each sock. Slip the sock over the patient's hand: put his thumb through the hole in the heel, his fingers through the cutoff toe. Then apply the splint.

The cotton absorbs perspiration better than knit material or a stockinette. And if you make two protectors from one pair of socks, the patient will always have one to wear while the other's being washed.
Beverly Walkling, RN

Padded socks
An elderly home care patient wanted some elbow protectors. I didn't have any with me, so I suggested she make them herself.

I told her to cut the tops and toes off an old pair of socks. She could then place a sanitary pad (with an adhesive strip) inside each sock, lengthwise over the heel. This makes a pair of comfortable, inexpensive elbow (or heel) protectors.
Angelina Elkin, RN

Ointment applicator
Add a disposable syringe (minus the needle) to your weapons for fighting decubitus ulcers.

Remove the syringe plunger, squeeze ointment into the syringe barrel, and replace the plunger. After cleaning the ulcer as ordered, squirt the ointment onto the ulcer. The pencil-thin ointment lines will allow you to target each crevice and fold.
Lynda L. Scherff, LPN

A healing sealing
When a patient has a decubitus ulcer on his sacrum or coccyx, I sometimes apply a hydrocolloid dressing. To provide a good seal, especially if the patient is incontinent, I apply strips of transparent polyurethane dressing around the edges of the hydrocolloid dressing. The waterproof strips can be wiped easily, and they keep the ulcer from becoming contaminated. Then I don't have to change the dressing so often.
Karen Gum, RN, MSN

No-drip irrigation
Cancer patients can get shallow excoriated lesions from radiation therapy. Daily irrigation with equal parts of hydrogen peroxide and sterile water can be cold and messy for the patient—when you use traditional irrigating equipment. So try using a sterilized spray bottle instead— the kind used for spray-on glass cleaner. You can deliver an adequate amount of solution, with a minimum of dripping and a maximum of comfort for your patient.
Joann Tervenski, RN, BS

Packing idea
To pack deep, large wounds after irrigations or dressing changes, use a roll of sterile stretch gauze instead of $4'' \times 4''$. Wearing gloves, hold the roll in one hand and a sterile hemostat in the other, releasing the dressing gradually and packing it in the wound. Since the stretch gauze is fluffier and smoother than $4'' \times 4''$, it packs better. And because it's all

one piece, the gauze can be removed easier and faster—a feature patients appreciate.

Marie-Lise Shams, RN

A thigh of relief

If your patient has a leg brace that rubs against the inner thigh of his other leg, avoid this irritation and possible skin breakdown by making a cushion for the normal thigh. Here's how:

Cut off one leg of an old pair of panty hose at midcalf and midthigh to give an open-ended nylon cylinder. Then sew a piece of furlike material (any soft fabric will do) on the cylinder's inner-thigh area.

Now your patient has a padded cylinder that slips on and off his leg easily, doesn't impair circulation, and best of all, protects his skin.

Etta M. Rosenthal, RN, BS, PHN

Clearing the ear

When a bedridden patient develops a decubitus ulcer on his ear, you're in for a big challenge, that is, trying to keep pressure off his ear so it can heal while he's lying in bed.

To meet this challenge, I use the following procedure: I make a pillow from foam rubber cut in the shape of a "C" and cover it with a pillow-case. (I fold and tape the case so it doesn't cover the cut-out section.) The patient can lay his head on the pillow with his ear in the cut-out section so no pressure is placed on the ulcer. Of course, I also keep the ulcer clean, dry, and infection-free to speed healing.

Delycia E. Feustel, RN, MS

Skin saver

One of my patients who had an ileal conduit developed skin breakdown

around his stoma. To help repair his skin, I used a heat lamp, a paper cup, and cotton balls.

First, I pushed out the bottom of the cup (leaving a smooth edge) and filled the cup with cotton balls. Then I had the patient hold the cup tightly over his stoma while I placed him under the heat lamp.

The cotton balls absorbed his urine, and, as they became saturated, I removed the cup and gave the patient a new one. The patient could stay comfortably under the heat lamp for about 30 minutes. After a few days of this treatment three times a day, his skin began to heal.

Lorraine Norem, RN

Thigh righting

One of my elderly patients, who had a hip arthroplasty, developed large blisters on her inner thighs from the abduction pillow she kept between her legs. To help heal the blisters and prevent future ones, I cleaned and dried her skin where it touched the pillow and applied a polyurethane adhesive dressing to the area. My therapy worked: the patient didn't get any more blisters, and she was much more comfortable.

Jill Quinto, LPN, SN

I.V. bags underfoot

To prevent decubitus ulcers from forming on the feet of patients who have sensory or motor deficits, we use 10-liter, fluid-filled plastic bags or I.V. bags. We cover each bag with a pillowcase or urinal bag cover before putting it under the patient's feet.

The bags could also be used to support a patient's neck and arms, and they make nice replacements for sandbags, water beds, and egg-crate mattresses. We've used the bags for 3 to 4 months before having to replace them.

Lucy Dalicancro, RN

Team up against decubiti

To prevent decubiti—and to treat them when they occur—Maimonides Hospital Geriatric Center, Montreal, Quebec, uses a team approach.

The nursing coordinator and the infection-surveillance nurse helped form a decubiti control team that includes themselves, an inservice educator, a doctor, a dietitian, and a physiotherapist.

The team meets twice a month to review data compiled by the infection-surveillance nurse. Team members then make rounds to assess the patients, their nutritional status, and the treatment plans. The team recommends changes in the patients' diets and the treatment plans as needed, and the staff nurses incorporate the recommendations into their care plans and document them on the patients' charts. Besides the usual means of treating decubiti, the team also recommends nonnursing techniques that may be helpful, for example, ultrasonography or infrared.

When the center first started using the team approach 3 years ago, most of the decubiti the nursing staff reported had already progressed to tissue loss. Now the nurses are reporting when they first spot a reddened area. Because decubiti are reported and treated earlier, healing time has been reduced: in most cases, ulcers that used to take months to heal now heal within a single month.

Margaret Bougie, RN, BSN
Judy Seri, RN

Jelly remover

Removing dried electrode jelly from a patient's skin can be difficult—espe-

cially if the patient has sensitive skin. Instead of using acetone, which is abrasive, use A and D Ointment.

Apply the ointment generously, and leave it on the skin for a few minutes before rubbing it in. With babies, apply the ointment before bathing them and remove it after their bath. Besides removing the jelly, the ointment also helps heal the skin.

Linda Milewski, RN, BSN

It's oil for the better #1

To remove the vernix caseosa from a newborn's skin, use mineral oil. Just soak some gauze or a cotton ball with the oil and wipe clean.

Irma Robinson, LPN

Tape remover

Use a little bit of alcohol to remove adhesive tape from a patient's skin. Saturate a cotton ball with the alcohol and rub it gently over the tape and skin until the tape loosens. Then continue moving the cotton between the tape and skin until all of the tape lifts off.

Betty Kapanak, RN

A removing experience

Here's an easy way to remove splinters embedded under fingernails and toenails. Instead of giving your patient an anesthetic (which is often as painful as the removal itself) and cutting through the nail, file the nail's *surface* with an emery board until the nail's paper thin. Then make a small cut into the nail with an iris scissors or scalpel. The splinter will be exposed and can easily be removed with forceps.

Susan B. Shipley, RN, MSN

Tick pick

To remove a tick from a patient's skin, cover the tick with petrolatum.

After a few minutes, the tick will suffocate and you can remove it painlessly with forceps.

Linda DeLuca, RN, BSN

Tarnished injuries
Some patients who come to the emergency department where I work have injuries covered with grease or tar. To remove the grease or tar without causing more pain or trauma, we gently wipe it off with gauze or cotton balls soaked in mineral oil. The oil cuts through the grease or tar quickly; then we can easily remove the oil with a liquid soap.

Kathleen Rohrer, RN

Painless removal of paint
To remove oil-base paint from the body, most people think first of using the solvent, turpentine. All well and good, but turpentine cannot be used around the eyes or mouth, for it can irritate and hurt. That doesn't help matters, especially with children, who are apt to have wiped their eyes with paint-covered hands anyway.

To solve this problem, use mineral oil. It's nonirritating and effectively removes paint.

Patricia L. Badowski, RN

Particle picker
When accident victims come to our emergency department covered with small glass particles, we remove the glass with our wall suction unit. We turn the unit on to medium or low and gently pass the suction tubing over the glass-covered area. Afterward, we throw away the tubing and carefully clean out the suction bottle.

Jerry Taylor, LPN

A glass act
Sometimes auto accident victims are covered with small glass fragments when they come to our emergency department. Brushing gently with a towel helps wipe away some of the fragments, but not all of them.

To remove the remaining glass, I wrap a piece of adhesive tape—with the sticky side out—around the fingers of one hand. Then I lightly touch the tape to the patient's skin. The glass lifts right off and doesn't fall onto the gurney or floor.

Nancy Jo Morgan, RN, BSN

It's oil for the better #2
You can use mineral oil (or baby oil) to remove fiberglass fibers from a patient's skin. Soak a cotton ball with the oil and coat the affected area. Then gently wipe the area with a terry-cloth towel to remove the fibers and ease irritation.

Susan Boisvert, LPN, SN

Vacuum cleaning
In the emergency department where I work, we use a hand-held, rechargeable vacuum cleaner to remove stones and dirt from patients' wounds. We also use it to remove glass particles from patients' skin, hair, and clothes without contaminating wounds or causing further injury.

Tom G. Bartol, RN

Thorn removal
We sometimes see patients in our emergency department who've fallen among cactus plants and have hundreds of small, hairlike thorns embedded in their skin.

If the patient shows no sign of a preexisting skin infection, we remove these thorns by applying a thin coat of white woodworking or household glue over the affected area with a tongue depressor. We allow the glue to dry for about 10 minutes and apply another coat. When this coat dries, we peel all the glue off in one sheet. With the glue come the pesky thorns. Finally, we scrub the area with povidone-iodine (Betadine) solution and apply an appropriate dressing.

William Ball, RN

A spirited cleanup

After removing a patient's cast, we wipe his skin with alcohol. The alcohol removes any dead skin and dirt that's accumulated under the cast, and it refreshes the skin as well. If the patient's skin is dry, we follow up with skin cream or lotion.

Connie Mongar, RN
Lisa Schill, LPN

Sting stuff

If you find yourself treating a lot of insect bites and stings, stock up on some Benylin cough syrup and Maalox. Just mix a small amount of the cough syrup with the Maalox and spread the mixture over the bite or sting area. It cuts down itching and pain and is soothing and cooling, too.

Jeannette Raschke, RN, BSN

Bath-time bolster

To keep skin pampered, pour some baby lotion into the water before bathing a patient. This eliminates the need to apply lotion after washing and drying (which patients appreciate if they're on complete bed rest). Also, baby lotion is an inexpensive substitute for bath oil. Diaphoretic patients especially will appreciate this.

Christy K. Greco, LPN

Blow-dry skin treatment

An extremely obese patient's deep folds of flesh present a real skin-care problem. After his bath, it's difficult to get the skin between these folds completely dry. As a result, the skin may break down.

To solve the problem, use a hair

blow-dryer. To be safe, set the dryer on a low speed and always keep it moving. Also test the airflow with your hand to make sure the patient's skin doesn't get too hot.

Besides preventing further skin breakdown, the blow-dry treatment gives the patient's medicated skin creams and powders a chance to work and keeps them from caking together.

Janet S. Ford, RN

Air fare

In the intensive care unit where I work, we recently had an unresponsive multiple-trauma patient with extensive skin breakdown and a *Candida* infection on both thighs and the perineum. To make matters worse, the patient was obese and flaccid, so we had difficulty exposing these areas to air.

To solve the problem, we put the patient in a supine position and applied padded restraints to her ankles. We flexed her knees, secured each ankle to the side rail, and put pillows between the rails and her ankles for padding and where needed for support. Then we draped a sheet over her knees and over a foot cradle (at the bottom of the bed). The patient was covered enough to maintain her modesty, yet her thighs and perineum got a good airflow, so her skin dried and healed quickly.

Cheryl Brown, LVN, SN

Preferred powder

Often, patients in our critical care units who are receiving steroids or have diabetes develop a yeast infection in the groin or under a pendulous breast. We apply powder to these areas to reduce moisture buildup and increase comfort.

But we've found that a cornstarch powder seems to make the infection worse, because the cornstarch and moisture from the skin act as a medium for yeast growth. Talcum powder, on the other hand, has a mineral base and doesn't promote yeast growth.

Doris K. Putland, RN, CCRN

It's a natural

To apply soothing, natural powder to moist, hard-to-reach areas of the body, get some cornstarch and two 4" × 4" gauze sponges. Unfold the gauze and place one on top of the other. Put about 2 tablespoons of cornstarch on the top gauze. Gather the corners and bind them together with a rubber band. Shake the pouch a few times until the cornstarch works its way through the gauze fibers.

This cornstarch pouch is an economic alternative for patients who can't afford expensive powder and puffs.

Alma G. Atkins

Soft and clean

For a quick, easy way to bathe a patient with dry skin, roll up one 6' long towel (cut from a bolt of terry cloth—it's less expensive that way), one regular towel, and two washcloths. Wet the towels and cloths in warm water mixed with 2 oz of a lanolin-based soap, then put them into a plastic garbage bag to keep them warm until you're ready to use them.

Place the large towel over the patient's body and massage gently. Use the smaller towel for back care, one washcloth for face care, and the other for perineal care.

The bath is warm and relaxing. And because no rinsing or drying is needed, you won't irritate the patient's sensitive skin.

Diana Lehmkuhl, RN

Oiled skin

A patient may balk at the discomfort of having his umbilical area cleaned. To prevent this, try using mineral oil. Apply the oil to the umbilicus before the patient's bath.

By the time you're finished bathing the patient, you can easily clean the umbilicus without scrubbing or causing him any discomfort.

Margery Lebel, RN, CCRN

Skin lotion potion

Cleaning dried fecal material from an incontinent patient is difficult. But a small amount of skin lotion applied with a soft cloth easily removes the material and prevents the dryness that soap can cause—even after rinsing with plain water. This technique is especially good for elderly patients and those with dry or fragile skin.

Elaine M. Neidert, SN

Peri-care(*fully*)

Some of the patients on our orthopedic unit are on complete bed rest for anywhere from several days to several weeks. I give the women perineal care this way:

I place a towel under the patient's hips and slide a bedpan under her, on top of the towel. Next I fill a clean container with warm soapy water, pour the water over the patient's perineum, and rinse with clear water. Then I remove the pan. (Applying a bit of lotion to the rim of the bedpan beforehand makes it slide out easily, without pulling the patient's skin or causing the water in the pan to spill.) Finally, I dry the patient with the towel and remove the towel.

Nurses and patients both like this procedure because it's easy to give— and to receive.

Allyson J. Maes, RN

A leak-proof bag

Sometimes patients undergoing peritoneal dialysis have a problem with
dialysate leaking onto their skin
around the catheter insertion site. We
solve this problem by cleaning the
skin, applying a Stomahesive wafer
around the insertion site, and applying a colostomy bag on top of the
wafer. We then pass the catheter
through the bottom opening of the
bag. Finally, we wrap rubber bands
around the bottom of the bag and
tubing to make it secure. The colostomy bag traps leaking dialysate
and protects the patient's skin.

Nancy L. Eder, RN

Rings on their fingers

Want to know a simple trick for
getting a ring off a swollen finger?
Use a few feet of string or silk suture.
Slip one end under the ring. Beginning next to the distal edge of the
ring, wind the other end of the string
toward the fingertip. The windings
should be close together to prevent
the swollen tissue from bulging
through. With the coils of string
tightly in place, take the short end of
the string on the proximal side of
the ring and pull it toward the tip of
the finger. This pulls the ring off
over the unwinding coil.

Evangeline Goodway, RN

Tongue depressors in hand

Some of my long-term care patients
have such severe hand contractures
that cleaning their hands is painful
for them and difficult for me. To make
the job easier and less painful, I
wrap some soft gauze around four
separate tongue depressors. Using two
of the depressors and some soap
and water, I gently insert them into
the patient's fist to clean the insides
of his fingers and palm. I use another
depressor to dry the area. With the
last depressor, I apply medicated
powder.

Cleaning the hands this way helps
prevent odor and infection without
too much discomfort for the patient.

Fe Perez, RN

Easy application

One of our patients recently had a
deep, sacral pressure sore. The doctor
ordered an ointment to be instilled
directly into the sore. But trying
to get the ointment from the jar to
the sore with a cotton swab proved
awkward.

To solve this problem, we asked
the pharmacist to put the ointment in
a tube. Then, to apply the ointment,
we put a new applicator tip from
a hemorrhoidal ointment preparation
on the tube. The pressure sore ointment went neatly into the sore, with
little waste.

Maria Schmitt, RN

Arm pads

When a patient has to wear an arm
splint for a long time, he could develop
pressure sores or skin breakdown.
To prevent such skin problems, pad
the splint with disposable sanitary
minipads. The pads cushion the skin,
absorb perspiration, and are inexpensive to replace.

Christine Destro, RN

Dressing guard

A sacral dressing can easily get
soiled if the patient is incontinent or
uses a bedpan. To keep the dressing
clean, simply tape a gauze sponge
to the edge. This way, fecal matter
will soil just the gauze, and you
can replace it without having to
change the whole dressing.

Sherman Hayhurst, LPN

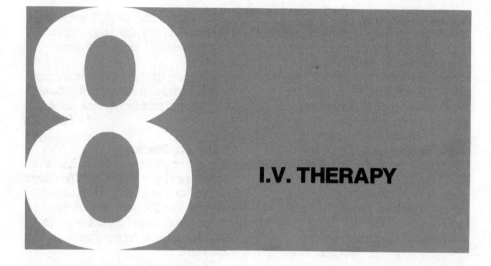

8 I.V. THERAPY

PREPARATION

Teaching first
Before performing venipuncture, consider patient teaching your first priority. Ask your patient if he's had an I.V. before. Tell him why he needs it, how venipuncture's done, and how much discomfort he'll feel.

Do your best to appear self-confident. Remember, patient anxiety can trigger vasoconstriction, making venipuncture more difficult for you and more painful for him.

Doris A. Millam, RN, CRNI, MS

A sticky problem
When starting an I.V. on a patient in isolation, you wear sterile gloves, of course. But the gloves may cause some problems.

For instance, the tape on the I.V. site can easily stick to the gloves instead of your patient's arm, and if you move your hand away, the I.V. could pull out.

To prevent this, wrap tape around each of your middle three fingers

over your gloves before you begin taping the I.V. in place. The tape on the I.V. site won't stick to your gloves as readily as before, the I.V. will stay put, and you—and your patient—won't have to worry about reinserting the I.V.

Terri Stambaugh, RN

Got you covered
On the pediatric outpatient unit where I work, I administer a lot of I.V. medications. Applying a tourniquet to the patient's arm before inserting the needle sometimes irritates the tender skin.

So for a pinchless venipuncture, I slip a disposable arm board cover over the child's arm, *then* apply the tourniquet. I roll back or cut a slit in the cover to expose the venipuncture site. Not only does the cover protect the patient's delicate skin, but the child also gets a kick out of his "instant sleeve."

Cathe Christo, LVN

Now, breathe deeply
Before inserting an I.V. needle, have

your patient practice a simple breathing exercise: inhale deeply through the nose and exhale slowly through the lips. Then, as you insert the needle, ask him to repeat this breathing technique. This will make him less tense, so the venipuncture will be smoother and less painful.

Sandra G. Ross, RN

Edema dilemma

Here's a way to insert an arterial or I.V. line into a patient's edematous arm:

Elevate the patient's arm and wrap it—from his hand to his shoulder—with an elastic bandage. Suspend the arm from an I.V. pole with another elastic bandage for 10 minutes. The edema will disperse and the forearm will return to normal size.

Then, with the sterile field and equipment prepared, quickly lower the patient's arm and unwrap his hand and lower forearm. Palpate the artery or vein, and you can insert the needle easily.

Lt. Melanie Thornton, ANC

Easy insert

Have to perform a venipuncture on a patient who has poor veins? Make it easier on yourself and the patient by using a blood pressure cuff. Put the cuff on the patient's arm and inflate it to about 100 to 120 mm Hg. This is low enough to avoid rupturing the vein but high enough to dilate it so you can easily insert the needle.

Immediately after you see a backflow of blood, thread the catheter about halfway, deflate the cuff, complete the threading, and securely tape the catheter to the patient's arm.

Cheri Knight, RN, BSN

Geriatips #1

Don't use a tourniquet to dilate a geriatric patient's veins before performing a venipuncture. His veins may look healthy, but they may actually be quite fragile; a tourniquet could cause a hematoma when the needle pierces the vein.

Instead, have the patient hang his arm at his side for a few minutes while he opens and closes his fist. Then lightly tap the area around the vein to dilate it.

If you must use a tourniquet, use only light pressure.

Karen L. Foster, RN

Squeezercise

If you have a patient with poor veins who needs frequent I.V. therapy, here's a simple exercise program to build up those veins.

Have the patient squeeze a small rubber ball in each hand as often as possible every day. In a few weeks, veins should protrude above the dorsal surface of the patient's hands, making the I.V. insertion much easier and less painful.

Jay M. Davis, MD, PhD

Put the squeeze on

Before starting an I.V. on a patient with poor veins, I have him squeeze a used grip from a pair of crutches. Squeezing makes his veins more visible and more easily palpated for successful venipuncture. And because the patient's concentrating on squeezing, the venipuncture is less painful for him.

Berna Knight, RN, BSN

Put the pressure on

If you have to insert an I.V. in the dorsum of a patient's hand and can't find his veins, simplify the search. Apply a blood pressure cuff to the patient's arm below the elbow. Then

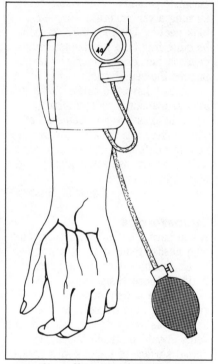

pump the cuff to 40 mm Hg and wait about 2 minutes for the small veins to appear on the hand.

The blood pressure cuff helps you locate veins better than a conventional tourniquet.

Larry K. King, RN

I.V.s in the bag
Our emergency department is always stocked with various kinds of I.V. start kits. We make them ourselves, using self-locking plastic bags filled with the following supplies:
• I.V. solution
• I.V. tubing
• I.V. angiocath
• tourniquet
• alcohol wipe
• bandage
• antibiotic ointment
• ½" tape.

In an emergency, the I.V. bags keep us from wasting time trying to find the supplies we need.

Eileen M. Suraci, RN

Venous equipment trayed
If you insert subclavian catheters frequently, set up a "Subclavian Tray." A simple, inexpensive plastic utility tray about 8" × 12" (the kind with a handle) holds all the necessary items:
• a prepackaged catheter
• sterile gloves and towels
• antiseptic skin preparation solutions
• gauze sponges
• syringes and needles
• paper tape and adhesive tape
• I.V. tubing and connecting tubing
• antibiotic ointment
• alcohol pads
• a CVP manometer.

Janeen Hendricks, RN

All boarded up
We used to have a real mess on our hands when our medication nurses were getting ready to set up I.V. medications. The I.V. bags would just lie in a heap at the nurses' station or on a medication cart while the nurses checked the information on the bags (patient's name, medication, dose, and route) against the doctors' orders. Now they hang the bags on a wooden I.V. board (which one of the nurses made) instead. The 23" × 11" board has 12 hooks (2 rows of 6 each) to neatly hold the bags while nurses check them and the orders.

Maj. Christina A. Santry, ANC

Getting it pegged
Don't waste time sorting through containers of I.V. additives and preparing I.V.s for patients. Instead, have the maintenance department make

a pegboard with long hooks to hang in the medicine room. Then, the pharmacist can prepare the additives, hang them on the hooks in the proper series order, and mark each hook with the patient's room number. Besides saving time, it also eliminates errors.

Espiranza Castellanos, RN

ADMINISTRATION

Making connections
When giving I.V. medication via a volume-control set, try securing the needle in the primary line's secondary port this way:

Cut a 3″ piece of 2″ wide adhesive tape. Fold over each end ½″ to make double-thick, nonadhesive flaps for easy removal. After inserting the needle into the port, center the tape (adhesive side up) under the connection, bring the tape ends up, and secure them to each other.

To remove the needle from the port, simply pull the flaps apart.

Joy Taurozzi, RN

No-fuss flush
When a patient is getting several incompatible drugs through one I.V. line, your work is really cut out for you: after each drug has been given, you have to draw up normal saline solution in a syringe, puncture the I.V. line, and flush the saline solution through the line.

To save time, use a piggyback set or Y-connector with a volume-control set to flush the line with normal saline solution from a hanging container. This way, you can start, stop, and control the amount of saline solution with a lot less fuss.

Anne E. Braun, RN, MSN

A pull tool
To remove a stubborn needle from I.V. tubing or a syringe, wrap one end of some Penrose drain tubing around the I.V. needle's hub and the other end around its adapter. As you twist in opposite directions, the Penrose tubing "grabs" the line to help you pull out the needle.

Nancy Perez Diatima, RN

A real loosener
Have you ever tried to loosen I.V. tubing or a distal port connector with a hemostat? If so, you know how easily the hemostat could slip and cause damage. Instead, use a flat tourniquet. Just wrap the tourniquet around the tubing or connector that needs to be loosened and twist. A tourniquet also works well in loosening tight lids on medication bottles.

Bonnie Forbes, RN

Getting disconnected
To disconnect stubborn I.V. tubing from the catheter hub, put a small piece of adhesive tape around the tubing and another piece around the hub. Twist firmly. The tape will give you enough traction so your fingers won't slip, and you can easily pull the tubing from the hub.

Andrea R. Mann, RN, MSN

It's a wrap
Occasionally you'll need to know an I.V. catheter's stock number or its length. Or you might quickly need the needle's size to determine whether you can administer blood through it. Of course, you could record this information on the I.V. tape, but if the tape gets wet, your notes will fade.

So save yourself some trouble and use the catheter's package label instead. Cut off the section that tells the needle's size, the catheter's length, and the stock number. You can mark the date and initials of the person starting the I.V. on this label and tape it on the I.V. dressing. Then you'll have a no-fade, ready reference for important I.V. information.

Charles F. Pike, Jr., RN

I.V. stop sign
When an I.V. is to be discontinued after the patient has absorbed all the fluid, tape a Band-Aid and a pack- aged alcohol swab on the I.V. bottle. Not only will this save time (no running to get these items when the I.V. stops), but it confirms at a glance the discontinue order.

Patricia Wilson, RN

I.V. flow formula
Here's a quick way to calculate the drops per minute in an I.V. flow rate when the drop factor is 15 gtt/ ml. Simply divide the hourly rate by 4. (When the drop factor is 10 gtt/ ml, divide by 6; when the drop factor is 12 gtt/ml, divide by 5.) The answer represents drops/minute.

For example, suppose the I.V. order reads "1,000 ml D_5W over 10 hours." (The hourly rate would be 1,000 ml ÷ 10 hours = 100 ml/hour.) To cal- culate drops per minute—given a drop factor of 15 gtt/ml—divide 100 by 4. The answer: 25 gtt/minute. Works every time.

Mangal Gupta, RN

Calculating fluid intake
Here's a quick way to calculate a patient's I.V. fluid intake. At the end of your shift, put a piece of paper tape on the I.V. bottle, then mark the date and amount of fluid in the bot- tle.

At the end of the next shift, the

nurse can simply subtract the amount of fluid still in the bottle from the amount marked on the tape. The result is the patient's I.V. intake for that shift. Then she can replace the paper tape with a new one so the next shift can measure intake.

Cynthia A. John, RN, BSN

Standardizing a heparin infusion
The doctor's order reads, "Heparin 900 units/hour I.V. diluted." Do you mix 50,000 units of heparin in 500 ml of D_5W and set the infusion pump at 9 ml/hour? Or mix 25,000 units of heparin in 500 ml D_5W and set the pump at 18 ml/hour?

Administer	Drops per min	Ml per hr
800 units/hr	16	16
850 units/hr	17	17
900 units/hr	18	18
950 units/hr	19	19
1,000 units/hr	20	20
1,050 units/hr	21	21
1,100 units/hr	22	22

If the hospital where you work standardizes its approach to heparin infusion, you won't have to decide. Northport (N.Y.) Veterans Administra- tion Medical Center uses a standard- ized approach. Doctors there write orders for heparin using only one standard format: "Heparin 25,000 units in 500 ml D_5W dose _____units/ hour." The pharmacy supplies the heparin in bags containing 25,000 units in 500 ml of D_5W. The doctor orders the dose and the nurses use the chart above to determine the pump setting that will deliver that amount/hour.

To further standardize the ap- proach, the nurses use only microdrip tubing that delivers 60 drops/ml through the infusion pump. In this way, the number of drops/minute set on the pump equals the delivery rate in ml/hour. Using this system, the nurse could let the same bag of heparin in D$_5$W hang for 24 hours before replacing it—even if the doctor changed the dose during that time. And any unused bags could be used for other patients because the mixture is always the same.

Nurses in the critical care unit (CCU) were very interested in improving heparin delivery. They started a research project to evaluate different delivery systems. All CCU nurses helped with the research, and the results were eventually adopted throughout the hospital. The new approach to heparin infusion is an example of nurses questioning and reviewing their practice—and making a change for the better.

Helen Weyant, RN, BS, CCRN

Warm and quick

When a trauma victim needs a blood transfusion, he needs it *fast*. But the usual ways of warming blood with hot water take up to 20 minutes. To save time, warm saline solution in a microwave oven and administer it— with the blood—through a Y set.

That's what they do in the emergency department (ED) at Geisinger Medical Center, Danville, Pa. When treating patients in hypovolemic shock, the ED staff members set their microwave oven (originally purchased for culinary purposes) to "high" and warm bags of saline solution in it for 2 minutes, raising the saline solution's temperature to 104° F. (40° C.).

When they administer the blood and the saline solution together, the saline solution warms the blood to about 84.2° F. (29° C.). This serves two purposes. First, it avoids problems caused by administering cold blood (for instance, hypothermia). Second, it decreases the blood's viscosity, making the blood run five to six times faster than it would if it were administered cold.

You wouldn't, of course, warm the blood itself in the microwave because the "cooking" would make the hemoglobin separate from the red blood cells.

Annals of Emergency Medicine,
April 1983

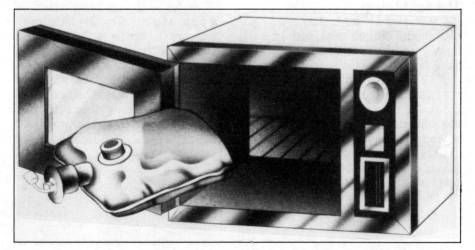

I.V. indicator

The self-adhering peel-back I.V. labels can save you time and effort. Here's one way to use them:

When you start an I.V., peel off the back of the right-hand side of the label and attach it to the I.V. bottle so the label markings align with those on the bottle. At the top of the label, mark the time the I.V. was started. This way, the label serves as a check on the absorption rate.

When the solution has been absorbed, remove the label, peel off the rest of the backing, and stick the label on the patient's chart. Besides the patient's name, the date, and room number, the label has space to write the fluids and medications administered. You can then complete the label information, adding when the I.V. was discontinued, the bottle number, rate of flow, and your signature. This completes the patient's record, eliminating the need for an I.V. stamp.

Labels are available for both 500-ml and 1,000-ml bottles.

Margaret E. Dunn, RN

The light touch

If you suspect I.V. infiltration in a patient with difficult veins, turn on a flashlight and hold it against his skin, directly over the suspicious site.

If I.V. fluid has infiltrated into the tissue, the beam will highlight the size of the infiltration. If no fluid has infiltrated, only a small halo will appear around the flashlight.

Using this trick can save you from having to do extra checks. Then, if necessary, you can stop the I.V. before the infiltration gets worse.

Betty Woodfin, RN

MAINTENANCE

Weight until the calm

The thrashing and pulling of confused, combative patients sometimes necessitates restarting I.V.s several times. So, after establishing an I.V., place a 5-lb sandbag under a standard arm board. Then wrap the sandbag, arm board, and arm with an Ace bandage. The weight of the sandbag, which can be varied as needed, keeps the arm immobile.

Ann Hensley, LPN

Gentle reminder

To remind a patient not to bend his hand or wrist when he has an I.V. inserted, try this. Cover a peri-pad with a washcloth, and tape the covered peri-pad to the patient's palm and forearm. This makes a soft, nonbulky arm board—a subtle reminder to the patient to keep his wrist or hand straight.

Lou Ann Jeffries, RN

PORTability

Say your patient has an intermittent I.V. device (such as a heparin lock or p.r.n. adapter). Try this technique to secure the needle to the port on the intermittent device.

Get a piece of adhesive tape and fold the ends to make tabs. Wrap the tape around the needle hub and port to hold them together. Bring the ends of the tape up so the two tabs

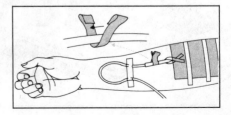

are free at the top.

Now the patient can move about without the danger of disconnecting his I.V. (For added security, tape a stress loop of tubing on the patient's arm.)

When the infusion is finished, grasp the tabs and pull the tape apart. You can remove the needle from the port without disturbing the intermittent device.

Sandra Ludwig Nettina, RN, BSN

Stretch to fit

Instead of swathing tape around a patient's forearm to keep his I.V. tubing and arm board in place, we use a piece of tubular stretch gauze bandage. After inserting the I.V. and taping the needle, we put a 10″

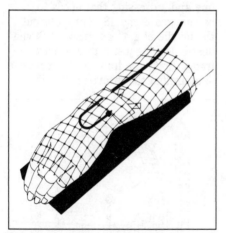

length of gauze over the I.V. site—from below the patient's wrist to his mid-forearm. Besides cutting down on tape, the stretch gauze provides extra protection for the I.V. site and can be rolled back for easy access to the site.

Patricia Varveri, RN, BSN

Free fingers

Next time you have to insert an I.V.

into a patient's finger or thumb, try immobilizing just the involved finger—not the entire hand—with a tongue blade.

Trim the tongue blade to the appropriate size, round the edges, and tape it to the finger. Or use a foam-padded aluminum finger splint, if one's available. Either way, the patient will be glad his hand is only minimally restricted.

Ann Neuser Lederer, RN

A stabilizing sandbag

If a pediatric arm board's not available when you're starting a child's I.V., tape a 1- to 5-lb sandbag to the child's arm or leg. The bag's weight limits movement of the extremity just as well as an arm board and stabilizes the I.V.

Jean A. Sandrock, RN

Improvised arm board

When you start an I.V. in a patient's lower forearm, wrist, or back of the hand, you may want to use something other than a conventional arm board for immobilization. An aluminum forearm splint works fine. It's comfortable, lightweight, and small enough to fit comfortably.

Darlene Lainchbury, RN

Boxed boards

If an I.V. arm board isn't available when you need one, just tape a washcloth or small towel around the empty I.V. tubing box and use that instead. The long, narrow box makes an excellent temporary I.V. arm board and saves you the time of looking for the real thing.

Carol Kenck Crispin, RN, MEd

A depressing splint

Children and I.V.s don't always mix

so well. For instance, even if a child resists the urge to pluck the I.V. out of his arm, he may bend his arm and inadvertently dislodge the I.V.

To prevent this, make a splint for the child's arm, using tongue depressors. Place some tongue depressors—enough to encircle the child's arm—side by side. Tape them together to make the splint. Cover it with a washcloth, and wrap it around the child's arm and the I.V. site. Tape the ends of the splint together, and it'll keep the child from bending his arm and dislodging his I.V. The splint's lightweight and easy to remove, too.

Dee Trottier, RN

Tape put-ons and take-offs

When taping a patient's I.V. needle to his arm, wipe the sticky underside of the tape (the section that will be next to his skin, not the ends that will attach to the arm board) with a cotton ball. Pieces of cotton stick to the tape, making a soft, nonirritating surface that can easily—and painlessly—be removed from the patient's skin.

Jeanine Whitaker, RN

Tug a tube

To protect a patient's Hickman catheter tubing against tugs or pulls at the catheter exit site, secure the tubing this way:

Loop a rubber band around the tubing and pin the rubber band to the patient's gown or pajama top. If the tubing is inadvertently pulled, the rubber band—rather than the catheter or patient—absorbs the pull.

M.I. Thomsen, RN, BSN

A gauze goody

In I.V. therapy, arm boards may present two problems: the adhesive tape used to anchor the board might irritate the skin, and, although multiple pieces of tape are used, the board may still be unsteady.

A solution is to place the arm board in the appropriate position and wrap 4″ gauze around the arm and board, securing the gauze with one piece of tape not in contact with the skin.

Besides saving the patient from tape irritation, the stability is particularly valuable when a patient is agitated or has to be moved.

Michele A. Cawley, RN, MN

Skin protection

Stomahesive can be used to protect the skin of a patient who has a central venous or Hickman catheter line and a dressing that needs to be changed every 48 hours. Cut out the middle of a 4″ × 4″ piece of Stomahesive, leaving just a thin, square frame. Apply the frame to the patient's skin around the insertion site. Then

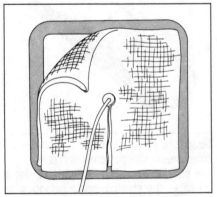

apply the dressing as usual (with a hole in the middle for the catheter or central venous line), and tape the dressing right to the frame. When you change the dressing, just pull the tape from the frame—not from the patient's tender skin.

Elizabeth Starkey, RN, BSN

Shower sleeve

The problem? How to keep an I.V. from getting soaked and becoming dislodged when the patient takes a shower.

The solution? Cover his arm with a long plastic bag that holds disposable drinking cups. Cut off both ends of the bag, slip it over his arm, and tape it at the wrist and upper arm with nonallergenic tape. The I.V. stays dry, and your patient can enjoy his shower.

Susan Freer, RN

Clean and dry

When a patient with an I.V. line in his hand or wrist wants to take a sponge bath, have him put on a sterile glove. The glove extends to about the mid-forearm, keeping the I.V. site clean and dry during his bath.

Cherri Bright Cronen, RN

Tender gloving care

If you use a heparin lock, instead of an I.V. line, to keep a patient's vein open, the lock and the dressing may get wet when the patient takes a shower. This will loosen the tape securing the I.V. needle, causing the needle to slip out.

Instead, keep the lock and dressing dry with an inexpensive, nonsterile examination glove. After cutting the fingers off the glove, slip it over the patient's arm. Fit the glove neatly over the lock and dressing, then wind hypoallergenic tape around the glove ends to seal the glove and affix it to the patient's arm.

Thanks to the glove, patients can take showers without worrying. And you don't have to waste time (and patients' money) reinserting I.V. needles and starting new heparin locks.

Sara M. Kerester, RN

Shower cap

Make showering easier for a patient who has a heparin lock: cut off the fingers (but not the thumb) from a plastic glove. Pull the glove over the patient's hand and wrist, covering the heparin lock with the thumb portion of the glove. Cover the insertion and dressing site with the rest of the glove and tape the ends of the glove to the patient's skin. The glove keeps the site dry and is easier to apply than plastic wrap.

Ann Damore, RN, BSN

Protected port

To stabilize a heparin lock in an active patient, use an eye bubble. After inserting the catheter and applying the dressing, tape the eye bubble over the infusion port and tubing. The clear plastic bubble protects the lock from accidental jostling, yet allows you to see the port. To inject medication into the port, just peel back the tape and remove the bubble. Replace the bubble when the medication's infused.

Lorrie Tatman, RN

Ideas that stick

Have you ever forgotten to readjust a patient's I.V. flow rate after the medication from his piggyback line has infused? Next time, try this reminder: tape a note over the dial on the infusion pump, reminding you to reset the dial to the proper rate.

Pam Kirk, RN, BSN

Quick trick for I.V.s

When the I.V. runs dry and you need to hang another bottle but air is in the tubing, here's a quick way to change bottles without breaking a closed system or introducing a needle into it. First, slide the drop regulator down the tubing as far as possible (usually to the Y-site) and close it. Remove the empty bottle and hang the new one. Squeeze the drip chamber to get fluid into it.

Then grasp the tubing just above the drop regulator, using your thumb and a hard object (such as your closed scissors or a pen) to compress it. Move your hand up the tubing, causing the fluid to push the air into the drip chamber. (Note: Your hand will slide easily if you first wet the tubing with an alcohol sponge.) Then release your grasp and turn on the I.V.

P. Seibel, RN

I.V. information
When checking I.V.s, use *one* master chart—just for I.V. information. The chart should have columns for the patient's name, age, room number, diagnosis, I.V. flow rate, type of solution, and amount left from the previous shift.

At the end of the shift, or during a slow period, transcribe the information onto the individual patient charts.

The master chart tells you at a glance which patients will need a new I.V. bag hung, and when. It saves time and steps.

Linda T. Dean, RN

Quick check for I.V.s
When you have several patients receiving I.V. fluids, a quick way to check on the absorption rate is to attach a piece of adhesive tape lengthwise to each bottle. At the top of the tape, mark the time the solution was hung. At the bottom of the tape, mark the time the solution should be absorbed. Midway between these two labels, mark the time when half the amount of the solution

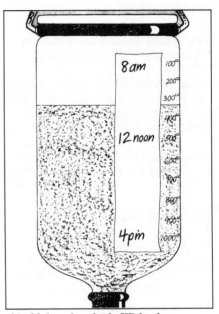

should be absorbed. With these markings, you'll be able to see at a glance whether the solutions are being absorbed on schedule.

Sylvia E. Platt, RN

I.V. check chart
Have you ever gone to check a patient's I.V. intake only to find the cardex in use? Do you find medicine cards too time-consuming to maintain? Then perhaps you'll like an I.V. chart.

It's easily made by cutting two pieces of cardboard to a size suitable for the number of patients' I.V.s you want to list, say $10'' \times 12''$ with enough room for eight patients. Cover both pieces of cardboard with attractive Con-Tact paper and cut the required number of holes about $2'' \times 3''$ in one piece. Using staples, tape, or paste, fasten the cut-out cardboard piece on top of the other, leaving space at the sides to insert small pieces of paper to show through the

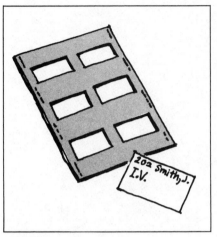

cut-outs.

Each patient's name, room number, and I.V. is put on a slip of paper. If a patient has several I.V.s, note each I.V. on a separate slip.

When a new I.V. is hung, place this slip in front of the old one. Thus, a quick glance at the chart tells what I.V. each patient has running at any specific time.

Nancy L. Scanlan, RN

Heparin lock(ed) in place

A heparin lock is inserted at such an angle that it may protrude and become dislodged. To remedy this, fill the space between the heparin lock and the patient's arm with some cotton or gauze. Place a piece of tape over the lock, leaving only the rubber port exposed. Now, no matter how active the patient is, the lock won't become dislodged.

Kathie M. Olney, RN

9

PREPARATION

Potassium pop
Ask your patient to try dissolving potassium bicarbonate (K-Lyte) tablets in a glass of lemon-lime soda instead of water. Disguised this way, the tablets' distinctive taste and effervescence may be more palatable.

Janice Kowalczyk, RN

Palatable potions #1
Patients who need to take potassium supplements usually complain about the bad taste of potassium powders and liquids. Mixing the potassium with equal parts of orange juice, ginger ale, and cranberry juice will make it a lot more palatable. For diabetics, use diet ginger ale and diet cranberry juice, and ask the doctor if orange juice is allowed.

Lilla Willey, RN

(Dis)solving the problem
Instead of waiting for a potassium chloride (K-Lyte) tablet to dissolve in a cold liquid such as orange juice,

try *warm* water. Put a small amount of water in a large glass. Add the K-Lyte tablet, and it'll dissolve immediately. Then add the orange juice or other cold liquid, and it's ready for your patient to drink.

David E. Riffel, LPN

Making medication tasteless
If your patient dislikes the taste of his medicine, tell him to suck on some ice for a few moments before you administer the medicine. The ice will numb his taste buds so the medicine will go down much easier.

Valerie Rubin Walsh, RN, BSN

Quick dissolve
If you have to administer tablets or capsules through a nasogastric tube because no liquid replacements are available, remember that the medication will dissolve more rapidly and completely in *warm* water. And since less warm water is needed to dissolve the medication, a patient on fluid restriction won't get too much liquid.

Barbara A. Matheus, RN, BSN

A valve in the vial

Filling a 50-ml syringe from several 10-ml vials is time-consuming— and frustrating. To speed up the process, insert a needle—minus syringe—and another needle with a syringe into the vial. The syringeless needle acts as an air valve, allowing air into the vial so the medication comes out faster.

Christine Masleid, RN, BSN

Get it on tape

When I have a lot of injectable medications to administer, I follow this procedure to prevent them from getting mixed up. First I prepare the syringes. Then I cut 1″ × 1″ pieces of adhesive tape. On each piece of tape I write the patient's name and room number, name of the medication, dosage, route of administration, and time he should receive it. I place each piece of tape on the appropriate needle cover so it doesn't obstruct my view of the barrel. Preparing and identifying all the injectables at once this way saves me time. And I'm sure I've got the right patient, the right drug, the right dose, the right route, and the right time.

Anne Casey, LPN

Twist-off cap off

If you're ever stuck with a hard-to-open pour-bottle of liquid medication, try wrapping any flat piece of rubber 1½ times around the cap. You'll find that the cap will unscrew with just a gentle twist.

Rubber tourniquets are ideal.

Diane Puta, RN

That's the breaks

Here's an easy way to break a scored pill in half. Just insert a sterile needle into the groove. The pill will break apart cleanly.

Barbara Birkenberger, RN

Scalped pills

Keep a disposable scalpel on your medication cart to cut pills in half. Just remember to clean the scalpel with a povidone-iodine or alcohol swab before and after each use.

Carol Brower, RN

Regular checkups

If you're a school nurse, checking expiration dates on vaccines and medications can be a tedious job. But it's a job that has to be done regularly.

To make the checking easier and less tedious, post a 3-year chart in your injection room. The chart should have a space for each month— from January 1986 to December 1988. When a new vaccine or medication comes in, record its expiration date in the appropriate month. Since you can see at a glance what medications will be outdated the next month, reordering is easier, too.

H. Irene Miller, RN

Medication refrigeration

Store aluminum hydroxide (Amphojel) in the refrigerator. When the medication's cool, it doesn't leave a chalky sensation in the patient's mouth. Also, the patient seems more aware of the drug's cool temperature than of its unpleasant flavor.

Penny Pica, RN

Special list

Before distributing medications from the unit-dose cart, quickly thumb through the medication sheets and make a list of other-than-routine administration times. Also list patients receiving hourly doses of a particular medication as well as patients receiving I.V. medications. Then use this list to ensure giving all medications at the time ordered.

Ellen Ludin, RN

Cold therapy

To reduce pain, irritation, and ecchymosis at the site of a subcutaneous heparin injection, place an ice pack on the injection site for 3 to 5 minutes before and after the injection. This helps most patients.

Marla Sandusky, RN

Cold comfort

Before giving your patient a rectal suppository, peel off the foil and place the suppository in a 30-ml plastic cup filled with ice chips for a few minutes. The ice keeps the suppository firm, and, as it melts, it lubricates the suppository for an easier, more comfortable insertion.

Sylvia T. Joseph, RN

Love the gloves

To warm a bottle of eardrops, fill a Styrofoam cup half full with very warm water. Stretch an examination glove over the rim of the cup with the fingers extending down into the water, and place the bottle in the glove. The eardrops will get warm, and the label will stay dry and intact. Also, you needn't worry about the eardrops becoming diluted.

Paula Breton, RN

ADMINISTRATION

Spoon-fed meds

Many of our geriatric patients have trouble taking a pill from a medicine cup. They can't tilt their heads back or open their mouths wide enough to swallow the pill.

So I drop the pill from the medicine cup onto a spoon, place the spoon in the patient's mouth, and lay the pill back on the patient's tongue. The pill is back far enough in the patient's mouth for easy swallowing. What's

more, the spoon helps prevent spills and unnecessary handling of the medication.

L.P. Brown, RN

Let them down easy

If a patient has difficulty swallowing a pill or capsule, dip the pill in maple syrup first. The pill will slide down the patient's throat more easily this way.

Dianne Charron, RN, BSN

Go with the flow

When a patient has trouble sipping water and can't swallow tablets or capsules, a squeeze bottle with a long, narrow curved spout (the kind athletes use for water) may help him.

Place the pill on the patient's tongue, direct a stream of water on the pill, and the pill will flow toward the back of the tongue. Then the patient can swallow the pill—without spilling any water on himself, his bedclothes, or the floor.

Barbara Naunchek, RN

What's the word?

When administering antibiotics through a heparin lock, do you ever have trouble remembering each step? Use this acronym to help remember the procedure:

*S*aline, 2 ml—to clear the lock
*A*ntibiotic—through the lock
*S*aline, 2 ml—again, to clear the lock
*H*eparin—to keep the lock patent.
"SASH" works fine, but you can make up your own reminder based on the procedure used at the hospital where you work.

Shirley Costanza, RN

Easy dose it

Babies and toddlers who've had

surgery are frequently given antibiotics by mouth because their I.V. lines have been discontinued. We've found a way to give these liquid medications without spills and dribbles. We cut the tip off a disposable nipple, pour the medication into the tip, and let the child suck on it. The baby gets an accurate dose, and we save time.

Susan R. Potts, RN

Syringe versus spoon

Oral antibiotics are prescribed for many of the babies brought to an emergency department. You usually administer the first dose, using a syringe to squirt the medication into the baby's mouth, then give the baby's mother the prescription for the remaining doses. But if the baby needs a second dose during the night—before the mother can get to a pharmacy—give her a single dose to take home.

A disposable syringe makes an ideal container for a single dose of oral medication. When you give the initial dose, show the mother how to use the syringe safely.

E. Rogers, RN

Let's pretend

Trying to get a 2 year old to take medicine can be a real battle. Before he has to take antibiotics or cough medicine, pretend to give some to a doll. After watching a "sick" dolly take the medicine, the child will happily take his dose.

Patricia Trefethen, RN

Hugging mommy

Here's a way to make preoperative injections less traumatic for young children, and for you, too. Have the child sit on his mother's lap and hug her while you're giving the injec-

tion. Hugging mommy gives the child a feeling of security and keeps his muscles relaxed while you're inserting the needle. If the child begins to fight back, his mother simply hugs him tighter. This is much nicer than having strangers hold the child while he's getting his injection.

Phyllis A. Smith, RN

Icing on the ache

One of my pediatric patients who required weekly allergy shots was absolutely terrified of the needle. I asked him to hold an ice pack against his injection site before I gave him the shot. The site became numb so he felt no needle stick or pain, and his fear subsided.

Now, although he still isn't happy about getting his weekly injections, he accepts them bravely.

William P. Taylor, CCFP

Muscle relaxer

Do you notice that a patient usually tightens his gluteal muscles in anticipation of an I.M. injection? If so, he's in for more discomfort than necessary.

To help divert his attention, ask him to wiggle his toes just before you give the injection. While he's concentrating on his toes, he won't tighten the gluteal muscles, so the injection will be less painful.

Kathleen A. Wallace, LPN

A rule of numb

To make immunizations and injections less painful for pediatric patients, place an ice cube on the injection site for about 15 seconds. Then quickly blot the skin dry with a tissue, clean the site with an alcohol preparation pad, and give the injection. The ice numbs the skin so the patient won't feel the needle's pinch. After this painless experience, most patients don't fear their next injection.

This icy tip works just as well on older patients who cringe a bit when an injection is ordered.

Mary Lu Rang, RN, BSN

Meds and mineral oil
When you administer crushed pills through a nasogastric tube, do you find that some of the medication sticks to the sides of the tubing? Here's a way to make sure all of the medication *really* goes down the tube.

If the doctor approves, mix a few drops of mineral oil with the crushed pills to form a paste. Add water or juice and pour this solution into the tube. The mineral oil keeps the medication from sticking to the sides of the tubing, assuring you that the patient gets his proper dose.

Angelina H. Fabello, RN

A fix on mixing
Administering a syrupy mixture of magnesium citrate and activated charcoal through a nasogastric (NG) tube can be really messy—especially when you have to pour the mixture into a 50-ml syringe first so you can inject it into the NG tube.

My solution is to pour the mixture into a tube feeding bag instead of a syringe. The bag, of course, has a larger opening than the syringe. I close the bag, shake it, and connect it to the NG tube with an adapter. Then I hang the bag and position the clamp to regulate the flow. The mixture is administered with no mess.

Barbara Doll, RN

Pick your flavor
If your patient dislikes milk of magnesia's taste, try adding a little of the flavoring designed for liquid dietary supplements. Some supplements offer pecan, cherry, lemon, orange, and strawberry flavors.

Whatever flavor your patient chooses, chances are it'll help his medicine go down easier—and with no unpleasant aftertaste.

Jocelyn Moritz, RN

Band it
Instead of using tape to secure a topical application of nitroglycerin (Nitrol) on a patient's arm, use a stretch terry cloth wristband. The patient won't have to remove and put on more sticky, irritating tape each time he needs another application.

Ruth Petkus, RN

Bags are better
To cover an application of nitroglycerin paste on a patient's arm, use a plastic sandwich bag instead of plastic wrap. With its bottom cut off, the bag fits over most arms like a sleeve and stays secure with just a bit of tape. Best of all, it doesn't snarl as easily as plastic wrap.

Sara Wister, RN

Down the straw
If a patient needs a nitroglycerin tablet but can't place the tablet himself—or even lift his tongue to let you place it—a drinking straw can help.

Just put one end of the straw under his tongue and drop the pill down the straw. Pull the straw back slightly, then lift the tongue with the straw to make sure the tablet's properly positioned. If everything checks out, remove the straw.

Zoe Margolis, RN, BS

Two 4″ × 4″s = convenience
A hint for the next time you need to

instill drops in a patient's eyes: First lay a sterile 4″ × 4″ gauze pad on your work surface to serve as a clean field. Put your supplies (bottle top, eye patch, or whatever) on the gauze pad. Wrap another gauze pad around your finger so you can easily clean and hold open the patient's eyes, remove secretions, and catch excess drops on the patient's cheeks.

Gail C. Skinner, RN

Single file

If you give many medications by I.V. push, you know these medications require various amounts and kinds of diluent and can be given safely at various speeds. However, if you can't take the time to read the detailed literature each time you give a medication, solve the problem with a recipe box. Keep a file card for each medication in alphabetical order. Each card should include information about dilutions, rates for pushing, alternate names, side effects, contraindications, and other pertinent information. This is a valuable tool for new nurses, especially in emergencies.

Ruth L. Horman, RN

Med trays made fun

Those plastic trays sometimes sold at fast-food restaurants can double as medicine trays for pediatric patients. They're durable, inexpensive, stackable, and have spaces for drinking cups, medicine cups, and syringes.

Best of all, the trays are brightly decorated with the fantasy, TV, and movie characters popular among children. And a familiar face (even if it *is* on a medicine tray) can do much to make a youngster more comfortable with unfamiliar hospital routines.

Donna Mahedy, RN, PNP

A speedy, safe way to identify drugs for cardiac arrest

Coping with cardiac arrest requires various drugs in syringes—quickly identifiable. And there's always a risk they might get mixed up. In some hospitals, the syringes are labeled by someone writing directly on the barrel with pencil or felt pen. Here's a way to do it quickly—and safely.

Take ½″ wide adhesive tape. On it write the names and dosages of various drugs needed in an emergency. Then cut the tape into separate labels and stick them on a sheet of clean X-ray film. This doesn't affect their adhesive property.

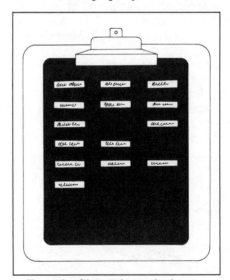

Keep the film and attached tape strips on the cardiac emergency cart. Then, in arrest, merely pull off the right label and stick it on the syringe.

This not only saves time—it always assures having a record of the drugs actually used during the resuscitation. It also simplifies figuring what drugs to replace afterwards.

Catherine A. Baden, RN, MS

DOCUMENTATION

Medication information

Here's a way to keep track of medications administered on a unit. Post a sheet of paper on the door of the narcotics cabinet. As each narcotic (sedative, pain-reliever, or whatever) is administered, record on the sheet the patient's name, room number, medication, and time it was administered. The sheet provides (1) a quick reference to indicate when a patient received his last medication, (2) a vital information list for the shift report, and (3) a checklist for the narcotic count at the end of each shift.

A.E. Siminski, RN

Charting campers' care

If you're a camp nurse, record the medications and treatments given campers on separate charts. Then for easy reference, tape the charts to the medication cupboard.

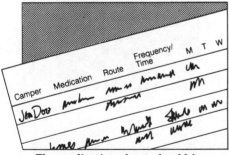

The medication chart should have columns for the campers' names, their medications, and the routes, frequency/time, and day of administration.

The treatment chart should have a column for the campers' names, plus columns for listing their complaints, treatments given, and comments.

These handy forms help you chart efficiently and accurately—even when hordes of campers report in at medication time or when they limp in with bruises and scrapes after sports time.

Susan Maurer, RN

P.R.N. list

Ever have trouble remembering to give p.r.n. medications? Just keep a p.r.n. list on the medication cart. The list should have columns for time of request, patient's name, medication requested, and medication given. Never fill in the last column until *after* you've given the medication.

Now you have a fast, accurate way to check the medications given if the narcotics count is ever off at the end of the day. And patients get faster service, too.

Vivian Hall, RN

Double check on drugs

To prevent drug interactions, you need to know what medications a patient is taking when he's admitted to the hospital and where those medications are being kept during his hospitalization. Recording this information on the back of the patient's cardex works well. The information is right at your fingertips whenever it's needed.

Doris Sedberry, LVN

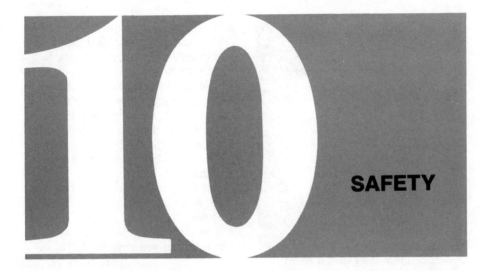

PATIENT SAFETY

Shock stopper
To protect patients with temporary pacemakers from electric shock, cover the pacemaker's unconnected wires with rubber tops from used Tubex syringes. The rubber tops ground the wires and can easily be removed when the wires are needed.

Bernie Stremikis, RN, BSN

Wrist watching
When a patient has I.V.s infusing in both wrists, what do you do with

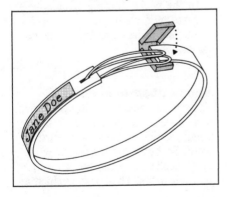

his wrist identification (ID) band? If the I.V. in the wrist with the ID band infiltrates, the wrist might swell, making the band too tight and impairing circulation.

To prevent this, make a slit in one end of the wristband before you put it on the patient. Put a rubber band through the slit, pull the two loop ends of the rubber band into the metal clasp, and close the clasp. Now you have a stretch wristband that will "grow" if necessary.

Sally Sumner, RN

Mouth guard magic
If a comatose patient with cerebral hemorrhage continually grinds his teeth and bites his lower lip, prevent further damage by using a football mouth guard. Soften it in warm water, and fit it over his lower teeth. Next, thread trach tape through the first hole of the guard's 6″ helmet strap. Finally, run one tape end over each ear and tie the ends behind the patient's head—loosely enough to be comfortable, but tightly enough to hold the guard in place if he coughs.

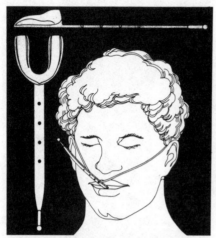

You can buy the guard at most sporting goods stores.

Tina Sykes, LPN

A lid latch

Do you find that a commode lid has a penchant for slamming shut just as you lower a patient onto the seat? Not only is this frustrating to you, but it's also dangerous to the patient. Here's a way to keep the lid raised.

Get a Velcro book latch (usually used to hold large chart pages open). As shown in the illustration, the

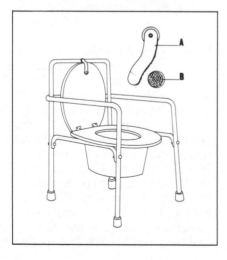

book latch has two parts: a long tab (A) and a circle (B). (Both parts have adhesive backs that stick to almost any surface.)

Attach the adhesive side of B to the underside of the commode lid. Then attach the adhesive side of A to the front of the commode frame with one end of the tab hanging down. (The tab's Velcro side should face backward.)

Before you help a patient onto the commode, lift the lid. Bring tab A up over the lid and secure it to circle B on the lid. The lid will remain raised until you undo the latch.

Ruth C. Flowe, LPN

Socks to swim in

While working at a camp for crippled children, I noticed a recurring problem when campers with spina bifida were in the swimming pool. Lacking sensation in their feet and legs, these children scraped their feet against the pool's side or bottom and got nasty abrasions, some of which became infected.

To prevent this, we put terry-cloth tennis socks on the children's feet before they went into the pool. This way they could splash to their hearts' content without scraping their feet. What's more, the socks didn't interfere with the pool's filtering system.

Next year, we'll add tennis socks to our list of camp clothing suggestions.

Pat Hunter, RN

Shock-absorbing sock

Some of my patients who take prednisone develop bruises on their arms when they do housework or yard work. So I suggest they wear white sport socks (with the feet cut off) on their arms. The socks cushion any impact and are easily hidden under long-sleeved shirts and blouses.

Techia McGrath, RN

Geriatips #2

Sometimes an elderly patient's skin is so fragile, thin, and dry that just a slight bump will tear it.

To prevent this, we cut stockinette into different lengths and put it over the patient's vulnerable areas (such as his forearms and elbows). The stockinette is like an extra layer of skin and really does decrease the incidence of skin tears.

Debbie L. Hill, LPN

Pad-a-tub

To keep our patients from slipping and falling in the bathtub on our unit, we put an egg-crate-like mattress in the bottom of the tub. The mattress gives the patients a sure footing when they get into and out of the tub. It also pads the tub, making it more comfortable to sit in. After a patient's bath, we either discard the mattress or squeeze the water out of it and let it dry for next time.

Joyce Kron, RN

Taped ties

For the patient who has a tracheostomy tube, aspirating a loose thread from the frayed ends of the ties is always a worry. But eliminating this worry is simple: just cover the ends of the ties with nylon tape. To further ensure the patient's safety (and comfort), knot the tie at the side rather than the back of his neck, so it won't cause irritation when he lies on his back.

Diana Contine, RN

Customized chairs

If a patient constantly gets his arms

and legs stuck in the side openings of a geriatric wheelchair, solve the problem by using plywood inserts to fit the chair sides. Make long, narrow pillows to pad the plywood. Then the patient has freedom of movement and can't get himself into dangerous positions. This idea can be adapted to other situations, too. For instance, make "bumper pads" from pillows to cover the side rails of the patient's bed.

Ruth Gault, RN

Emergency necklace

A patient who has a fractured mandible that's wired and banded should always keep wire cutters nearby in case of an emergency. But remembering to carry the wire cutters with him can be a problem. That's why we make a "necklace" from tracheostomy tape and put the wire cutters on the tape. The patient wears the necklace wherever he goes (except to bed, when he leaves it on his bedside table) so the wire cutters are always handy in an emergency.

Vicki Cornish, RN, BSN

Crash bag

When we transfer a critically ill patient from our emergency department to a critical care unit, we send a monitor and defibrillator along with him. But we also send along a plastic drawstring bag filled with alcohol wipes and prefilled syringes of atropine, epinephrine, lidocaine (lignocaine), and sodium bicarbonate. If the patient should need life-support measures during the transfer, these necessary supplies will be right at hand.

Later, the plastic bag is sent back to the emergency department. We refill it and hang it on a wall hook for the next time.

Kathleen Rohrer, RN

Finding yourself
As you go from one patient's room to another, you can easily forget which room you're in if the number's not posted inside. This could cause a delay if you had to call a code or call for help.

To prevent this problem, mark each room's telephone (or some other central object) with the room number on fluorescent tape. Or use a fluorescent marker or crayon to write the number on white paper, then tape it to the phone.

Whichever way you choose, the room number will be clearly visible—even in the dark.

Margaret Beckert, RN

A scale tale
Some of our nursing home residents are afraid of falling when they step on the scale to be weighed. To ease their fears, I put a walker behind the scale—with the handgrips extending toward the front of the scale. Now the residents just have to hold onto the walker for a surefooted step up. (For an accurate weight measurement, the walker mustn't touch the scale, and the resident must let go of the walker once he feels secure on the scale.)

Susan R. Poliski, LPN

Milk out, syringes in
I tell my home care patients who have diabetes to discard their used syringes in empty milk cartons. They can drop the syringes into the carton through the spout, then tape the carton shut before throwing it away.

Disposing of syringes this way

keeps children and others from hurting themselves with loose needles and (especially in high-crime areas) conceals the fact that syringes are available in the home.

Mary K. Hill, RN

Evac-pack
When we have tornado warnings, we have to evacuate patients from our alcoholism rehabilitation unit to an underground tunnel. Sometimes we have to stay in the tunnel for as long as an hour or more, and the patients get restless.

To alleviate their boredom and to be prepared in case of an emergency, we've prepared a "tornado pack." These items—stored in a wash basin and enclosed in a plastic bag—are included in our pack:

alcohol swabs	name bands
ammonia ampuls	pens
Band-Aids	plastic cups
battery-powered	playing cards
radio	prepackaged
blood pressure cuff	towelettes
emesis basin	safety pins
flashlight	stethoscope
hard candy	tissues
Kardex with patient	tongue blades
census	

The pack is always ready to move whenever we are.

Terry Clayburn, RN
Rita Biggs, LPN

Wheelchair safety
To stress wheelchair safety and make it enjoyable, nurses at Memorial Hospital of Southern Oklahoma, Ardmore, offer a special class in wheelchair safety and award a "driver's license" to employees and volunteers who complete the class.

Personnel assigned to transporting patients in wheelchairs attend a 1½-hr class where they learn how to ascend and descend a ramp with an occupied wheelchair; how to use footrests; how to comfortably secure a helpless patient in a wheelchair; and more. After the class, participants receive a driver's license.

The director of inservice education at the hospital, says she plans to put the "rules of the halls" on the back of the license. For now, though, personnel are proud of their driver's license—and their proven skill in transporting patients.

Lenna Lee Davidson, RN, MPH

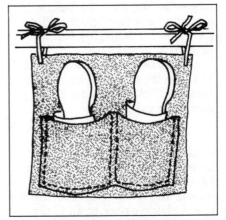

keep them handy at all times.

Linda Barr, RN, CCN

Slipper holder

Do your patients' slippers seem to play hide-and-seek under their beds? Retrieving these slippers is not only a nuisance for you, but also a danger for patients, especially the elderly and those with balance problems or limited vision.

Make a slipper holder. All you need is a piece of heavy-duty cloth or canvas, about 16" wide × 10" long. Stitch two pockets—about 6" × 8" long— to the front of the cloth. Attach strings to the upper corners so the holder can be tied to the side rail or frame of the bed.

Becky Schroeder, RN

A pedigreed clamp

I teach my patients who have indwelling central venous catheters to use bulldog clamps instead of plastic or padded Kelly clamps, which are not only awkward but may damage the catheter. The bulldog clamps are small, lightweight, inexpensive, easy to handle, and don't need to be padded. And they fit easily on neck chains or bracelets so patients can

Remote control

If you worry about patients who smoke in bed without supervision, you may be interested in the *Smoker's Robot*, a "long-distance" cigarette holder.

You place the heavy chrome-plated base on a flat surface away from the patient, then put a lit cigarette in the holder on the base. A 38" long

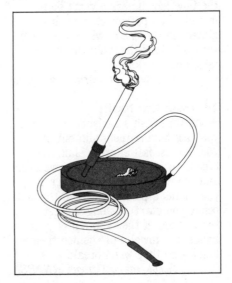

tube extending from the base is capped with a mouthpiece for the patient. Ashes fall safely into the base's tray.

The *Smoker's Robot* is available for $10 from the Cleveland Orthopedic Company, 3957 Mayfield Rd., Cleveland, Ohio 44121.

Diane M. May, RN, MS

A glass assignment

A patient's eyeglasses can easily be knocked off his bedside table and broken. To prevent such an accident, I tape a plastic emesis basin to the table and write the word "glasses" on

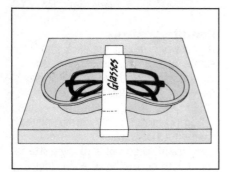

the tape (so the basin won't be removed). The patient can put his glasses in the basin, where a sudden jolt won't send them sliding off the table and breaking.

Laurie Roper, LPN

To towel the tooth

When you wash a patient's dentures, you risk having them slip out of your hands, fall into the sink, and break. To prevent this expensive loss and the resulting inconvenience to your patient, place a towel in the sink before you start washing the dentures. Then, if they slip out of your hands, the towel will cushion their landing so they won't break.

Cheryl Hanka Darsow, RN, BSN

Denture dots

Has the "lost denture epidemic" struck the hospital where you work? You know the causes: a patient removes his dentures and puts them on his meal tray or beside his pillow instead of in his denture cup. Later, when the tray is taken away or the bed is changed, the dentures are inadvertently thrown out or they fall on the floor and break.

We've halted this epidemic by placing a self-adhesive red dot on the headboard of the bed of each patient who wears dentures. We put another red dot on the patient's cardex. The dots remind staff to look carefully for stray dentures on meal trays before removing them, among linens when changing beds, and in tissues and cups when straightening the bedside tables. When the patient leaves the hospital, the red dot is removed from the bed and the cardex.

Our red dot prevention program has saved our hospital a lot of money—no more lawsuits against the hospital for broken or lost dentures, no more staff time spent looking for lost dentures. And it's saved our patients the inconvenience of being without their dentures.

Barbara S. Vosburgh, Patient Relations Service

Cup 'a loot

In the emergency care center where I work, we ask patients who have midarm or hand lacerations to remove their rings, bracelets, and watches from the affected arm or hand. To make sure these valuables don't get lost, stolen, or misplaced, we put them in a small, clean specimen container or sputum cup with a lid. Then the patient can hold the cup, and we're all sure that his valuables are safe.

Cindy Sue Goertz, RN

NURSE SAFETY

Red = Caution
While transferring a patient with a halo apparatus from his bed to a wheelchair, the metal rods on the apparatus may stab you in the head or chest.

To prevent this, cover each protruding rod end with a red rubber stopper from a blood-collection tube, then secure the stopper at its base with tape.

The bright red stoppers warn you to keep your distance from the rods, and if you still get too close, they cushion the blow. They also serve as conversation starters and tension relievers, encouraging patients and their visitors to smile and make the best of a difficult situation.

Margaret Capitelli, RN

Ampules—just in a case
I always carry ammonia ampules with me for patients who feel faint. To prevent the ampules from getting crushed in my pocket, I carry them in an empty plastic thermometer case. Two ampules fit in the base and one fits in the cap. When I need one, I can easily remove the ampule with my fingers or a hemostat.

Sylvia T. Joseph, RN

A high-rise bed
How can you raise the head or foot of a heavy hospital bed to place shock blocks under the wheels without injuring yourself in the process?

Ask the maintenance department to cut notches on the ends of two 18" broad-based blocks of wood. We call

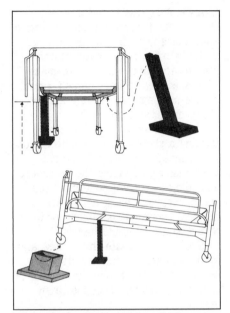

these blocks "high holders." Then raise the *entire* bed as high as it will go. Place one high holder under each side of the bed frame (next to the frame's crossbar, for added support) at the head or foot of the bed, depending on which end you want to elevate (see first illustration). Be sure the bed frame is resting securely in the notch of each high holder and that the patient is lying still; then lower the bed to its lowest position. The wheels on the end you want elevated will be raised off the floor. Now place the shock blocks on the floor under these wheels (see second illustration).

Again raise the bed as high as it will go. This will take the weight off the high holders so you can remove them easily. Then, lower the bed again so its front (or rear) wheels are resting on the shock blocks.

Denise Emerson, RN, BSN
Timothy Rice, NA

Check out the moves

When a staff member recovers from a sprain or strain (frequently suffered while lifting a heavy patient) and returns to work, we want to make sure she doesn't hurt herself again. So the nursing supervisor does a "body mechanics review."

She observes the employee performing a procedure similar to the one that caused the injury. If the employee isn't performing the procedure according to correct body mechanics, the supervisor refers her to the physical therapy department for instructions in body mechanics.

Staffers appreciate this review and so does hospital administration— because it helps reduce the number of repeat injuries and time lost from work.

Joanne Breden, RN

Traction protection

Bars protruding from a traction setup are not only a nuisance, but also dangerous to staff and visitors. Make them injury-proof by placing soft sponge rubber balls on the protruding ends. The balls cushion any contact with the sharp ends. And, since you use bright red balls, people see them from a distance *before* coming in contact with the bars.

Della Anderson, RN

Handle-with-care packet

Nurses in our hospital who administer I.V. antineoplastic drugs get a "chemotherapy administration and disposal packet" from the sterile supply department.

The packet comes in a heavy polyethylene bag and includes:
• a card with written instructions for the use and disposal of the packet's contents

• two polyethylene disposal bags
• a 3" × 2" label printed with the word BIOHAZARD
• one disposable, water-repellent gown with elastic cuffs
• one face mask
• latex examination gloves
• preparation mat (made of absorbent material and coated with plastic on the back).

After the drugs are administered, all chemotherapy materials are placed in one of the disposal bags, double-bagged in the other one, and discarded.

The packet is an inexpensive, convenient way to make sure hazardous drugs and equipment are disposed of properly.

Sandra G. Jue, PharmD

Needles: Take cover

Here's an easy way to prevent unwanted needle jabs when you set up a piggyback I.V. line. After you attach the needle to the tubing port, tape the needle cover to the I.V. pole. Later, when you're ready to discard the needle, put the cover back on it. This way, you won't get stuck by the discarded needle.

Barbara Birkenberger, RN

Protection *capability*

Add one more item to the stash in your uniform pockets: the protector cap from an irrigation syringe. Use it whenever you have to snap open a glass ampule. Just insert the top of the ampule into the protector cap and snap the ampule open. No more worry about cutting your fingers on shreds of glass.

Liz Barnes, RN

An ampule opening

To safely and easily open glass medication ampules, use a foil alcohol-wipe envelope.

Open the envelope and remove the wipe for later use. Insert the top of the ampule into the envelope, break the ampule, and remove its bottom portion, which contains the medication. The envelope's foil and plastic lining will protect your fingers from glass slivers.

Then discard the envelope and the rest of the ampule.

Susan L. Irwin, RN

Pop top protection
When giving medications, how often do you find yourself in such a hurry that you pop the top off an ampule without using gauze or cotton to protect your fingers? A solution is to carry a nipple in your pocket. Just place the nipple over the ampule and snap the top off—no more nicked or cut fingers. You can easily clean the nipple with alcohol to prevent cross-contamination.

Harold L. Hardgrave, LVN

For openers
Next time you break open a medication ampule, protect your fingers from the glass with a rubber diaphragm from an I.V. bottle. Wrap the diaphragm around the ampule, then break off the ampule's top. Also, with a diaphragm, you don't risk getting alcohol in the medication, as you would if you used a foil alcohol preparation packet.

Sue Evers, RN

COST AND TIMESAVER TIPS

EQUIPMENT

Resuscitated manikin

When your resuscitation manikin wears out, here's how to replace the body. Remove its head and shoulders and disengage its chest mechanism. Then make a small slit inside the shoulder insert. Through this slit, tightly stuff Dacron batting (purchased at a local upholstery store) into the manikin's arms, legs, and abdominal area. After replacing the chest mechanism, continue stuffing until the manikin is filled. Put a vinyl patch over the slit in the shoulder to seal the stuffing securely.

Finally, reattach the manikin's head and neck band, and it is as good as new—but at a fraction of the cost of a new body.

Ann P. McClellan, RN, BSN
Gerry Tadlock, RN, BA

Cover story

The recorder and metronome switches on manikins for cardiopulmonary resuscitation instruction get a lot of use—and abuse. Not only do the knobs sometimes break off in the middle of a class, but they're very hard to replace.

Here's how to make your own replacement knob: Break off the needle of a disposable (preferably 25G) needle at the hub. Trim the plastic hub at the syringe site, leaving the cover intact. Fit the cover over the broken switch, and you'll have a durable, inexpensive replacement knob.

Susan Schulmerich, RN

Handy holder

If you need a bedside dispenser for nonsterile cotton balls, try a plastic soft-margarine container. Cut a hole in the lid large enough to pull a cotton ball through. Then, fill the container with cotton balls and snap on the lid.

Besides being inexpensive, the dispenser's easy to use at a patient's bedside. Also, because it holds unused cotton balls in one place, it helps keep the patient's room neat.

Mariann Markan, BSN

Paint protector

To keep the cast from scraping paint off the toilet seat or gouging it, cut a piece of heavy vinyl into an oval shape—the same shape as the toilet seat. Sew Velcro tabs to the sides of the vinyl oval. Before the patient sits on the toilet seat, he can place the vinyl on the seat, lift the seat, and attach the Velcro to itself underneath each side of the seat.

Mary S. Duff, RN, CCRN

A flip tip

Each time a patient's bed linens are completely changed, or at least twice a week, the mattress also should be flipped. Flipping the mattress preserves its life and makes for greater patient comfort.

Charles Koltz, RN

Wall saver

Have you ever moved a bed with a horizontal overhead traction pole and accidentally gouged the wall with the pole? To prevent such wall damage, cut an old tennis ball in half and slip the halves over the ends of the pole. (The ball may fit snugly without tape, or you may want to tape it in place for additional security.) A tennis ball also makes a great cushion for the top bar of a Hoyer lift.

Melinda Crawford, RN

Card-carrying tubes

Since counter space is at a premium in patients' rooms, their get-well cards usually wind up taped to the walls. But a nicer way to display cards (and to prevent tape damage to the walls) is to punch a hole through each card and string a piece of used, clean I.V. tubing through the holes. Tie the tubing to two out-of-the-way objects in the room (from a lamp to the headboard, for example). Then each time the patient gets a new card, he can simply untie one end of the tubing, add his new card, and retie the tubing.

Mary L. Malone, RN, BSN

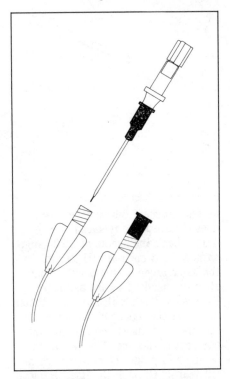

Cath patch

To patch a cracked hub in a Swan-Ganz catheter, thread a 20-gauge angiocath into the hub's porthole, then remove the angiocath needle. (Don't pierce the Swan-Ganz tubing with the needle.) The angiocath will wedge tightly in the porthole and form a seal, bypassing the cracked hub.

Debra C. Davis, RN, MSN

Mending matters

Here's how to fix the cut or damaged balloon-inflation (cuff-inflation) of

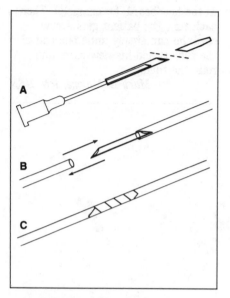

an endotracheal tube so the tube
doesn't have to be replaced.
1. Pull back the needle of a 20-gauge
catheter and cut the catheter at
the same angle as the needle. Then
slide the needle forward again so
its bevel is flush with the cut catheter.
2. Cut off the damaged portion of
the line, and insert the catheter into
one part of the line. (The submerged
needle will guide the catheter, without tearing through the line.) Remove
the needle from the catheter and
cut the other end of the catheter at
an angle. Insert this end into the
other part of the line.
3. Tape the connections securely.
    Now you've repaired the line with-
out causing the patient unnecessary
discomfort or expense.
Randy H. Finley, RN, BSN

A scope scoop
The diaphragm on my stethoscope
would crack every month or so,
it seemed, and I'd have to replace it.
So now I cover it with the cap from

a vitamin bottle (after first popping
off the child-proof part of the cap). To
protect the stethoscope's bell, I cover
it with a snap-on plastic cap from a
medicine bottle.
    The caps provide good protection
and can easily be removed.
Candy Henson, RN

IDeal idea
To keep your scissors, stethoscope,
and other equipment from disappearing, give them permanent identification (ID)—metal dog tags.
    The dog tags, which are available
at any pet store, are easier to keep
clean than tape and plastic wristband
IDs. And unlike other identifiers,
dog tags can't be washed, peeled, or
cut off.
Sue Grant, RN

A key note
To prevent your medication keys from
rubbing against and fraying the
lanyard, try this. Untie the lanyard
and thread it through a piece of clean
I.V. tubing. Then, thread the tubing
through the holes on the keys. This
way, the keys will rub against the
tubing instead of the lanyard.
Trish Zapf-Reid, RN

SUPPLIES

Cost horizons
What would you guess your hospital
spends annually for examination
gloves? Or incontinence pads? Nurses
at Burdette Tomlin Memorial Hospital
in Cape May Court House, N.J.,
learned the cost of these and other
items in a most unusual way during a
recent "Cost Awareness Day Contest."
    The contest was part of a cam-
paign to make nurses and other employees more aware of the staggering

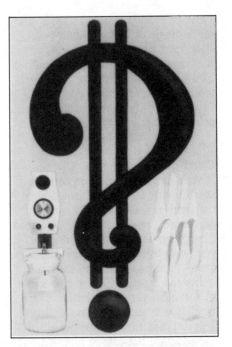

costs involved in running a hospital. Members of a Cost Containment Committee set up a table outside the employees' cafeteria, displaying various items—suction bottles, restraints, and so forth.

To enter the contest, employees had to fill out an entry blank. For all but one of the displayed items, the entry blank listed several figures as the amount of money the hospital spends annually on the items. The employees had to match each of these items with the figure they thought was the correct amount. For the remaining item, no choices were given; the employees had to guess the correct amount. If more than one employee got all the multiple-choice questions right, the employee who came closest to guessing the annual cost of the last item would be the winner. (The prize was dinner for two at an area restaurant.)

The assistant coordinator of inservice education said the nurses were surprised at some of the costs—almost $10,000 annually for examination gloves and close to $13,000 for incontinence pads, to take just two examples. As a result, they're more cost conscious and less likely to waste supplies. They've even come up with ideas of their own to help cut costs. For instance, the hospital had been using different kinds of tubing for hyperalimentation systems. After the contest, one nurse suggested that the hospital order a standard tubing that fits all systems. It's saved money and has made the nurses' work easier.

The hospital plans to hold a Cost Awareness Day Contest every other month. The next one will focus on the medical records department and its costs, such as file folders and microfilming charts.

Nancy Dougherty, RN

Every little bit helps

If the crunch to contain costs has hit the hospital where you work, you may want to try the plan nurses at Nebraska Methodist Hospital, Omaha, use to help their hospital avoid replacing supplies unnecessarily.

Here's how the plan works. Each unit has a "clean your pockets" box placed where nurses will remember to use it: in the nurses' lounge or on top of the time clock, for example. At the end of each shift, nurses empty their pockets of such supplies as alcohol and povidone-iodine wipes, aspirin packets, hemostats, needles, syringes, and unused urinalysis test tubes.

The box is a friendly reminder to return items the nurses may inadvertently take home. A staff development nurse at the hospital says emptying pockets has helped reduce waste and trim the supply budget.

Mary Wolcott, RN

Homemade ice packs

Here's an effective, inexpensive substitute for commercial ice packs.

Simply soak a sponge with water, and place it inside a plastic sandwich bag or zip-lock bag. Then put the bag into a freezer.

One caution: If you use a twist tie to lock the sandwich bag, be careful that the twist tie doesn't inflict injury.

Lorraine E. Lemus, RN, BSN

A credit to patients

To make sure a discharged patient gets credited for any unused medication, we follow this procedure.

When our unit clerk learns that a patient is to be discharged, she stamps a discharge sheet and an empty bag with the patient's nameplate. Then she tapes the sheet and the bag on the patient's door.

When the patient is ready to leave, we fill out the discharge sheet and take his leftover medications out of the medication cart and put them into the bag. Then we take the bag to the pharmacy so his account will be credited.

Elizabeth Foronjy, RN

Multipurpose covers

Don't discard those plastic covers from 50-ml syringes. They can be used in many different ways at home or in the hospital.

Paint them brightly, for instance, and children will use them as crayon holders, sandbox castles, or bathtub submarines. Adults can use them to house crochet hooks or to organize sewing-basket spools. They're also

great for storing sinkers, screws, and other tackle or toolbox items.

So next time, before you toss out the covers, consider their possibilities. How about using them to hold your toothbrushes when you go camping? Or to file all those coins you've been collecting. Or....

Phyllis A. Smith, RN

Card guard

If your hospital's isolation cards identify only the type of isolation on the front and have specific isolation procedures listed on the back, to read the precautions on the reverse side, you must tear the card from the door—perhaps destroying the card.

Instead tape or hang on the door a 6" × 9" clear plastic pocket envelope (available in most stationery stores). The isolation card can be placed in the envelope but can be removed for reading without being destroyed.

Louise M. Land, RN, BS

Recycled socks

Worn-out tube socks can find new life as elbow protectors. Just cut off the leg portion and fold it in half to create a slip-on elbow guard.

These recycled socks contour to fit the patient's arm snugly, helping prevent skin irritation or possible ulceration from bed linens. Not only are they less expensive and more comfortable than disposable elbow protectors, they are also cooler and easier to wash than sheepskin protectors.

Elizabeth A. Farmer, RN

Tube therapy

Don't throw away leftover pieces of Penrose drains; give them to the occupational therapy (OT) department. In OT, patients with arthritis or those recovering from strokes can cut the pieces of tubing into various sizes. Such therapy not only exercises patients' hands but also provides the hospital with a supply of strong, flexible rubber bands.

Joseph Glinsky, ORT

Glucose testing strips

In the doctor's office where I work, we cut the costs of blood and urine glucose tests by cutting reagent strips in half. Even cut in half, the strip has enough reagent to give an accurate reading.

Donna Priestly, GN

Exposed but not disposed

X-ray film has a diverse potential afterlife—after it's been exposed, that is. I use it as a notebook divider for patient profiles, narcotic books, and charts. I also write notes on it with a grease pencil. Later, I erase my notes with a clean gauze pad or cloth and use the film over again.

Lt. Jeri L. Hoover, NC, USN

Improvising transparencies

Are cost controls on audiovisual aids hampering your inservice style? Here's one way to fight back: Use X-ray film (with the coating removed) instead of costly overhead transparencies.

The film's light-blue color and sturdy composition make it a perfect substitute for a transparency. You can use either permanent or washable felt-tipped markers on the film. And if you cut the film to fit into your copying machine, you can copy more detailed pictures and graphs right onto the film.

Teresa Gentry, RN
Charlyn Cassady, RN

Tough tape

Paper measuring tape often ripped when I tried to measure a patient's abdominal girth. So now I put a strip of adhesive tape on the "inches" side of the measuring tape (we read the "centimeters" side). This makes the measuring tape—strengthened with the adhesive tape backing—almost indestructible.

Mary Fourth, RN

Mattress manipulation

Here's a number of ways to recycle a Stryker foam mattress after a patient no longer needs it. First, send it to the laundry, where it is washed and dried. Then cut and use it in various ways.

Here are some:
—pads for wheelchairs (they take a lot of pressure off sore hips).
—wedges the size of a child's leg. Taped just above and below the knee, they serve as a restraint during clysis. They are soft and the child can still move his legs.
—pillows for positioning patients.
—strips that can be rolled to fit a patient's hand and used for exercising in physical therapy.

Jane Rayburn, RN

Good to the last drop

Sometimes the last half of a bottle of liquid wart remover would become so hard that I couldn't use it, and I'd have to throw it away. Then I found that putting the bottle in the refrigerator keeps *all* the liquid in it at the right consistency.

Tirrel C. Kinchen, RN

A calamine find

Instead of using a new cotton ball each time you apply calamine lotion for sunburn or minor skin irritation, try using—and reusing—an old roll-on deodorant bottle. Just clean and dry the empty bottle, fill it with calamine lotion, and roll the lotion onto the patient's affected skin. The rolling ball spreads the lotion evenly—without wasting cotton balls. After each application, snap off the bottle's ball for cleaning.

Joanne Krisko, RN

Padded pull sheet

When you're making the bed of a bedridden patient who needs a disposable under pad, prepare his bed as you normally would—with one exception. Instead of placing the pad on top of the pull sheet directly under the patient, sandwich it between the pull-sheet layers.

This technique will mean fewer soiled bottom sheets, thereby saving you time and cutting your hospital's linen consumption. It'll also add to your patient's comfort, because paper from the pad won't cling to his skin.

Janet Markey, RN

A spec of organization

Our emergency department (ED) stocks four sizes of disposable ear and nasal speculums in one box on a shelf. Whenever we need a speculum, we reach up, rummage through the box, and invariably come up with the wrong size, so we discard it.

To avoid this needless waste, I bought a small, plastic, rectangular container, inserted dividers, and sorted the speculums in the container according to size. I marked each space on the outside of the container with the speculum size (3, 4, 5, and 9) and the type of patient who'd use that size speculum (infant, pediatric, adolescent, and adult).

The speculum container has not

only saved money by cutting down on wasted supplies, but it's also helped us get a bit more organized, and that's always a help in the fast-paced ED.

D. Whipple, RN

Saving 4″ × 4″ gauze pads

When my 3-month-old daughter had to wear a hip brace, I taped 4″ × 4″ gauze pads to the sides of the brace to protect her skin. Because she had frequent bowel movements, I had to change the gauze pads often—too often, since the gauze and tape were expensive.

Then I decided to try using thin sanitary pads, cut to size, instead. I found the pads cheaper to use than gauze, and since they have an adhesive backing, I didn't have to buy adhesive tape anymore, either.

Maisie Hubbard, RN, MSN

Cost-cutting care #1

When my grandfather needed a new colostomy irrigation bag, I went shopping for it at the local drugstore. I came away with an inexpensive alternative: a douche bag. The douche bag does the job as well as a colostomy irrigation bag, but it's sturdier and costs only about one third as much.

Linda Harrish, LPN

Irrigating? Think small

When a patient has a small fistula or wound that needs to be irrigated frequently, don't use a big 1,000-ml bottle of normal saline solution. It just clutters the patient's bedside table, and later, the unused solution will have to be discarded.

Use 5-ml vials of normal saline solution instead. A few vials are usually sufficient for each irrigation.

Mary E. Anderson, RN, MSN

A pointer on catheterization

When learning how to insert a urinary catheter into a woman patient, a student sometimes contaminates several catheters just trying to locate the meatus. To cut down on catheter waste, I have the student open a package of sterile cotton-tipped applicators onto the sterile field. Then she puts on her gloves, picks up an applicator, and points to where she intends to insert the catheter. If she needs help, I can use another applicator to show her where the catheter should be positioned.

Using applicators saves the time and money of repeated catheterizations. But most of all, it saves your patient the embarrassment and discomfort of a prolonged catheter insertion.

Connie Norehim, RN, BSN, MSEd

Cost-cutting care #2

I cut costs in giving perineal care by using small plastic sandwich bags, cleansing solution, and toilet paper squares instead of prepackaged perineal care packs and gloves. Here's how.

I put a sandwich bag over each hand and secure it at the wrist with a rubber band. The bag is roomy enough so I can move my thumb and fingers easily. Then I perform perineal care with the cleansing solution and toilet paper squares.

When finished, I just turn the bags inside out, place them and the soiled paper squares inside a clean plastic bag, and throw everything away.

Sharon McMahon, BSN, MEd

Foam and fortune

The hospital where I work used to spend a lot of money replacing damaged fetal monitor transducers. And no wonder. When the transducers weren't being used, they were just stored loosely in a drawer where they could roll around, increasing the chance of breaking the sensitive heads and connectors.

To solve the problem, I made slits in a $12'' \times 4''$ piece of packing foam and inserted the transducers into the slits. This works so well that we haven't had to replace a single transducer since we started using the foam.

Mary Marchel, RN

TIME

Finding lines

When patients have multiple I.V. and pressure-monitoring lines, you may have trouble figuring out which line is which.

So color-code the lines. For instance, arterial lines can sport a piece of red tape, pulmonary artery catheter lines may have green tape, central venous pressure lines will bear yellow tape, and each medication line will have a different colored tape marker.

The coding system helps you find the line you need quickly—especially important in an emergency.

Carol Steinruch, RN

Boxed boards

If an I.V. arm board isn't available when you need one, just tape a washcloth or small towel around the I.V. tubing box and use that instead. The long, narrow box makes an excellent temporary I.V. arm board and saves you the time of looking for the real thing.

Carol Kenck Crispin, RN, MEd

Heard, but not seen

When several I.V. infusion pumps are running on our unit at the same time and one starts beeping, we're never sure which room the signal is coming from.

To save time and steps, we put a small piece of colored tape next to the call button of each patient who has a pump. We also put a piece of tape on the door of each room that has a pump.

When we hear beeping, we call patients in the marked rooms on the intercom to find out which controller is signaling us. Then we go right to that room.

Marsha Miller, RN

Twist and tape

I like to carry a rubber tourniquet with me, but it doesn't fit neatly into my already overcrowded uniform pockets. So I wind the tourniquet—like a spiral—around the tubing of my stethoscope and tape the tourniquet's ends to the stethoscope. The tourniquet stays in place neatly, is always at hand, and I never have to rummage through my pockets looking for it.

Sr. Doreen Casey, RN, BSN, MA

Measuring made easy

If your patient has a pulmonary artery catheter and needs to have his cardiac output measured frequently, do you disconnect the catheter's proximal lumen hub from the I.V. tubing to inject iced saline solution each time? That's a time-consuming procedure. Instead, connect the hub to the I.V. tubing with a three-way stopcock. Then, you can push the iced saline solution through the stopcock. You'll not only save the time of disconnecting the tubing, but you'll also

decrease the possibility of contaminating the line or introducing air into it.

René R. Guild, RN

Solutions on ice #1

In our 10-bed cardiac/intensive care unit, we never know when we'll need to measure a patient's cardiac output with the thermodilution technique. To make sure we're prepared, we keep a 500-ml bottle of D_5W in our refrigerator. When we have to fill syringes for a cardiac output measurement, the injectate is already chilled and doesn't have to be iced.

The nurse who takes the bottle of D_5W from the refrigerator is responsible for replacing it. And we all check the bottles' expiration dates periodically.

Lorna E. Stern, RN

Emergency baster

When we're called to an accident scene or a private home to assist a victim in cardiac arrest, we frequently find that the victim has vomited and needs to be suctioned immediately. Our suctioning equipment is packed in the ambulance and not always handy. So I carry a turkey baster in my jump kit, which I can tote with me wherever I go. Because the baster has a $5/16''$ hole at the tip, I can quickly suction the victim and begin resuscitation while another paramedic gets the rest of the equipment from the ambulance.

Ann Hauser, BA, EMT-P

Kits, carts, and emergency care #1

I work in a newborn nursery, but I'm frequently called to the delivery room or emergency department (ED) to give emergency care to a newborn in distress. Taking the crash cart along with me is difficult, time-consuming, and frequently unnecessary since I usually don't need all the supplies on it.

To save time and effort, I made a newborn emergency kit—a fishing tackle box stocked with the drugs and supplies I usually use in emergencies. Now when I get a call from the delivery room or ED, I just grab the emergency kit, and off I go.

The kit has worked so well that other nurses in the hospital have adapted it for diabetic patients: they stock a tackle box with supplies needed for hypoglycemic reactions.

Mary Lu Rang, RN, MSN, CRNP

Kits, carts, and emergency care #2

In our intensive care unit, we've simplified storing and transporting emergency supplies. We use two small, mobile carts that roll right up to the patient's bedside. One cart holds supplies for starting any kind of line—I.V., arterial, total parenteral nutrition, Swan-Ganz, or cutdown. This cart also holds arm boards, tape, alcohol wipes, dressing change kits, and povidone-iodine ointment.

The other cart holds supplies for gastrointestinal bleeding—nasogastric tubes, gastrointestinal tubes, saline bottles, large irrigation syringes, Chux pads, and so on.

The carts save us the time of collecting supplies from the supply room and carrying them to the patient's bedside. What's more, new staff and pool nurses who aren't familiar with our unit don't have to worry about hunting for supplies in an emergency.

Lt. Linda P. Massimiano, RN

Precalculated precaution

Would you know what dose of atropine to give to a 27-lb pediatric patient in an emergency? Or would you lose time having to calculate the dose on the spot?

We save time by calculating dosages for emergency drugs *when each child is admitted* to the intensive care unit. Then we record them on a "resuscitation medications sheet."

The recommended dose/kilogram for a number of drugs is preprinted on the sheet in the first column. Then we calculate the dose for the patient and enter it on the sheet in the next column in red ink. Other preprinted columns include: route of administration, dosage interval or rate, maximum dose, and dose preparation (dilution requirements, if any).

We tape the sheet to the head of the patient's bed, where it's readily available for reference in an emergency. Besides saving valuable time, the sheet greatly diminishes the chance for error.

Patricia Fuchs, RRT, SN

I.V. grab bag

To save time during a code, a nurse at Spencer (Iowa) Municipal Hospital prepares "I.V. drip bags" containing

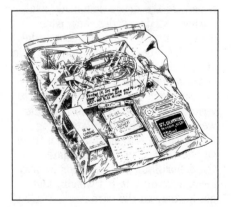

all the equipment needed to start an I.V. drip.

The bags are the kind oxygen supplies come in : 10" square plastic with a zip-lock top. The equipment inside each bag includes:
• a 250-ml bag of D_5W (or normal saline solution)
• prefilled syringes of medications in the necessary doses (for example, lidocaine and dopamine)
• medication labels marked with the drug names and doses to attach to the I.V. bag after mixing
• an I.V. tubing set
• 2 alcohol preparation pads
• a 19G 1" needle.

Now, during a code, a nurse simply grabs one of the bags and has everything she needs to quickly mix and hang the I.V. medications.

Melodie Kinsley, RN

Saving time in a pediatric code
Precious seconds can be lost calculating drug dose and defibrillator watt-seconds during a pediatric code. That's why the staff of the pediatric intensive care unit at Wilford Hall Medical Center, Lackland Air Force Base, Tex., developed resuscitation cards.

Listed on a 9" square of white paper are the drugs commonly used during pediatric codes, how each drug is supplied, and the dose in ml or mg/kg. The list is laminated onto a 10" cardboard square.

When a patient's admitted to the unit, a nurse uses a grease pencil to write on the card his name and his weight in kg. She calculates drug doses for his weight and marks them on the card. She also calculates the defibrillator watt-seconds he may need, according to his weight, and marks that on the card.

Name __Jim Gavin__

Weight __32__ _____kg

Cardiovascular Resuscitation Drugs for Children

Sodium Bicarbonate: __32 – 96 mEq__
1-3 mEq/kg

Epinephrine 1:10,000: __3.2 ml__
0.1 ml/kg of 1:10,000 solution

Calcium Chloride 10%: __3.2 ml__
0.1 ml/kg

Atropine Sulfate: __3.2 ml — 6.4 ml__
.01-.02 mg/kg
(dilute 1 ml of 1 mg/ml in 9 ml NS = .1 mg/ml)

Lidocaine 2%: __1.6 ml__
1 mg/kg of 2% solution (20 mg/ml)

Dextrose 50%: __32 ml__
1 ml/kg up to 50-ml dose

Defibrillation: __64 watts__
2 watt-seconds/kg

Every patient has a resuscitation card hung at the head of his bed. When he leaves, the card's wiped clean so it's ready to use for another patient.

The cards save valuable time during a code by supplying the necessary information. A nurse there found the cards so helpful that she now uses them in a regular pediatric unit. For any patient who's seriously ill, she completes a card and hangs it on the emergency cart. She says that during a code the card is literally a lifesaver.

Capt. Debbie Gammage, USAF, NC

Crash cart convenience
After working many years in the intensive care unit and recovery room, I finally found a way to neatly and conveniently store endotracheal equipment on the crash cart.

First, I measured the depth, width, and length of the crash cart drawer and bought a flat piece of upholstery foam cut to that size. Then I laid all the endotracheal equipment (blades, handles, extra bulbs and batteries, forceps, and so on) on the foam and traced their outlines with a felt-tipped pen. Next, I removed the equipment and, using my tracings as a guide, cut out their shapes in the foam with a scalpel blade, leaving a thin layer of uncut foam at the bottom of each shape. When finished, I placed the foam in the crash cart drawer and put the equipment in the cutout "pockets."

Now the equipment is easily visible and accessible, so I save time finding what I need during an emergency. And I can see immediately what's missing when I check the cart.

Susanne T. Smith, RN, BSN

Not carting disaster

Crash carts are necessary equipment in every hospital, of course. But because they're used less often than other equipment, our staff members weren't always able to locate the items in the cart quickly in an emergency. And sometimes certain items were missing from the cart.

To solve this problem, we took pictures of the inside of each fully stocked drawer. Then we pasted each picture and a list of that drawer's contents on separate pages in a looseleaf binder. We laminated the pages for durability.

To ensure that the cart stays fully equipped, we banded each drawer so the band breaks if the drawer is opened.

We urge all staff members, and especially new employees, to periodically study the loose-leaf binder. Consequently, they're more familiar with the cart's contents and can function better in an emergency. Banding the drawers assures them they'll be able to find all the necessary equipment when they need it.

Chris Chytraus, RN, BSN, CCRN

Code tool

During a code, every second counts,

so don't waste precious time looking for the proper size endotracheal tube. Have the linen department sew an expandable tube holder (similar to a silverware holder) out of muslin. Make a pocket for each tube and mark the tube size in large numbers on each pocket. Fasten a tie string on each end so you can roll the tube holder into a compact bundle and tie it, ready to use for the next code.

Chris McSharry, RN

Solutions on ice #2

Recently, we had several patients on our unit with GI bleeding. We spent so much time doing iced lavages that we decided we had to be better prepared for them. So we put a few large bottles of normal saline solution in the refrigerator. Now whenever iced lavages are needed, the solution is already cool. We just have to get the ice and replace the used saline solution with a new bottle.

Bonnie Handerhan, RN, BSN

Hooray for the flags

With a little imagination, the "flags" on charts for stat orders can be used in many different ways. For instance, use them for evacuation drills. Put one—gray side out—on the outside door frame of the resident's room, then, during a drill, after making sure the room is empty, switch the stat flag to the red side.

Sr. Sean Damien, RN

Cupboard ID

If your department has many cupboards, locating a particular item can involve a long and annoying search. Here's a way to identify the contents of each cupboard at a glance. Cut the labels from cartons, or the names of products from the literature that accompanies them, and paste these labels on the outside of the door. Now you can quickly find an item just by looking at the labels on the door.

Naomi Jones, CRNA

Color-coded cards

To keep instructions for preparing patients for X-ray procedures right at your fingertips, list them on 3″ × 5″ cards and keep them in the cardex. Color-code each index card according to procedure: intravenous pyelography on a yellow card; gallbladder test on a green card; barium enema on a blue card; and so on. Now, when a procedure is ordered for a patient, just flip through the cardex until you find the proper color—a great timesaver!

Cheryl Boehly, RN

Step saver

Ever have to break isolation to get admission items? Or call another nurse to bring the items to the room entrance? The admission procedure can take too much time, too many steps, and too many nurses.

To save time, steps, and nurses, make an admission cart that can be wheeled right to the door. The cart can be an old wooden filing cabinet. Simply add wheels and paint it a bright color. Then you have all the admission items right at the patient's door.

Heather Hay, RN

Snag solution

Many postoperative patients wear elastic abdominal binders for support in coughing, deep breathing, and ambulating. The binders' Velcro linings are great for adjusting the binders to fit properly, but the lining causes a problem for some women. After surgery, they like to wear their own nylon nightgowns; but the Velcro catches and snags the material, ruining the gowns.

To solve this problem, cover the exposed Velcro with gauze. Besides eliminating needless wear and tear on the patients' nightgowns, the gauze guides you in reapplying the binder after a dressing change or ambulation. A timesaver for you—no more readjustments for proper fit—and a gownsaver for patients.

Janet Pospy, RN, BSN

Band-edged cast

Petaling the perineal area of a hip-spica cast with adhesive tape is tedious: you have to cut the tape in strips, round off the edges so a sharp corner won't poke the patient's skin, and apply the tape petals all around the edge of the cast.

A quicker way to do this is with small round Band-Aids. Unlike adhesive tape, these plastic bandages don't have to be cut, they have a small pad for extra comfort, and they peel off easily for replacement.

Sydney Anne Gambill, RN

The write holder

You know that a pen lurks on your medication cart somewhere, but where? In the drawer? Clipped to the chart? Or perhaps hidden under some papers?

To avoid this seek-and-find-the-pen game, make a pen holder for your cart. Tape a plastic cover from a 35- or 60-ml syringe to the side of the cart. The syringe cover is wide and deep enough to hold several pens, pencils, and other necessities.

Lisa Elvin-Geyer, RN

Conference coordination

Coordinating a conference, workshop,

or seminar involves a lot of work. The following checklist helps me organize the details.

1. Choose topic and title ☐
2. Obtain speaker ☐
3. Choose date ☐
4. Confirm location ☐
5. Reserve audiovisual machines ☐
6. Make up brochures and send to participants ☐
7. Arrange publicity ☐
8. Compile list of registrants ☐
9. Confirm date and time with participants ☐
10. Develop and print handouts ☐
11. Prepare slides and other audiovisual material ☐
12. Confirm date, time, and topic with speaker ☐
13. Prepare conference packages for participants ☐
14. Pick up and set up audio-visual machines (have spare bulbs on hand) ☐
15. Circulate attendance list ☐
16. Obtain evaluation forms from participants ☐
17. Return audiovisual machines and tidy up room ☐
18. Compile evaluations ☐
19. Send thank-you note to speaker ☐
20. Pay conference costs, if any. ☐

Nicole Florent-Legare, RN

Reference bound

Our staff members frequently find certain articles in professional journals that they want to refer to over and over. But they don't always remember which article was in which issue of which journal.

To help keep track of these articles, each staff member photocopies articles of special interest to her. She keeps the copied articles in her own three-ring binder.

This system of individual reference books has saved us all a lot of time in recall and research.

Marion B. Dolan, RN

Keepsake copy

As a special memento for new parents, make another copy of the baby's footprints for them. The footprint form also has space to list the baby's vital statistics—birth weight, length, time of birth, and so on. On the other side, use a rubber stamp to record visiting hours, mother's room number, and phone numbers.

Not only do parents appreciate the keepsake copy, but you're spared having to repeat the same information over and over, so it's a timesaver for you.

Maryann McNamara, RN

FORMulating shift report

When I was a new staff nurse on a medical/surgical unit, I was surprised and frustrated with all the note taking expected of me during shift report. Having to write name, room number, diagnosis, vital signs, and so on for patient after patient took a lot of time and kept me from listening attentively to report. So with suggestions from my co-workers, I designed a form for use during report that looks something like this:

Room	101	102	103
Patient	Smith		
Dx	M.I.		
IV/I&O	D5/LR@ 125/hr.		
V.S.	4ᵖ & 8ᵖ		
Treatments	telemetry		
Lab results	cardiac enzymes		

The form was enthusiastically adopted by nurses on my unit. But it can also be easily altered to reflect specific needs of any nursing unit.

Sandra D. Andrew, RN, BS

Generic is here

Tired of rewriting entries in your hospital's procedure manual every time you get a new piece of equipment? Adapt a generic format that separates the purpose of a procedure and its rationale from the instructions for operating specific pieces of equipment.

A student nurse in Avon, Conn., devised the generic format. Here's an example of how she used it: For the entry in the procedure manual on chest tube drainage systems, she described the purpose of the procedure and its rationale. Then, on a separate sheet of paper, she wrote the instructions for operating the Pleur-evac system. Should the hospital start using a different chest tube drainage system, she would simply discard the Pleur-evac instructions and replace them with instructions for operating the new system. She wouldn't have to rewrite the purpose of the procedure and its rationale.

Patricia Fuchs, SN, CRTT, RRT

Handouts: Ready and set to go

Nurses in our hospice and home health agency used to spend a lot of time researching, assembling, and photocopying patient-teaching materials for each of their patients. Then we discovered that sometimes two or three nurses would be preparing materials on the same subject at the same time.

To eliminate this duplication of effort, we developed standard handouts on frequently taught subjects such as catheter care and irrigation, diabetes and diabetic diets, anticoagulant therapy, foot care, and energy-saving techniques. We circulated them among our nursing and medical advisors for review and approval.

Now we're sure that all our patients are getting standard information on their conditions and certain care procedures. And we save a lot of time, since the handouts are already prepared and ready to go.

Sandra Caban, RNC

Notes on education

As head nurse on a special care unit, I'm responsible for keeping a record of my staff's continuing education efforts, including staff development classes, outside seminars, and home-study programs. To help me do this, I've asked each staff member to record her own continuing education information in a notebook at the nurses' station. This gets the job done without extra effort for me or the staff.

Margery Lebel, RN, CCRN

What *is* that dosage?

In our small intensive care unit, we often have patients receiving medications in dosages calculated on μ/kg of body weight. Our pharmacist has prepared a standard dosage chart for frequently administered medications such as nitroprusside (Nipride) and dopamine (Intropin). But sometimes we need to double or even quadruple the strength of a medication, and this can be confusing as well as time-consuming during an emergency or critical period.

To avoid confusion and not waste precious minutes, we've devised this procedure. We weigh the patient each morning and recalculate his medication dosages according to his new weight and the strength ordered. The calculations are always checked by two nurses. Then we write on a piece of paper the patient's name, his weight, the date, the name of his medication and dosage ordered, and the number of ml per hour he's to be given. We tape the paper to the I.V. pole above his infusion pump. If an emergency arises and the doctor asks, "What is that dosage?", we'll know—at a glance.

M. Cecilia Wendler RN, CCRN

Point of reference
I like to index the articles in *Nursing* so I have a handy reference for any information I might need. Here's how I do it.

After reading each article, I write the title, issue, page number, and a short description of the article on an index card. In the upper right-hand corner of the card, I note the topic of the article. (If the article covers more than one topic, I make another card for cross-referencing.) Then I file the card alphabetically according to topic.

Although I always order the year-end indexes that *Nursing* publishes, my card index allows me immediate access to any article I need.

D. Lynn, LPN

Figure on this
Does figuring end-of-shift intake and output totals and balances leave your head in a whirl? Then use a mini-calculator. It's inexpensive, accurate, and fits right in your uniform pocket. And because it can do complicated mathematics quickly, you'll have more time to devote to patient care.

Barbara Steininger, NA III

12

PERSONAL GROOMING

PATIENT GROOMING

A hair piece

Here's a neat and easy way to wash the hair of a bedridden patient:

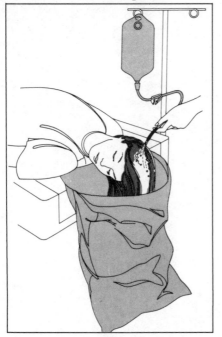

Position the patient near the head of the bed and put incontinent pads under her shoulders and upper back. Then drape a large plastic bag over the head of the bed. Open the bag, fold the lower open edge onto itself to make a lip, and place the patient's head on the lip.

Next, fill an enema bag with water and hang it on an I.V. pole. Use the bag's tubing as a hose to direct the flow of water onto the patient's head. (Adjust the clamp to control the amount of water.) One bag of water is usually enough for a shampoo and rinse.

Hair washing, a la this no-mess method, leaves the bed and patient dry—most of the excess water drains into the open bag. The remainder is caught in the lip of the bag and you can brush it into the bag with your hands.

Annette Bourgault, RN

A hair bin

One of my biggest problems in caring for my bedridden mother after her stroke was how to wash her hair without getting water all over the bed and floor or causing her unnecessary discomfort. A plastic, stackable vegetable bin (with a half-circle cut out from the rim on one side), a large plastic trash bag, one heavy towel, and one hand towel helped solve the problem.

I put the plastic trash bag under my mother's head and the heavy towel over the bag. Then I padded the cutout section of the vegetable bin with the hand towel. I placed the bin under her head with her neck resting on the cutout section. To wash her hair, I poured a pitcher of warm water over her hair into the bin and applied shampoo. I removed and emptied the bin as needed. After rinsing, I removed the bin and dried her hair with the heavy towel.

My technique works: while my mother got a refreshing hair wash, she stayed comfortable and her bed stayed dry.

Connie Davis, RN

Hair care
Here's a tip for a patient with very oily hair who can't have it shampooed. Sprinkle powder through his hair. Then push the teeth of a comb through an open 4″ × 4″ gauze pad and comb the patient's hair. The powder absorbs much of the excess oil, and the 4″ × 4″ collects the powder. The patient's scalp will smell cleaner. And the best part is it costs much less than dry shampoo.

Tara Hummel, RN

Dripless hair wash
Here's a tip to pass on to the parents of a pediatric patient who's recently had a myringotomy. It's a way to give the child a shampoo without getting water in his ears.

First, dampen his hair with a wet, wrung-out washcloth. Then work a small amount of shampoo into a lather in your hands, and apply the lather to the child's hair. Wash his hair as you normally would, being careful not to let the lather run into his ears. To rinse, wet the washcloth in clear water, wring it out, and wipe the lather from the child's hair. Continue rinsing this way until all the lather is gone.

In fact, this is a good way to shampoo the hair of *all* small patients who fuss when water drips into their eyes or ears.

Barbara Weinstock, LPN

Removes hair tangles
If you have difficulty combing tangles from patients' hair, try this: rub the tangled strand of hair with an alcohol-saturated cotton ball, then comb. The tangles are gone and the alcohol evaporates quickly.

Irene Evans, RN

Fork over the tangles
To remove tangles from matted hair, apply a small amount of rubbing alcohol on the hair, then "comb" the hair with a plastic fork. These forks are inexpensive, readily available, and can untangle hair better than a regular comb. Be careful, though: if you don't comb gently, some of the fork prongs could break. To avoid this (or if a plastic fork isn't available), use a stainless steel fork.

Connie Pardee, RN, CNRN

Portable beauty parlor
If you've ever wanted to wash a bedridden patient's hair but couldn't find the plastic tray used for hair washing, here's a slick substitute. The materials to make it are always close at hand.

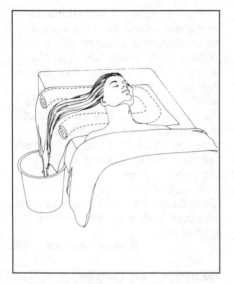

Open a bath blanket to its full length and roll it into a log. Fold the rolled-up blanket into a U-shape and place it inside a large plastic bag (such as those used for contaminated waste). Put the bottom of the "U" at the bottom of the bag.

Then put the bag at the head of the bed, with its open end hanging over the edge. The bag thus becomes a three-sided basin. Put a bucket on the floor under the open side of the basin to catch the water as it drains out.

Now position the patient with his head in the basin and his neck over the rolled blanket, and scrub away. The patient will enjoy the relaxing shampoo, and you'll love the job's ease. Best of all—the bed will stay dry.

Janice Petersen, RN

Soft and smooth
Before shaving a patient who has a coarse beard or sensitive skin, try coating his face and neck with lubricating jelly. Let the jelly stand a

minute or so, apply shaving soap or cream, then shave and rinse as usual. This will soften the patient's skin and hair and let the razor blade glide more smoothly over his face.

A word of caution, though: Don't use the jelly with electric razors.

Brenda M. Sands, RN

Close shave
If you need to shave a patient but don't have any commercial shaving cream, you *could* use plain soap and water. Often, though, this irritates the patient's skin. Instead, try this inexpensive, readily available substitute. Mix about a tablespoon of water-soluble lubricant with an equal amount of body lotion. This combination softens the beard, moisturizes the skin, and prevents irritation.

Sandra Meyer, RN

Brush a beard
In the trauma unit where I work, we see a number of patients with facial injuries. When those patients have beards, we have a problem. Sometimes we have to shave off the beard, but when it can be left on, we have a hard time cleaning the dried blood and debris from it.

What works best, we've found, is to gently scrub the beard with a toothbrush and a solution of warm water and hydrogen peroxide. The warm solution softens the crusted material, and the toothbrush allows us to scrub without applying too much pressure.

Ellie Franges, RN

Tongue tonic
Patients on ventilators often get a hard white caking on their tongues. To remove this caking, we gently scrub the tongue with a gauze pad

moistened with a clear soda. Besides keeping the tongue pink and moist, the soda scrub leaves no unpleasant aftertaste.

Diane Atkins, RN

Clean, covered collar
When a patient has to wear a cervical collar for a long time, I suggest he cover it with a 1' piece of stockinette to keep it clean. The stockinette cover also keeps the collar odor-free and can be easily removed for washing.

Mary Kennedy Eggen, RN

Skin care tips
Before shaving a male patient's beard, apply Dermassage to the stubble and leave it on for 5 minutes. This softens the beard and allows for an easy and painless shave.

Rose A. Briley, LPN

Sponging off
For patients who have one arm or one hand immobilized, using a washcloth is difficult. A sponge is easier for such patients to handle. It fits right into the hand, can be wrung out easily, and doesn't require folding as a washcloth does. Patients feel more independent, giving their own sponge baths.

A sponge is also effective for arthritic patients, since the squeezing action helps loosen up stiff joints.

Vicki Prechenenko, RN

A body (odor) guard
How can you help a patient who suffers from body odor that defies soap and deodorants? Try washing his offending feet or underarms with mouthwash, full strength or diluted. Or if the area's difficult to wash (a clenched fist, for example), just gently press a mouthwash-soaked washcloth against it for 10 to 30 minutes, then pat dry—no rinsing needed.

Suzanne D. Shutze, RN, CCRN

An odor shield
Perspiration can cling to the edges of a body cast and create an odor. To help ease this problem, I attach dress shields over the edge of the cast with a small piece of moleskin. The shields, which can be changed, washed, and reused, help the patient feel and smell fresh.

Leslie M. Hautz, RN

Coming clean
A patient who wears a shoulder immobilizer may develop body odor because he can't wash under his arm or apply deodorant. To solve the problem, give him this tip.

Drape a damp, soapy washcloth around a tongue blade. Carefully place the washcloth and tongue blade under the armpit. Remove the tongue blade, and clean the armpit by gently pulling the washcloth back and forth. Rinse and dry the same way.

Then apply spray or roll-on deodorant to a clean, dry washcloth. Fold the washcloth in half, drape it on a tongue blade, and place it under the armpit. Remove the tongue blade, but leave the washcloth under the armpit to absorb moisture and control odor.

Gladys M. Thorsell, RN

A help for hands
Giving skin and nail care to elderly patients who have contractured hands can be painful for them. Soaking hands in Vaseline first helps remove dead skin and clean under the nails with less discomfort to the patient.

Put a rubber examining glove

on your own hand and coat it with Vaseline. Then pull the glove off, turning it inside out, and put it on the patient's hand. Do the same for the patient's other hand. After an hour or so, remove the gloves, wipe the patient's skin clean, and give him nail care. The softening effect of the Vaseline is a help to the patients and to you.

Ruth Gibson, RN

Manicure

You can make nail care part of your patient care. At bath time, soak the patient's hands in the bathwater to loosen debris from under his fingernails. Then break a wooden tongue depressor in half lengthwise and gently scrape dried or caked material from under his nails. You can push the cuticles back with the rounded edge.

Since the depressor is disposable and provides manicures for two patients, it's sanitary and economical, too.

Louise Gore Grose, RN, MSN

Finger fresheners

I use toothpaste, too—for my patients who get fecal material under their nails. I put some toothpaste on a soft child's toothbrush and brush their nails until they look and smell clean.

I also use toothpaste to clean cigarette stains from their fingers.

Ruby Tetreault, RN

Swab those toes

When even a vigorous soap-and-water scrub can't remove the incrustation from a patient's toes and nail beds, try a glycerin-and-lemon swab instead.

A single application will gently remove debris, without causing discomfort or tissue damage.

Rosemary Ragonese, RN

A hair-razing lift

One grooming practice to enhance a mastectomy patient's self-image is shaving her legs.

Have her use this easy way to get a smooth shave without using soap or shaving cream, or having to rinse off with water. First, have her wet her legs with a washcloth. Then apply a thin film of lotion or baby oil and proceed to shave.

This procedure is simple enough for you to do on patients. But the patient shaving her legs herself makes her feel better than having someone else do it for her.

Linda S. Bates, RN

NURSE GROOMING

Stain stopper

Does your hospital use I.V. solutions that come in plastic bags? If so, save the small blue rubber stoppers that you remove before attaching I.V. tubing to the bags. You can use the stoppers to cap your pen and pencil points so your uniform pockets don't get stained.

Sheila Langille, RN

Uniformly clean

To remove a bloodstain from your uniform, rub the stain with a piece of cotton soaked with hydrogen peroxide. Rinse with alcohol or water, and the stain will disappear.

Ruth L. Nermal, RN, BSN

A fantastic idea

To remove povidone-iodine or tincture of benzoin stains from your uniform, spray the stain with Fantastik spray cleaner. Then wash your uniform as usual—and the stain will disappear.

Janet Meyer, RN

Stain 'n' scuff paste

To remove ball-point pen ink from your uniforms, wet the stained area and rub in some toothpaste. Rinse, then wash your uniform as usual.

Helen Bosch, RN

On-the-spot solution

Do you get ball-point pen ink spots on your uniforms? Here's a way to remove them. Wet the stained area, then pour a small amount of 70% isopropyl rubbing alcohol on the ink spots. Give the material a quick rub, and the spots will disappear.

Lucy Dalicandro, RN

Spot check

Here's another way to get rid of those seemingly indelible ink spots that adorn your uniform pockets—the products of uncapped pen points. Just saturate the spot with hairspray, then wash your uniform with your usual detergent. The result is a truly "spotless" uniform.

Cheryl Diorio, LPN

Scuff stuff

When your white shoes get deep scuffs or scratches, coat the marks with white typewriter correction fluid. The fluid will fill in the scuff, permanently hiding and sealing it. And it's waterproof and durable besides.

Pamela R. Numbers, LPN

Shoes like new

Toothpaste will clean your white shoes. Just rub a dab over the scuff marks with a moist tissue or rag. Then polish with a dry tissue, and your shoes will look good as new.

Kathy Anderson, RN

Spotless shoes

You know those black spots that even soap and water won't erase from your work shoes—spots that still show through the white polish? Here's a way of handling them.

Next time you clean your shoes, remove the spots first with nail-polish remover. It really works, and you'll almost believe you have new shoes.

Susan Ketcham, RN

Polish plus

Do you find that polish alone just can't cover those black scuff marks on your nursing shoes? Try spraying the marks first with a prewash laundry spray and rubbing them with a damp cloth. Then polish as usual. They'll be clean and professional looking once again.

Pam Hietbrink, RN

Shoe biz #1

I keep my new duty shoes white by applying a coat of clear floor wax to them before wearing them. The wax helps prevent scuff marks, so I don't have to polish them as often.

Claire Mendenhall, RN

Shoe biz #2

To keep my old duty shoes looking like new, I use baby powder. First I apply white shoe polish as usual and wait until it's just about dry. Then I liberally sprinkle the powder on the shoes. When the polish is dry, I gently buff the shoes until they look as white and clean as new.

Mona Kuroki, RN, BSN

Shoe biz #3

Now that your shoes are white, what about the laces? To clean them, place them in a bowl or jar of warm water and add some dishwasher detergent. Agitate the laces in the solution, let them soak for 1 or 2 hours, then rinse and air-dry. Your laces will look as white and clean as your shoes.

Janet Widman, RN

Runs? Recycle
When your panty hose get a run, you don't need to run to throw them away. Instead, recycle them.

If you have two pairs of panty hose, each with a run in *one* leg, cut off the bad leg from each pair. Put on the panty and remaining good leg of one pair. Then put on the panty and good leg of the other pair. Now you have a "new" pair of panty hose.

When these panty hose get runs, cut them in pieces and use them as stuffing for pillows, quilts, or toys.

Verna Honsaker, RN

Lotioned legs
Before putting on support hose, apply a generous amount of body or hand lotion to both your legs. And if you want to slow down absorption by the skin, mix a little glycerin with the lotion.

Either way, you'll be surprised at how much longer your hose stay up—and how comfortable they are.

Hilda Swanson, RN

More support
If your support hose aren't being very supportive, try this:

After slipping your feet and ankles into the stockings, lie down and raise your legs to at least a 45-degree angle. Stay in this position for a minute or two, then pull the hosiery on the rest of the way. You'll be amazed at how much more supportive your hose can be.

Shirley A. McGuire, RN

Tear repair
If you get a tear in your white stock-

ings at work and can't change to a new pair, try taping them.

Just cut two pieces of white nonallergenic tape the same size. Slide one piece adhesive-side-up under the tear, then align the tear edges and affix the tape. Affix the second piece over the tear, matching edges with the first tape.

The tape keeps the hole from getting bigger and running, and it blends well with your stockings.

Sandra L. Turner, RN, MEd

Mix and match
After laundering several white pantsuit uniforms together, you may have difficulty matching the tops and bottoms correctly. Sew a small clump of colored thread inside the collar and waistband, using a different color for each uniform. Then, after washing and drying, simply match the colored threads.

Ellen L. Badger, RN

Fuzz busters
Do fuzzy little balls of lint decorate your old uniforms? If so, redecorate—with a safety razor. Just shave off the lint balls, and your uniform will look like new again.

Margery Lebel, RN

White again
Rust stains ruining your whites? Squeeze some lemon juice on the stains, sprinkle a generous amount of salt over the juice, and place the uniform in the sun until it's dry. Then wash as usual and—voilá!—your whites are white once again.

Etta M. Rosenthal, RN, BS, PHN

Cling no more
Do your noncling slips persist in clinging and creeping despite your using antistatic additives in your

wash? Here's a simple solution. When applying hand lotion, just wipe the excess lotion on your hose. No more will slip and skirt cling to your knees.

Beverly Gault, RN

Toothpaste on hand
To get fecal odors off your hands, try some toothpaste. Just rub a small amount into your hands, and the odor will disappear.

Mary Payne, RN

Soda for odor
To control odor in your duty shoes, sprinkle baking soda in them before putting them on each day. You can easily store the baking soda in a grated-cheese shaker or any container with large holes in the lid.

Susan Appleby, LPN

Eradicating losses
School pins and nameplates occasionally come undone and drop off unnoticed. As a safety precaution, use a small cube of rubber, cut from an eraser.

Push the spike of your pin through the cloth of your uniform, and then slide the eraser cube onto the spike before clasping. Then, if the clasp comes undone, the cube prevents the spike from slipping through the cloth. When the cube becomes too loose, simply cut a replacement.

Virginia Davis, RN

Firm backing
Did you ever lose a name pin because it fell off your uniform unnoticed?

To prevent this, rummage through your jewelry box for the back of an earring for pierced ears. Then put your pin on as usual, but before clasping it, slide the earring back onto

the pin shaft. If the clasp opens, the earring back will keep the name pin firmly attached to your uniform.

Kathleen Williams, RN, CCRN

On guard
I like to carry my hemostat with me, but I *don't* like the holes it pokes in my uniform pockets. So I cover the ends of the hemostat with a *rubber* needle guard. The needle guard protects my pockets—without affecting the hemostat's clamping action.

Betty Francis, LPN

Sew-sew organizer
Uniform pockets do get crowded— what with the hemostats, scissors, pens, and other items you must carry. To solve this bulky problem, sew some dividers right into your pockets.

For each pocket, cut a strip of white bias seam binding—as long as the pocket is wide. Place the seam binding along the top *inside* of your pocket. Stitch up and down at each end of the binding and at different intervals to make holders for each item you carry. Then simply slide the blades of your instruments through the holders so the handles catch on the upper edge. Slide your pens through the holders, clipping them to the binding.

Now, you have a pocket divider-organizer that's less bulky and less expensive than the plastic version. And these sew-on organizers don't have to be transferred from one pocket to another as you change uniforms.

Jacqueline Meister, RN

Pockets make perfect
If your white pantsuit uniforms have no pockets in the pants, you can sew a pocket on them from any available white material. These pockets

take the pressure off regular blouse pockets, which always seem to become overloaded. They also provide an excellent place to carry a notebook, tissues, scissors, keys, and whatnot. What's more, your blouse covers the pocket, so you don't have to worry about imperfections.

Ruth Thesing, RN

Pocket protector

To keep pencils from smudging your uniform pockets, cover each pencil point with a rubber tip from a Vacutainer needle. The tips protect the pencil points and keep your pockets clean.

Norka Vélez Ramos, RN

A pen pointer

If you like to keep two different colored pens on hand together but need a penholder that protects your uniform from unsightly ink spots, try this:

Measure and cut some used I.V. tubing about 20″ from the drip chamber. Then cut the drip chamber in half. Cover the points of two pens with the drip chamber and wrap the rest of the tubing between and around the pens to prevent unraveling.

This penholder keeps your pens together and keeps the points covered. Best of all—no more ink-soiled uniforms to worry about.

Eva Tapoler, RN

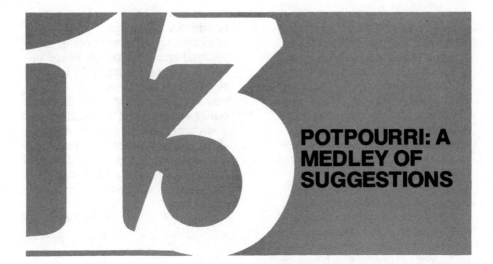

POTPOURRI: A MEDLEY OF SUGGESTIONS

Traction tree

The traction room is often cluttered and disorganized. Here's a space-saving, no-cost way to store traction equipment: make a "traction tree." Using extra traction bars, make a trunk, branches, legs, and feet. The trunk is an overhead traction bar, the branches are corner bed pins, the three legs are 18″ bars, and the feet are short bars of different lengths.

Hang all traction bars on the branches, putting the heaviest bars on the bottom. Because the trunk is slightly off the floor and the legs staggered one above the other, the tree is stable and freestanding. For extra stability, though, attach the tree to a wall with a long traction bar.

Scott Goodrich

Hooked on hooks

In our hospital nursery, we recycle the metal hooks from Pleur-evac units. We hang them on incubators and crib frames to hold clipboards for our daily worksheets and graphs. We also hang mobiles on them to give the babies visual stimulation.

Patricia Homola-Portuondo, RN

How to beat aching feet

Do you dread having to break in a new pair of work shoes because they pinch your toes? Stuff damp wash-cloths in the toe of each shoe and leave them in overnight. The next day the pinch will be gone.

Patricia Kleve, LPN

Bag the unit

Have you ever had to prepare a patient for telemetry monitoring, only to discover that you were out of telemetry pouches? If so, you might be interested in this solution: a piece of tubular stretch bandage.

Measure and cut a length of bandage the same size as the telemetry unit. Tie a knot at one end. Thread a long piece of twill tape through the gauze bandage down one side, across the knotted end, and up the other side. Thread a second piece of tape across the bottom knotted end only. Tie the first piece of twill tape around the patient's neck and the second piece around his waist in a comfortable position so the telemetry unit and pouch hang securely on his chest.

Janet R. McMillan, RN

Binder benefits

If you're a visiting nurse, use looseleaf binders to maintain patient records.

The benefits of a binder over traditional charting are many. For instance:

• The binder lies flat when opened, and notes can be conveniently and neatly transcribed onto the charts.

• Notes can readily be written on both sides of a page, which cuts the pages per record.

• Preprinted tabs can be attached to the dividers, allowing quick access to record sections.

• Pages can be rearranged easily or added as needed.

• When a binder is full, parts of a patient's record can be removed and filed in a manila envelope, which can then be labeled for easy retrieval.

Lucille Gress, RN

Christmas treats

Even patients on liquid diets won't have to pass up Christmas cookies—if they're made of gelatin, that is. Here's how to make them:

Combine four envelopes of unflavored gelatin with three 3-oz packages of cherry- or lime-flavored gelatin. Add 4 cups of boiling water and stir until the gelatin is dissolved. Pour the mixture into a 13" × 9" cookie sheet and chill until firm. Then cut out shapes with Christmas cookie cutters.

The "cookies" will help patients keep to their diets *and* enjoy some Christmas treats.

Eileen Laudermilch, LPN

Cushiony creations

Used egg-crate–like mattresses, as you well know, can be cut up and recycled in numerous ways. For example, you can use them as wheelchair cushions. You can cut a hole in the center and use them as commode seat cushions. You can place a piece of the mattress under a patient in a tub chair so he won't slide forward. And you can cover a piece with sheepskin to pad a patient's coccyx and hips.

Edna Begun, RN

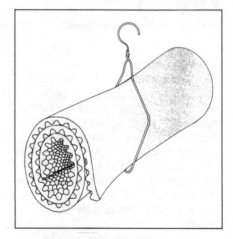

Crating the egg crates

Many patients want to take their foam egg-crate-like mattresses home with them when they're discharged. We're happy to oblige them, but getting the mattresses packed is a problem. We've tried rolling the pads, then taping or tying them with gauze strips. The tape doesn't hold, and the gauze is unwieldy.

We finally discovered that a wire coat hanger was the answer to our problem. We pull the long straight edge down, away from the hook, to make a large, diamond-shaped opening. Then we roll up the mattress and push it through the hanger's opening.

The hanger keeps the mattress rolled up neatly and even has a ready-made handle for easy carrying.

Shari Katz, RN
Terry Friedrich, RN

Take snow chances

I work for a home health agency in a rural area. Most of our nurses travel about 100 miles a day on narrow, two-lane roads that become dangerous to drive on when winter weather arrives. So late each fall, we prepare for the oncoming snow and ice storms by holding a "weatherproofing" staff development session.

We're reminded to pack all the items we'd need if we were stranded on the road or stuck in traffic. For instance, boots, socks, gloves, scarf, hat, blanket, and white fabric for an emergency flag should go in the car. A gallon of water, a deicer, a windshield scraper, and carpet squares for traction on ice (they're easier to carry than sand) should also be packed. An empty coffee can, a candle, and matches could be used in two ways: either we can anchor the candle in the can and light it for warmth or we can fill the can with snow and melt the snow with the candle for water.

Although we never willingly take a travel risk, our annual weatherproofing session helps us feel better prepared for unexpected bad driving conditions.

Winnie Bowen, RN

A line on leads

We keep lead wires for our cardiac monitors neat, unraveled, and ready to use with the help of a stick figure made from tongue blades. We glue snaps from lead patches onto the stick

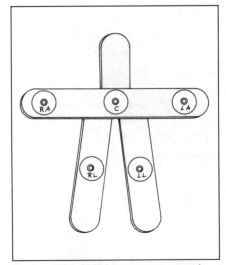

figure and label the snaps appropriately: RA (right arm), LL (left leg), and so on. Then we snap the corresponding leads onto the stick figure.

Now when we need to connect a patient to the monitor in a hurry, the leads stay untangled, and we can quickly tell which lead goes where on the patient.

Jean Ballenthin, RN

A lead on lines

We use a tongue blade to organize the ports on a patient's Swan-Ganz catheter. We secure the tubing right above each port to the tongue blade with a piece of ½" adhesive tape. Then we place another tongue blade on top of the first one and wrap a piece of tape around the ends of the two blades to keep them together.

Finally, we wrap a piece of tape around the middle of the blades, fastening the ends together to make a tab. We put a safety pin through the tab and pin it to the patient's gown or bedclothes, loosely enough to prevent tension on the line.

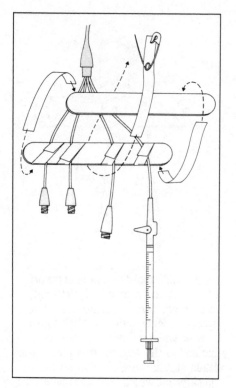

This helps us keep track of the many lines this patient has.

Jean Ballenthin, RN

Job sharing

Each month in our intensive care unit, each nurse is assigned a different job: one nurse is responsible for maintaining our floor stock; another for assembling the Swan-Ganz setup; another for checking the arterial line setup, the cut-down setup, and so on.

This work-assignment rotation keeps the nurses familiar with *all* of our emergency equipment setups and eliminates the panic of assembling scattered emergency equipment at the last minute.

Katherine Link, RN

A better way to float

Floating, pulling, temporary reassignment. These words strike dismay in many a nurse's heart. But not nurses from Research Medical Center (RMC), Kansas City, Mo. RMC expects nurses to float only within their specialty—but it also foots the bill for orienting them to other specialties so they can float to other areas if they choose.

Here's how the floating system works: Nursing service at RMC is divided into six specialty departments, and the nursing skills and knowledge needed for units within each specialty department are similar. For example, the inpatient surgical care department has six units. Nurses from each surgical unit are oriented to all other surgical units. They then feel comfortable and competent if they're floated to another surgical unit.

Nurses can refuse to float without fear or retaliation by the medical center. But, since they can receive orientation to other specialties at the medical center's expense, many choose to do this, providing RMC with more nurses to float to different areas.

The director of the intensive care unit says the new system decreases nurses' anxiety and resentment because they're not floated to unfamiliar areas.

Gail Poelker, RN, MA

Wristwatch in isolation

When working with isolation patients, do you miss being able to use your watch? Try slipping it into a plastic sandwich bag before entering the patient's room. That way you can see it, but it won't become contaminated.

Irene Evans, RN

Reducing ICU stress

Job dissatisfaction, emotional fatigue, and overdependence on supervisors can develop within the staff of any unit. But intensive care unit (ICU) nurses are even more susceptible to these "occupational hazards."

To combat this problem, the ICU supervisor at Mansfield (Ohio) General Hospital invites staff nurses to serve on a voluntary basis as ICU charge nurses. She rotates the assignment weekly, and also rotates the staff nurses through the three ICU areas (surgical, medical, postcoronary) every 2 to 6 weeks.

The ICU nursing instructor at the hospital is in a unique position to evaluate this new approach and says the nurses are now more understanding when someone else is in charge. They are showing an increased interest in management and decision making. One nurse, as a result of this experience, even joined the professional standards committee.

Jan Vinson, RN, BSN, CCRN

Pick a job, any job

Thanks to a "job jar," those repetitive, tedious—but necessary—tasks needed to keep the unit running smoothly can get done promptly.

Type task descriptions on separate slips of paper, fold the slips, and place them into the jar. Each nurse picks a slip from the jar, completes the designated task, and tacks the slip on the bulletin board. One nurse removes the slips from the bulletin board and recycles them as often as necessary.

Besides allowing nurses to share the load, the job jar adds an element of surprise to the unit: you never know which job you'll pick next.

Joni L. Ulman, RN

A bright idea

If you're repeatedly going home from work with the narcotics cabinet keys still in your pocket, try this.

Attach the keys to one end of a long, brightly colored thick string or rope. Make a loop on the other end to slip over your head.

If the string's long enough, the keys will reach comfortably into your pocket. If it's bright enough, you'll be reminded not to take the keys home with you.

Patricia Dubovec, RN

Keys keeper

From time to time, a nurse on our unit would forget to empty her pockets at the end of a shift and go home with the narcotic keys in her pocket.

So now we account for the keys on the controlled drug disposition record—the sheet on which we account for the drugs we've used during that shift. With this system, the keys stay on the unit where they belong.

Nancy Evans, RN

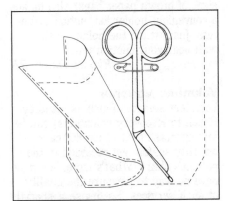

A pin point

To keep my scissors from falling out of my uniform pocket or sliding to the bottom of my pocket (where I could never find them in a hurry), I pin them in place.

I pin a safety pin to the inside of my uniform pocket and slip the blades through the pin. Now the scissors stay in one place with the handles in an easy-to-grasp, upright position.

Ramona Dekrey, RN, BSN

Knee pads

Cardiopulmonary resuscitation (CPR) students and instructors used to complain about sore knees after a practice session spent kneeling on the floor next to the manikin. To save their knees, we got free samples of foam rubber products (such as egg-crate-like mattresses) and cut them into $2' \times 2'$ squares. We placed the squares inside pillowcases to keep them clean. Now everyone can kneel on a pad and concentrate on the CPR instructions—instead of on how much his knees hurt.

Sande Jones, RN, MS

Not left holding the bags

A commercially available paper bag holder (usually used to hold various sizes of brown paper bags) also makes a convenient holder for suction catheters. Just attach the holder to the wall near your suction unit.

Eleanor Vinson, RN

Volunteer voucher

Volunteer services (such as visits by Reach to Recovery volunteers) can be an important part of patient care, but they seldom get recorded in the patient's chart. What's more, you may have no way to measure the quality of such services. So devise a special "chart" for the volunteers.

Use a gummed label, which the volunteer fills out after visiting the patient and gives to the head nurse, along with a verbal report of the visit. The head nurse can paste the label on the nurse's notes and write a summary of the volunteer's report.

The label includes space for the patient's name, his illness or disability, the date of the volunteer's visit, and the service provided by the volunteer (such as prosthesis, exercises, and so on). The label can also have room for comments and for the volunteer's and doctor's signatures.

Mary E. Corcelius, RN

Pictures? Perfect

Our hospital rooms are brighter and more cheerful than they once were. In fact, they're quite picturesque, thanks to our efforts at fund-raising. Here's how we do it:

We sell inexpensive "chances" to our hospital staff members, offering three money prizes. Then we buy pictures for the patient rooms with the money left after the prizes are awarded. To date, we've bought over 50 pictures—everything from peaceful landscapes to children at play. The patients appreciate our efforts at making the hospital rooms more cheerful: some have even donated their own artwork (framed needlework and photos) to the collection.

Wendy M. Farmer, RNA

Stay-put strips

We used to tape a patient's EKG rhythm strips in our nurse's notes. But we found that when the notes were microfilmed later for hospital records, the tape sometimes obliterated pertinent information. We tried doubling the tape to itself and applying it to the back of the strip, but strips taped this way sometimes fell out of the nurse's notes.

So now, instead, we rub the back of the strips with a glue stick and press the strips into our nurse's notes.

The strips stay put, and *all* the information on them gets microfilmed.

Pat Kaldor, RN, MSN

Rhyme saves time

We use color-coded electrodes (white for negative, black for positive, red for ground) with the cardiac monitors in our intensive care unit (ICU). Remembering where to place each of them on a patient's chest used to be a problem for me until I learned the phrase—"White on right and smoke (black) over fire (red)."

Now, even in emergencies, I'm sure that the white electrode goes on the upper right side of the patient's chest, and the black electrode goes on the upper left side of his chest, "over" the red electrode on the lower left side of his chest.

Virginia Rodgers, RNC

Organized storage

In our emergency department, shelf space is at a premium. To keep us from overstocking certain items or storing unnecessary supplies, we've drawn up a quota for each item we need to stock (for instance, four boxes of hypoallergenic tape, three boxes of I.V. catheters, or a certain number of artificial airways).

To make sure we never run out of supplies, we put a red label on the last box of every item in stock, reminding us it's time to reorder. This keeps space, storage, and supply problems to a minimum.

Della Whipple, RN

Stretcher storage

If your recovery room patients need an emesis basin or some tissues—stat—but these items aren't close at hand, ask the maintenance department to make and attach small metal trays under the head of each stretcher. Then store supplies on the trays, and they're always within reach, p.r.n.

Emily Nickles, RN

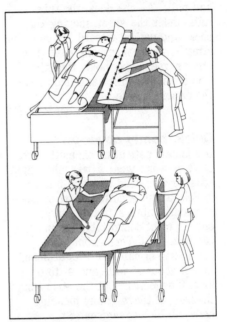

Tubes to move on

You've heard of moving pictures and moving day? Well, how about *moving tubes*? To us, a moving tube is an invaluable tool when transferring an immobile, postoperative, or obese patient from his bed to a stretcher.

We make a moving tube by sewing a piece of $60'' \times 36''$ synthetic material (the slippery, shiny kind used to make lightweight windbreakers) into a $60''$ long tubular shape. When we have to transfer a patient, we place the moving tube lengthwise under the patient's untucked bottom bed sheet. We bring the stretcher next to the bed and place the rest of the moving tube across the stretcher.

Two nurses then take their positions: one stands on one side of the stretcher; the other stands opposite the first nurse on the far side of the bed. The nurse next to the stretcher reaches across the stretcher, grabs the untucked bottom bed sheet, and pulls. As she does, the tube rolls under the sheet, moving the sheet and patient toward her onto the stretcher with surprising ease. The other nurse simply holds the other side of the bed sheet and makes sure the patient is safe.

Trish Zapf-Reid, RN

Quick, comfy cover-up

If a female patient on chemotherapy can't or won't wear a wig, she might consider this head cover-up instead.

Fold or cut a cotton scarf or piece of material into a triangle large enough to fit comfortably around the patient's head. Then, from a wig, cut a strip of hair (with its attached lining) about 1" wide and 4" to 6" long. (Suggestion: Cut the strip from the back of the wig; any mending here will be less noticeable.)

Center and sew the strip to the inside of the triangle's longest edge, allowing the hair to protrude like bangs. On each end of the same edge, attach a strip of Velcro tape, one inside and the other outside. When fastened together, these strips will hold the cover-up securely in place.

This cover-up will flatter the patient's face and give an illusion of hair without the bulk of a regular wig. It's great for keeping her head warm at night and handy to have around when unexpected company drops in.

Michelle Griffin, RN

School sleuths

If you're a school nurse, teach the home economics and physical education teachers how to spot shoulder and hip disproportions—sewing classes and locker rooms are ideal places to spot scoliosis.

Sherry French, RN

No ice tubes

If a patient needs a rubber nasogastric tube, don't rush out looking for ice to stiffen the tube. Instead, place a packaged tube in the refrigerator's freezer for about 5 minutes. By the time the patient's prepared, the tube's ready for insertion.

Hermila Villarreal, RN

Flower holder

Many times visitors arrive with cut garden flowers to brighten a patient's room, but no vases are available. Here's how to make a substitute vase.

Take two paper cups (wax-coated or Styrofoam), place them with mouths together, and fasten with a strip of 1" adhesive tape. Cut a hole in one end large enough to accommodate the flower stems. Fill the vase with water to just below the taped area. Then add the flowers.

These vases are not only sturdy, but also can be made in seconds from supplies kept on the floor.

Marilee E. Harrison, RN

Pass the towel, please

Ever have difficulty passing intubation equipment to the doctor, piece by piece?

Gather all the intubation equipment—laryngoscope with blade, endotracheal tube with stylet and inflation syringe attached, oral airway, lubricant, and roller gauze—and wrap it in a disposable sterile towel. Then pass the whole bundle to the doctor with nothing getting lost. This is also handy when the equipment is needed outside the arrest area—

the bundle is compact and easily transported.

Yvonne M. Lesiak, RN

Other plaster problems

Always use cold water for easy removal of plaster from patients and instruments after a cast has been applied. If you get plaster on your uniform, let the plaster dry, then brush it off.

Since working with plaster can dry your hands, keep a bottle of hand lotion nearby and use it frequently.

Let mothers soak the serial casts off their babies. And add a little vinegar to the water to aid removal of the casts.

Elsie Hajdics, RN

Pretty cool solution for several problems

There's a simple, enjoyable way to solve certain problems: ease bleeding of cut lips or tongue of crying children...ease swelling gums of cranky oldsters after dental procedures... administer fluids to patients of any age apt to vomit. It's a *Popsicle.*

It's a valuable item, especially for children, when the doctor wants to start certain patients on fluids by mouth, as after acute gastroenteritis or surgery, or when ordinary fluids are apt to precipitate vomiting. And, needless to say, patients almost invariably enjoy the cold treat.

Adelaide Rosen, RN

Cent-saving scent

Have you ever wished you had an effective, pleasant, continuous room deodorizer—for example, when you're caring for new ostomy patients or cancer patients? For such situations, mechanical deodorizing sprays can

be overpowering at first and then dissipate quickly. Time-released sprays are expensive.

Oil of cloves can be used as a pleasant, effective, long-lasting deodorizer. Here's how: pour a small amount of oil of cloves into a glass test tube (the solution eats through plastic). Then dip a 1″ wide gauze wick into the solution and pull one end out over the rim of the test tube.

For the best effect, prepare two such test tubes. Tape one to the foot of the patient's bed and the other to the bathroom wall.

You may also use oil of wintergreen, but it's not as long-lasting and its fragrance is harsher than oil of cloves.

4 West Nursing Staff
University of Colorado
Medical Center

A hint of mint

Here's how to absorb strong odors caused by a patient's draining wound or profuse bleeding.

Take three or four cotton balls and put a few drops of peppermint oil on each ball. Then put the balls in a plastic medicine cup and place the cup in the patient's room, usually on a windowsill.

Change the balls every day, so the peppermint oil keeps the patient's room smelling fresh.

Sr. Frederica, RN

Extra-large tourniquets

Do you find that a regular tourniquet isn't long enough to wrap around a large arm? You can make an extra-large tourniquet by simply attaching two tourniquets together. The Velcro fasteners make it easy.

Henry Schneiderman, MD

A tote-all success

When you're transporting a critically ill patient from the emergency department to the intensive care unit, you often have to tote along his personal possessions, a cardiac monitor, and charts. If you've ever wished for three more arms at times like these, you might try placing a long backboard under the mattress on the stretcher. Position the board so that it extends out about 2' from the foot of the stretcher. Put the patient's personal items and the equipment on the end of the board; they'll be counterbalanced by the patient's weight on the stretcher.

Now, with your arms free, you can concentrate on getting the patient to the intensive care unit safely.

Kimberly A. Stotts, RN, BSN

Photo IDs

Imagine trying to find a particular nursing home patient (one you've never met) at medication time. He could be anywhere in the facility—game room, garden, visiting area—*and* you don't know what he looks like.

Finding and identifying him would be a lot easier if you had a photograph (taken when he was admitted) attached to his medication file. Of course, when you did find him, you'd have to be sure you had the right name, right drug, right dose, right route, and right time.

Sandee Campbell, RN, BSN

EKGs to go

When a patient is discharged from our coronary care unit, we give him a copy of his last electrocardiogram

(EKG) rhythm strip and suggest he carry it in his wallet. It could save him an unnecessary hospital admission later.

For instance, at some future time the patient may have another EKG run that shows some abnormalities he's being treated for. If his regular doctor isn't available to interpret the results, another doctor might want to admit him to determine whether these abnormalities are new or old findings. The rhythm strip in his wallet will provide the information immediately, and the patient won't have to be admitted.

May Edwards, RN

The straw that broke the bad habit

When one of my patients is trying to quit smoking, I give him a plastic straw cut to the length of a cigarette. The straw becomes a cigarette substitute: the patient can hold it like a cigarette to keep his hands busy. And to satisfy his craving for a smoke, he can even "inhale" the straw just as he would the real thing.

Linda Tate, RN, BSN

Ready when you are

To keep your hemostat handy when you're working with a patient who has a central I.V. line, do this. Wrap a piece of tape around the I.V. pole, bringing the ends together to make a tab. Clip your hemostat onto the tab, where it'll always be ready when you need to change solutions and tubings, obtain blood samples, or whatever.

Diana E. Contine, RN

A friendly word

For some of my elderly patients, English is a second language. Their first language is Polish or Italian or German. Although I can't speak these languages, I can communicate with my patients.

On a sheet of paper, I've written some common English words and phrases, with the foreign equivalents opposite them. I post the paper on the patient's bedside bulletin board when he's admitted to my unit.

The patients appreciate hearing a friendly "good morning" in their own language: gin dobre (Polish), buon giorno (Italian), guten Morgen (German). They also respond appreciatively when they're told it's time to eat, take medicine, or turn to the side.

Fe Perez, RN

Leading questions

I have many patient-teaching opportunities on our short-stay surgery unit. For example, when doing preoperative assessment of a pediatric patient, I might weigh the patient and say, making sure his parents are listening, "I see you weigh 33 pounds, Justin. You must still be riding in a car seat."

The parents usually respond to such a comment, giving me the chance to review local car-seat regulations.

Rose Coalson, RN, BSN

Stick-to-itiveness

When clipping a patient's eyelashes before eye surgery, try putting some K-Y jelly on the blades of the scissors. The eyelashes will stick to the blade, making it easier for you to clip them. And the clipped ends won't fall on the patient's face.

Katherine Link, RN, BSN

Cupped hands

To prevent flexion contractures of the hands, place a plastic juice cup in each of your patient's hands. If he's making a tight fist and you can't get the cup in his palm, gently flex his wrist forward and his hand will relax.

The cup's firm surface inhibits and relaxes the flexors. If the cup falls out of the patient's hand, use Montgomery straps to hold it in place.

Lois A. Kolada, PT

Bed changing—an easy weigh

The best time to change bed linens for a bedridden patient is after you've weighed him with a bed scale and recorded his weight. While he's still on the scale, place a pillow under his head and a cover over his body. Then change the linens. When you're finished, lower the patient back to his clean bed, and see that he's in a comfortable position.

By doing these tasks while the patient is on the scale instead of in his bed, you'll have saved the patient a lot of needless and uncomfortable turning.

Lorretta A. Debus, RN

Take-out menus

I suggest to my patients that they take their hospital menus home with them. After discharge, they'll find it helpful to review the diet exchange lists and sample menus.

Karen C. Stowe, RN

INDEX

A

abduction pillow, 143, 170
abrasions, 71, 94, 196
active learning sessions, 30
activity level cards, 23
adhesive tape, 171
admission procedures, 16
affection, 80
aging, education about, 31
airflow, skin healing and, 173
airway, artificial, 67
allergy
    identifying patients with, 6
    injections for, 101
ambulance, 8, 104
ambulation, 58, 59, 64, 158
ammonia, fainting episodes
        and, 201
Amphojel, storage of, 189
ampules, safety precautions for
        opening, 202, 203
anaphylaxis kit, 79
anatomy
    of heart, 40
    renal, 24
anesthetic antiseptic, 75
antihypertensive drugs, 42
antiseptic, anesthetic, 75
anxiety, 12
aphasic patient, communicating
        with, 3
arm boards, 182, 184, 211
arm exerciser, 63
armrest, pressure from, 142
arm splint, 71, 175
arrhythmias, 39
arteriovenous shunt, clamps
        for, 79
art gallery, in-house, 83
arthritic patient, 78, 112, 121
aspiration, prevention of, 197
assessment
    fracture, 126
    heel, 125
    leg pain, 131
    lung, 127
    neurologic, 125
    nighttime, 127
    of patient, 123
    patient-teaching aids, 33, 34
    postpartum, 128
    skin, 125
assignment sheet, 18

B

baby, progress report for, 13
balloon-inflation line, fixing,
        205
bandage, elastic, 165
bathing
    with heparin lock, 185
    with I.V. line, 185
    one-handed, 223
bathtub, safety precautions for,
        197
beard, care for, 222, 224
bed cradle, 114
bed linens, 144, 145, 239
bed making, 76
bedpan, 147, 148
bedridden patient
    bowel habits of, 149
    changing linens of, 144, 145,
        239
    feeding aid for, 56
    hair washing of, 220, 221
    moving of, 142
    raising head of bed for, 112
    self-lifting aids for, 111
    sling for positioning, 142
bedside commode, 149
bereavement visits, 14
binders, abdominal, 216
bleeding
    oral, 118
    reporting amount of, 130
blind patient
    clothes coding for, 117
    medication aids for, 108, 109
blood
    specimen, 157, 158
    stains, 224
    warming, 181
blood pressure, 73, 131
body heat, preventing loss of,
        95
body odor, 223
boredom
    prevention of, 84
    relieving, 90, 91
bottle caps, 189
bowel patterns, 10, 149
bowel resection, 22
breast examination, 128
breast-feeding
    alternating breasts for, 122
    reducing discomfort during,
        121
    teaching, 28

breast prosthesis, 119
breast shield, 121
breast support, 59
breathing exercises, 86, 92
Broviac catheter, 74
bruising, prevention of, 196
bulldog clamps, 199
burn patient, maintaining fluid
        intake of, 57

C

calamine lotion, 87
calendars, as memory aids, 5,
        6
call systems, 1, 2, 61, 80
cancer, oral, 134
Candida albicans, prevention of,
        93
cane, retrieval of, 111
carbonation, elimination of, 57
cardiac arrest
    drugs used during, 193
    staff preparation for, 79
cardiac board, 103
cardiac monitor, lead wires for,
        231, 235
cardiac output, measurement
        of, 212
cardiopulmonary resuscitation,
        34, 39, 234
care kit, 120
cast
    care of, 21, 71, 98, 111, 116,
        117, 205, 216, 223
    removal of, 94, 173
catheter
    Broviac, 74
    condom, 164
    Foley, 64, 145, 158, 159,
        160, 161
    Hickman, 22, 48, 184
    holder for, 234
    ports, 231
    storage of, 149
    Swan-Ganz, 205, 231
catheterization
    conserving supplies for, 211
    of female patient, 146
    of male patient, 146
central venous pressure lines,
        199

cerebrospinal fluid, managing drainage of, 152
cervical collar, 71, 223
chafing, prevention of, 93
chart
    camp nurse's, 194
    neurovascular check, 124
chemotherapy
    drugs, 42, 202
    head cover-up after, 236
chest percussion, 96, 99
chest tubes, 52, 64
child, unresponsive, 92
cigarette, straw as substitute for, 238
circulation, collateral, 23
circumcision
    comfort measures for, 95
    dressing, 165
cleft palate, feeding infant with, 86
coccyx, decubitus ulcer on, 169
code blue
    during patient transfer, 197
    responsibilities, 18
collection devices, easing discomfort of, 162
colostomy, cleaning of, 115
colostomy bag, 154, 210
comatose patient, positioning of, 141
commode, 196
communication
    nonverbal, 13
    system, 3, 4, 239
computed tomography scan, 6
conference coordination, 216
confused patient, I.V. maintenance in, 182
contact lenses, removal of, 135
continuing education, 218
contracture, hand, 175, 239
controlled-relaxation techniques, 66
contusions, measurement of, 129
cotton balls, 204, 209
cranial nerves, 51
craniotomy patient, head covering for, 60
crash cart, 39, 79, 80, 214, 215
crib mobiles, 91

croupette, filling ice chamber of, 97
crutches, retrieval of, 111
cuff-inflation line, 205
cystostomy tubes, 154

D

debilitated patient, head support for, 143
decubitus ulcer, 169, 170, 171
dental floss, 134
dentures, 200
deodorizers, 114, 237
depressed patient, encouragement for, 83
diabetes, teaching about, 24
diabetic patient
    diet for, 35
    injection practice for, 26
    insulin preparation for, 108
    schedule adjustment for, 5
    skin care for, 117
diagnosis, lunch as tool for, 126
dialysate, preventing leakage of, 175
diapers, 146
diarrhea, 115
diary
    for baby, 12
    for ventilator patient, 2
diet
    for diabetic patient, 35
    hospital menus and, 239
dietary supplements, 53, 54
discharge instructions, 32
distal port connector, 179
distraction techniques, 101
doctor, questions to ask, 5, 15
doctors' orders, 19
drainage bag, urinary, 161
drawsheet, 144
dressings
    abdominal, 166
    anal-perianal resection, 61
    Broviac catheter, 74
    hip wound, 165
    incisional, 117
    leg, 121
    sacral, 175
    thigh, 165
    torso, 97

drugs
    antihypertensive, 42
    for cardiac arrest, 193
    identification of, 123
    incompatibility of, 179
    information on, 42, 43
    labels for, 31
drug samples, labeling of, 31

E

ear
    irrigation of, 136, 137
    piercing, 116
    speculums for, 210
eardrops, 190
edema
    of arm, 177
    stretchable identification band for, 195
egg-crate-like mattress, 230
EKG strips, 234
elbow protectors, 60, 169
elderly patient
    education on aging for, 31
    skin and nail care for, 223
    urine specimen from, 156, 158
electric shock, 195
electrode jelly, 171
elimination, 97
emergency
    medication for, 43
    practice for, 39
    suctioning, 212
    supplies, 79, 212, 213
emergency cart, 104
emergency department, 11
emesis basin, 115
emotions, 81
endotracheal tube, 127, 163, 164, 215
enema, 151
environment, 11
episiotomy, 167
epistaxis, 137
equipment
    endotracheal, 214
    loss of, 206
    orientation, 47
evacuation drills, 215
evacuation shelter, 198
examination
    rectal, 68
    vaginal, 68

excoriated lesions, 169
exercise
    postmastectomy, 63
    postoperative breathing, 92
    postpartum, 116
exerciser
    arm, 63
    hand, 64, 92
    hip 71
    leg, 63
expiration dates, 189
eyecup, 135
eye drops, 34, 192
eye examination, 128
eyeglasses, 200
eye irrigation, 135
eyelashes, 239
eye pads, 102, 103
eye patch, 136
eye surgery, communicating after, 61

F

fainting
    ammonia for, 201
    visitors and, 80
falls, prevention of, 197
fecal material, cleaning of, 174
fecal odor, 227
feeding tubes, 116, 137, 138
fetal development, 29
fever, 62, 95
fiberglass fibers, removal from skin, 172
finger, immobilization of, 183
fingernails
    care for, 223
    cleaning, 224
finger soak 89
finger splint, 118
fire, prevention of, 199
fire drill, 15
first-aid kit, homemade, 119
Fleet enema, 151
flexion contractures, 239
floating, unit-to-unit, 232
flotation mattress, 76
fluid, self-dispenser of, 116
fluid intake
    maintaining, 54, 55, 57, 85, 86
    measurement of, 116, 128
fluid restriction, management of, 54, 57

foam-rubber pad, 61
foot cradle, 72, 113
foot drop, 143
foot soaks, 168
foreign-speaking patient, communication with, 4, 239
fracture
    assessment of, 126
    pain, 73, 147
frequency, urinary, 115
frightened child, diversions for, 87

G

Gastrografin, 67
gastrointestinal studies, 69
gastrostomy tube, 60, 162
gauze pads, 210
geriatric patient, caring for, 45, 190
glass particles, removal of, 78, 172
glucose testing strips, 209
Gomco suction machine, 153
gravity drainage, measurement of, 132
gravity tube, preventing leakage from, 152
grease, removal from skin, 172
grief, 83
grip, checking patient's, 112

H

hair, infant, 105
hair care, 220, 221
halo apparatus, 201
Halo-Tibial traction, 93
handicapped patient
    feeding aids for, 56
    swimming precautions for, 196
    walking instructions for, 93
handouts, patient-teaching, 218
hand soak, distracting child during, 90
hand splint, 72
hand washing, 44
head cover-up, 236
head dressing, 95
head support, 143
head ulceration, prevention of, 73
healing, promotion of, 99
health maintenance programs, student, 37

heart, anatomy of, 40
heat loss, preventing, 95
heel, assessment of, 125
heel sticks, 157
helpless patient, transferring of, 141
hemodynamic monitoring, 40
hemostat, 227, 238
Hemovac
    ambulating patient with, 64
    drainage measurement, 132
heparin infusion, 180
heparin injection, 190
heparin lock, 185, 187, 190
hernia, comfort measures for, 95
Hickman catheter, 22, 48, 184
hip disproportions, 236
hip-spica cast, 147
hospital
    costs, 206, 207
    credit for unused medications, 208
    open house, 35
    orientation programs, 36, 104
    procedures, 48
    rooms, 234
hot packs, 140
hot-water bottles, 137
Hoyer lift, 76
hypospadias surgery, managing elimination after, 146

I

ice bags, 120, 137, 139
ice lavage, 215
ice pack, 77, 87, 136, 140, 167, 208
ice trauma, 139
incision
    sacral, 99
    ureterostomy, 154
incontinent patient, disposable diapers for, 146
identification
    infant, 11
    wristband, 195
incentive spirometer, 89
incompatible drugs, I.V. administration of, 179
incontinent male patient, 148, 158

infant
chest percussor, 99
hair, as keepsake, 105
measurement of, 129
premature, 96, 99
tracheostomy patient, 2
infection
prevention and control, 44, 116
signs of, 30
urinary tract, 43
infiltration, assessment of, 182
information sharing, 43, 49
infusion pump, 212
injection
aids, 27
distraction techniques for, 101
intramuscular, 191
of multiple medications, 189
for pediatric patients, 191
practicing for, 26
site rotation, 89
ink stains, removal of, 93, 225, 228
insect bites and stings, treatment for, 173
inservice sessions, reminder cards for, 50
instruments, information about, 47
insulin, 27, 108, 119
intake, oral, 55
intake and output, calculation of, 219
intensive care unit, 81, 233
intermittent I.V. device, 182
intubation equipment, 236
invasive monitoring lines, 40
irrigation
ear, 136, 137
for excoriated lesions, 169
isolation
admission procedure, 216
cards, 208
children in, 104
precautions, 7
reminder, 66
sterile technique for, 176, 232
itchiness, 71

I.V.
absorption rate, 186
administration, 180
ambulating patient with, 64
bottles, 185
catheter, 179
equipment, 51, 213
flow rate, 180, 185
indicator, 182
information, 186
lines, 185, 211
maintenance in confused patient, 182
medications, 176, 178, 193
needle insertion, 176, 177, 184
test, 48
tubing, 50, 179, 183

J
jejunostomy tube, feeding with, 54
job sharing, 232
jogging, 8

K
K-Lyte tablets, 188
knee immobilizer, 143
knee pads, 234
Kodel sling hip exerciser, 71

L
labor pain, 70
lacerations, measurement of, 129
lapboards, 77
laryngectomy patient, emergency phone messages for, 118
larynx, artificial, 1
laundry costs, 210
lead wires
maintenance, 78, 231
placement of, 235
leg brace, 103, 170
legs, shaving of, 224
librarian, nurse as, 46
limb restraints, 65
liquid diet, treats for patients on, 230
lithotomy position, 144

logbook for staff communication, 19
lung, assessment of, 127

M
magazine articles, reference system for, 16, 217, 219
manicure, 224
manikin, 204
mastectomy
exercises for, 63
skin care, 59
surgical measures, 57, 58
mattress, 205, 209
measurement
abdominal, 130
of drainage, 132
of pupils, 130
sputum output, 131
stool, 131
urine output, 131
of wounds, 129, 130
medical antishock trousers, preventing contamination of, 138
medication
administration, 189, 190, 192
ampules, 202, 203
board, 124
cart, 216
charts, 86, 105, 120
containers, 108
documentation, 194
dosage calculation, 218
for emergencies, 43
expiration dates, 189
identification, 109, 124
information on, 42, 43, 218
keys, 206
pediatric, 213
recording of, 16
regimen, 32
schedule, 106, 107, 108
tasteless, 188
tray, 193
medication cards, 124
memory aids, 5, 6, 47
milk of magnesia, 192
monitoring, hemodynamic, 40
monitoring lines, invasive, 40
Montgomery straps, 158, 166
mother's milk, 121

mouth
  blood in, 134
  care of, 134, 135
muscle relaxer, 191
music, promoting sleep with, 74
myringotomy, 120

N

nameplates, 227
narcotic keys, 233
nasal cannula, 74
nasal speculum, 210
nasal surgery patient, oxygen
    mask for, 58
nasogastric drainage, measure-
    ment of, 132
nasogastric tube
  clamping of, 162
  insertion of, 66
  medication administration
      through, 188, 192
  preparing for insertion, 236
  securing of, 161, 162
  unclogging of, 152
neck surgery patient, gown for,
    59
needle
  preventing jabs with, 202
  removal of, 179
needs of patient, 9
nerves, cranial, 51
newborn
  information for parents
      about, 217
  mouth examination of, 94
new patient, locating room of, 6
nipples, easing soreness of, 70
nitroglycerin, 192
Nitrol, application of, 192
normal saline solution, 210
NPO patient, providing comfort
    for, 57
nurse assignments, identifica-
    tion of, 16
nursing assistants, 9
nutrition, educating children
    about, 38, 87
nutritional supplements, 53

O

obese patient
  comfort measures for, 173
  hospital gowns for, 67
  skin treatment for, 173
  transferring of, 141
  weighing of, 141
obstetric/gynecologic examina-
    tion, comfort measures
    during, 68
obstetric patient
  home follow-up service for,
      29
  information for, 28
odor
  body, 223
  cast, 223
  control, 154
  coping with, 75
  elimination of, 137
  fecal, 227
  shoe, 227
ointment, applicator for, 169
operating room, procedural aid
    for, 47
Op-Site, 161, 163
oral cancer, mouth care for,
    134
oral hygiene trays, 135
oral surgery, application of ice
    packs after, 167
orientation programs, 46
ostomy, care of, 45, 148
ostomy appliances, deodorizing
    of, 114
otitis media, 35
outpatient, stool collection for,
    156
output, cardiac, 212
output and intake, calculation
    of, 219
over-the-bed table, 114
oxygen mask, 58, 74

P

pacemaker, transvenous, 65
pads, postpartum, 114
pain
  contralateral relief of, 77
  distracting child in, 90
  gas, 61
  labor, 70
  leg, 131
  postdelivery, 70
paint, removing from skin, 172
paralysis patient, improving
    holding ability of, 112
paraplegic patient, positioning
    of, 141
parents
  information for, 28, 35
  teaching aids for, 31
patient
  care of, 15
  comfort of, 69, 70, 71, 76
  condition of, 7
  diabetic, 27
  education, 31, 239
  information on, 8, 9
  needs, 8
  positioning of, 141, 143
  records, 230
  restless, 65, 67
  unmotivated, 83
  with walker, 109, 110, 112
patient-teaching
  aids, 33
  assessment, 33, 34
  handouts, 218
  nurses' guides to, 46
pediatric code, 214
pediatric patient
  decreasing boredom of, 89,
      90
  explaining procedures to, 90
  lessening fear of injections
      of, 191
  locating of, 10
  medication administration for,
      190
  medication charting for, 86
  reducing pain of injections of,
      191
  transporting of, 92

pencil smudges, 224, 228
Penrose drain
    evaluation of, 133
    recycling of, 208
perineal care, 174, 211
perineal surgery, 61
personnel, temporary, 20
petroleum jelly, 100
photographs, 6
pillbox, sliding, 106
pills
    administration of, 190
    breaking of, 189
plaster, removal of, 237
Pleur-evac units, 229
Popsicle, therapeutic use of, 237
postmortem care, 66
postoperative information, communication of, 17
postsurgical patient, warming of, 60
postural drainage, 120
potassium supplements, 188
povidone-iodine, stains from, 224
powder, application of, 174
premature infant
    promoting buttocks healing of, 99
    seat for, 96
preoperative instructions, group, 22
pressure sore, ointment for, 175
privacy, protection of, 65, 67, 69
p.r.n. list, 194
procedure
    manual, 16
    timed, 17, 67, 99
prosthesis
    aid in dressing with, 117
    breast, 119
pulse taking, 102
pupils, measurement of, 130
puppets, for rewarding children, 104

Q
quadriplegic patient, call system for, 1, 2

R
radiation therapy, orientation to, 32
records, patient, 230
rectal surgery, 61
reference file, personal, 49
refrigerator doors, 111
relaxation techniques, 101
reminiscing, 82
respiratory care, review of, 41
restraining pants, 65
restraints
    for children, 98
    limb, 65
    stockinette, 64
resuscitation
    cardiopulmonary, 34
    mouth to stoma, 41
retina, reattachment of, 60
rheumatoid arthritis patient, bathing, 113
rhythm strips, 39
ring
    removal from swollen finger, 175
    securing preoperatively, 62
room deodorizers, 237
room numbers, remembrance of, 198
rust stains, removal from uniform, 226

S
sacrum, care of decubitus ulcer on, 169
Salem sump tube, easing insertion of, 152
sanitary belt, avoiding skin ulceration from, 72
sanitary pad
    for baby's comfort, 100
    as incisional dressing, 117
    as nursing pad, 114
scales, infant, 94

scalp laceration, suturing, 61
school pins, preventing loss of, 227
scissors, pinning of, 233
self-treatment procedures, instructions for, 30
semicomatose patient
    transferring of, 141
    weighing of, 141
Sengstaken-Blakemore tube, 79
sensory-impaired patients, identification of, 11
shaving, 222, 224
shift report
    addendum to, 17
    formulation of, 217
shock, electric, 195
shock blocks, 201
shoes
    cleaning of, 225
    discomfort when new, 229
    odor prevention for, 227
shoulder disproportions, 236
shunt, arteriovenous, 79
"Sick Child Care Kit," 120
skeletal traction, exercise during, 92
skin
    abrasions, 71, 196
    assessment of, 125
    breakdown, 169, 170
    care of, 117, 172, 173, 223
    irritation, 115, 170
    itchiness, 71
    lesions, 130
    lotion, 77
    protection of, 184
    tears in, 197
    testing, 90
    ulceration, 72
slide presentation, 46
slip, preventing clinging of, 226
slippers
    bedside holder for, 199
    disposable, 62
    nonslip, 62

smoking, prevention of fires
    during, 199
snacks, 53
snow, emergency measures for,
    231
soaking, 121
soaking solution, 89
socks, recycled, 208
sound transmission, assessing
    child's needs by, 12
specimen, handling of, 7
speculum, nasal, 210
sphincter muscle, relaxation of,
    151
splint
    arm, 71
    hand, 72
    incisional, 61
    skin breakdown from, 169
splinters, removal of, 171
splinting, 61
sprain, recurrent, 202
sputum output, measurement
    of, 131
staff
    camaraderie, 16
    communication, 15, 18
    development, 45
    education, 48
    messages, 16
    updating of, 19, 49, 50
stains, removing from uniform,
    224, 225
sterile field, avoiding contami-
    nation of, 156
stethoscope, repairing, 206
stockinette restraint, 64
stockings, care for, 226
stoma
    leaks, 118
    resuscitation through, 41
    skin breakdown around, 170
stool
    collection, 156
    measurement, 131

strain, prevention of, 202
stress, reducing in intensive
    care unit, 223
stroke patient
    positioning of, 56
    shoes for, 62
student health, maintenance
    programs for, 37
study aid, tape recorder used
    as, 50
stump, practice in bandaging,
    51
subclavian catheter tray, 178
suction bottles, 137
suctioning
    artificial airway, 67
    emergency, 212
supplies
    emergency, transporting of,
        212, 213
    locating of, 215
    shelf space for, 235
supply orientation, 47
supply quotas, use of, 235
support, abdominal, 60
suppository, rectal, 190
surgery
    nasal, 58
    neck, 59
    oral, 167
    rectal, 61
surgical services, 17
suturing, scalp laceration, 61
swallowing difficulties, 56
Swan-Ganz catheter, 205, 231
swelling, postdelivery, 70
syringe
    covers, 208
    disposal of, 198
    filling of, 189

T

tape, removal of, 73
tape measure, 209
tar, removal from skin, 172
tasks, repetitive, 233
teeth, preserving for replanta-
    tion, 103

telemetry pouches, 229
telemetry units, 73
telephone, explaining proce-
    dures by, 14
tennis socks, preventing
    scrapes with, 100
TENS, 72
thorns, removal of, 172
throat, sore, 75
throat soak, 101
ticks, removal of, 171
toe
    care of, 224
    warm compress for, 166
tongue, care of, 222
tonsil suction tip, 137
tourniquet
    carrying of, 212
    oversized, 237
towel bath, infant, 100
toys, identification bands for,
    104
tracheostomy
    cannula, 164
    care, 48, 62
    communication system for pa-
        tient with, 3
    faceplate, 74
    oral intake with, 55
    prevention of aspiration with,
        197
    tube tie, 101
traction
    bars, 202
    beds, 205
    cord spools, 63
    skeletal, 92
    tree, 229
    weights, 98
transcutaneous electrical nerve
    stimulator, 72

transferring
    of patient, 141
    patient's belongings, 76, 238
    procedures, 16
transfusion, warming blood for,
    181
transparencies, 209
trauma, oral, 195
treatment modes, charting of,
    10
tub bath, infant, 87
tube
    abdominal, 52, 153
    chest, 64
    endotracheal, 127, 163, 164,
        215
    feeding through, 54
    nasogastric, 66, 236
turning schedule, communica-
    tion of, 11

U

ulceration, skin, 72
umbilical cord, promoting heal-
    ing of, 96
umbilicus, cleaning of, 174
under pad, maintaining position
    of, 66
uniform
    care of, 226
    cleanliness of, 224, 225
    pocket, 224, 227, 228
    preventing damage to, 227
    stains, 224, 225, 226
unit orientation, 40
unmotivated patient, encourage-
    ment of, 83
unresponsive child, hand exer-
    ciser for, 92
ureterostomy incision, manag-
    ing drainage from, 154
urinal, comfortable use of, 147
urinary frequency, 115

urinary tract infections, 43
urine
    contamination, 147
    drainage bag for, 154
    filtering of, 115
    output, 131
    pouches, 160
    specimens, 154, 155, 156,
        158

V

valuables, ensuring safety of,
    200
vase, 236
Velcro
    opening medication bottle
        with, 108
    retrieving cane with, 111
venipuncture
    kit, 178
    pinchless, 176
    preparation for, 157, 177
ventilation
    preparation for, 79
    teaching of, 23
ventilator patient, 1, 2
vernix caseosa, removal of, 171
visiting hours, 8, 14
visual stimulation, infant, 89
vital signs, communication of, 9
voiding, difficulty in, 146
volume control set, 179
volunteer services, 234
vomiting, inducing, 66

W

walker, 109, 110, 112
walking
    practice in, 113
    teaching handicapped toddler
        in, 93

warm compress, 166
wart remover, 209
water rings, 73
waveforms, creating, 40
weighing
    infant, 94
    reducing fear during, 198
wheelchair
    abduction pillow for, 109
    bedpan use with, 147
    independence using, 109, 110
    positioning patient on, 142
    safety precautions, 197, 198
    using drainage bag with,
        109, 161
wire cutters, 197
wound
    abdominal, 165
    buttocks, 165
    cleansing of, 172
    condition of, 10
    drainage, 133
    dressings, 22, 165, 168
    healing of, 21
    home care of, 118
    packing, 169
    understanding about, 21
wristband, stretchable, 195

X

X-ray
    film, 209
    procedures, 216

Y

yeast infections, care of, 173
young patients, communication
    system for, 4

NOTES

NOTES

NOTES